COMPLEX REGIONAL PAIN SYNDROME

PAST, PRESENT AND FUTURE

Pain and its Origins, Diagnosis and Treatments

Additional books in this series can be found on Nova's website
under the Series tab.

Additional e-books in this series can be found on Nova's website
under the e-book tab.

COMPLEX REGIONAL PAIN SYNDROME

PAST, PRESENT AND FUTURE

NADER D. NADER

AND

OGNJEN VISNJEVAC

EDITORS

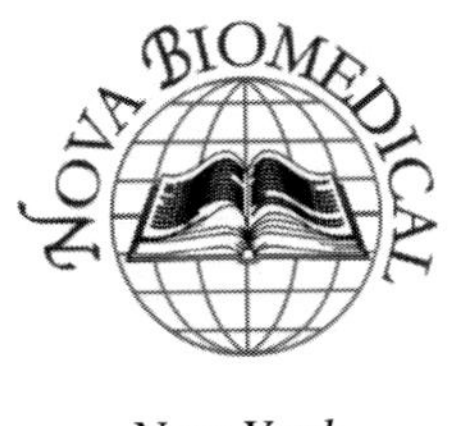

Nova Biomedical

New York

NOTICE TO THE READER

Library of Congress Cataloging-in-Publication Data

ISBN: 978-1-63483-130-7
Library of Congress Control Number: 2015942059

Published by Nova Science Publishers, Inc. † New York

CONTENTS

PREFACE

Complex regional pain syndrome (CRPS) has had many names over the past several centuries. Rooted in an incomplete understanding of the pathophysiology of this syndrome and confounded by a plethora of diagnostic strategies used by clinicians and researchers, it was not until 1993 that the current diagnostic criteria for CPRS began establishing itself. Although refined since then, these criteria have allowed for an explosion of more focused research regarding the etiological, pathophysiological, molecular, and immunological mechanisms involved in CRPS development, treatment, and prognosis. Nonetheless, this remains a difficult-to-treat pain syndrome dependent on current and future research to provide new strategies for treatment and prevention, as well as to establish an evidence-based paradigm for current treatment options.

The next few decades hold immeasurable promise in many areas of future research for CRPS. Although not discussed in great detail, one of the most valuable potential areas of future research would be the development of reliable and translatable animal models for CRPS. The variable phenotypic nature of CRPS makes the development and reproducibility of animal models difficult, and several models may be necessary to reflect various pathologic processes present in CRPS. Current model-derived data is often obtained from neuropathic pain models and may not accurately reflect human CRPS pathophysiology, thereby inherently limiting the reliability and significance of findings. More recently, a CRPS-specific animal model has been proposed, but it has not been widely utilized.

Moreover, special consideration and attention should be made for CRPS in children. Unfortunately, there is a paucity of data regarding pediatric CRPS, providing an expansive arena for future research opportunities. While the course, treatment response, and presentation of pediatric CPRS often differ from that of the adult CRPS population, suggesting that pediatric CRPS may have unique pathophysiological components, perhaps the first significant milestone to be sought is the development and validation of formal pediatric CRPS diagnostic criteria. In addition to allowing for sharing of data and findings between various research groups, use of such universal diagnostic criteria will allow for the incidence of pediatric CRPS to be effectively investigated for the first time.

Lastly, while the authors and editors herein believe they have undertaken a thorough and exhaustive review of literature pertaining to this syndrome, readers must recognize that this textbook is up-to-date as of 2015 and its contents should be taken in this context.

Nader D. Nader
Ognjen Visnjevac

Dept. of Anesthesiology
SUNY at Buffalo
3495 Bailey Ave,
Buffalo, NY, US 14215

nnader@buffalo.edu
ovisnjevac@yahoo.com

April 2015

In: Complex Regional Pain Syndrome
Editors: Nader D. Nader and Ognjen Visnjevac

ISBN: 978-1-63483-130-7
© 2015 Nova Science Publishers, Inc.

Chapter 1

HISTORY AND EPIDEMIOLOGY

Remek Kocz, MD, MS*

Clinical Instructor, Anesthesiology, University at Buffalo, Buffalo, NY, US

HISTORY

Complex Regional Pain Syndrome (CRPS) has had many faces and many names throughout its documented history, and these are likely to change again. Moreover, like all diseases prior to their discovery, CRPS was apt to have been observed long before it was first described. The earliest mentions appeared in the 16th century. In the centuries to follow, authors almost exclusively discussed injuries suffered during wartime, reflecting the tragic opportunity that the brutality of war offers to physicians seeking new methods of treatment for those wounded in combat. Subsequently, more formal reports emerged in the 19th century and, by 20th century, a variety of treatments were described.

The first known description of CRPS is from the 16th century report of the French barber-surgeon, Abmroise Paré (1510-1590), who served in that capacity at the royal court of Kings Henry II, Francis II, Charles IX, and Henry III. His considerable talent as a surgeon led to his eventual appointment as *Maître-Chirurgien* [2]. Considered one of the fathers of surgery, along with development of new surgical techniques, Paré was a pioneer in battlefield medicine and treatment of wounds. His description of phantom limb pain, which was later to be named as such by Silas Weir Mitchell, was the first in medical literature. He described contractures and continuous pain that King Charles IX felt after a curative blood-letting procedure in his work, *Of the Cure of Wounds of the Nervous System*. He was also first to observe the presence of chronic pain subsequent to injury of the peripheral nerves in wounded soldiers [3, 4].

The famed English surgeon, Sir Percivall Pott (1714-1788), who was the first physician to describe a connection between an occupational hazard and cancer in the contemporary chimney sweeps, made a mention of "certain painful afflictions of nerves" as they related to injuries of the extremities [5]. John Abernethy (1764-1831), another English surgeon, was aware of Pott's observations, and himself described a similar case that resulted from a

---

* Email: rkocz@buffalo.edu.

venesection. Other early 19th century cases included descriptions by Charles Bell in 1812 and Antonio Scarpa in 1832 [6].

First reported case of CRPS I is credited to the English naval surgeon, Alexander Denmark (Figure 1). During his appointment at the Royal Naval Hospital Haslar as the Physician to the Mediterranean Fleet, he cared for soldiers wounded during the Peninsular War. Denmark came upon a patient named Henry Croft who was injured on the last day of the British siege of the Spanish town of Badajoz in 1812. A musket ball had penetrated his triceps extensor cubiti muscle above the inner condyle of the humerus. Although the wound healed uneventfully, Croft developed pain so severe that it was unresponsive to the largest doses of opiates given. Denmark's diagnosis pointed to radial nerve involvement and a resection of the injured portion of the nerve was offered to Croft, who refused fearing that an unsuccessful resection would necessitate another surgery. Croft instead chose to undergo an amputation of upper limb, which was carried out successfully, providing immediate relief from pain. He "was discharged cured in three weeks, having, in that time, rapidly recovered both his health and strength" [7, 8].

In 1838, a surgeon named John Hamilton from Dublin, Ireland, published a report that consisted of a series of three cases in which a peripheral nerve injury was sustained to be followed by severe pain along with exquisite tenderness, contraction of the limb, and frequent redness and swelling. In each case, the symptoms ultimately abated and resolved, having been unresponsive to a variety of treatments. Hamilton also compares his cases with those of his contemporaries, debunking the view held by some that the condition is particular to anxious females. Countering that the condition then should spontaneously develop in these women, rather than as a consequence of a direct nerve injury, he posits that a "peculiar irritable inflammation is set up in the wounded nerve, and its branches conveying morbid impressions in the brain and spinal marrow" [9]. He notes that the curative procedure for the condition, in the absence of spontaneous resolution, tends to be a nerve resection.

Timeline of CRPS History

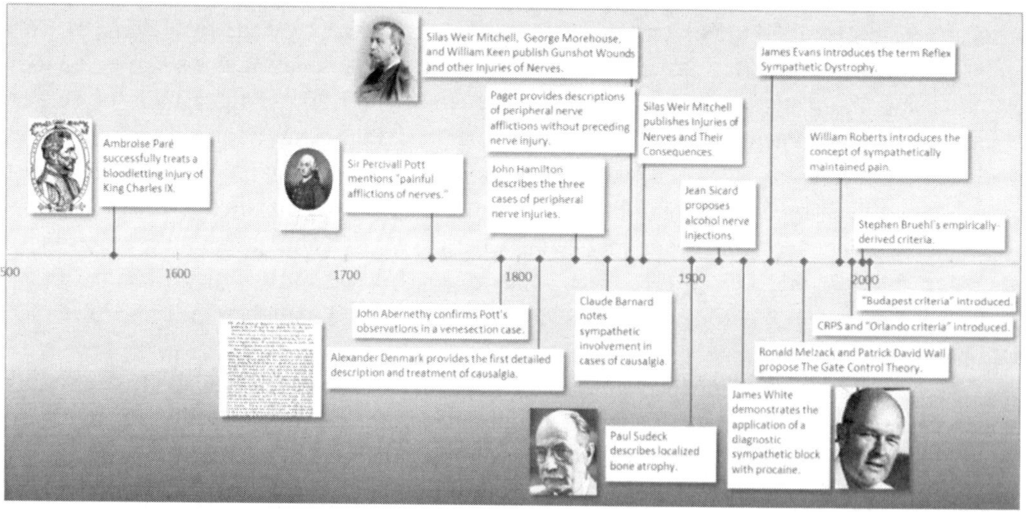

Figure 1. Historical timeline of people and events that have notably contributed to the body of knowledge currently known as CRPS.

In 1851, Claude Bernard (1813-1878), the French scientist who is considered to be one of the founders of the field of physiology, noted the association of sympathetic nervous system in the regulation of the body's internal environment. He was the first to identify a pain syndrome that was tied to a dysfunction of the sympathetic nervous system [10, 11].

On February 6th, 1864, James Paget (1814-1899) delivered a lecture in which he described a number of cases of local paralysis secondary to a peripheral nerve injury. He spoke of them as rare cases in which a total paralysis of the limb was present along with wasting and neuralgia, with all symptoms being out of proportion to the injury and without a sign of brain or spinal cord injury [12].

The vast scale of the American Civil War (1861-1865) was marked by significant weapons advances that contributed to a large number of wounded. This is especially notable in the form of the Minié Ball, a type of ammunition that resulted in better range and accuracy of rifles. Nerve damage resulted from direct contact with the bullet, from the surrounding tissue damage and deformation during the traversal of the bullet through the body, or through fragmentation upon impact. Silas Weir Mitchell (1829-1914) was an American physician who, at the time of the Civil War, volunteered to treat the Union wounded in Philadelphia. Working at the Filbert Street Hospital, he took interest in the patients with nerve injuries. Along with George R. Morehouse and William W. Keen, Mitchell was instrumental in the opening of the Turner's Lane Hospital where he focused on gunshot injuries of peripheral nerves, while his aforementioned colleagues studied their respective interests [13]. Together, in 1864, they published the book *Gunshot Wounds and Other Injuries of Nerves*, which documented their experience in caring for the Union Army soldiers with nerve injuries. There we find the first full description of the disorder that later came to be known as CRPS II, or causalgia. In 1872, Mitchell, this time by himself, followed up with *Injuries of Nerves and Their Consequences*. By that point the term "causalgia" was already in increasing use. Interestingly enough, for approximately a century its origin was unclear. It was commonly assumed that Mitchell coined the word "causalgia" in one of his books and 19th century authors deferred to him. However, a careful reading of the 1864 monograph revealed a complete absence of the term, while the 1872 volume does contain the word, where it is used throughout the text undefined, suggesting an already accepted usage. Voices of uncertainty began to be heard early in the 20th century, with M. Leriche expressing his regret in being unable to ascertain the precise year of causalgia being named on the pages of *La Presse Medicale* in 1916, while W.H. Coupland in an 1918 letter to *Lancet* asked readers for assistance in clearing up the mystery [14]. As late as 1958, Sir James Paterson Ross noted the obscure nature of the derivation of the word in his *Surgery of the Sympathetic Nervous System* [15]. Ten years later, in 1967, in a *Medical History* journal article, R.L. Richards finally solved the mystery. There he presented an excerpt from the *United States Sanitary Commission Memoirs*, published in 1867, in which a passage from Mitchell's contributory chapter reveals the background of the term. S. Weir Mitchell approached his friend, Professor Robley Dunglison, to help him coin a more convenient name than merely using the phrase "burning pain." Dunglison, a professor of medicine at the Institutes of Medicine in the Jefferson Medical College of Philadelphia, a student of philology and a medical lexicographer, suggested causalgia, from the Greek words *kausos* (heat) and *algos* (pain). In the posthumous edition of his Medical Dictionary in 1874, Dunglison first formally introduced the word causalgia, but rather than concretely defining it, he simply provided the linguistic origin of the root words [8, 16-18].

Mitchell also coined the term erythromelalgia, in reference to a disorder the lower extremity, notable for its symptomatology consisting of redness of the feet, pain, burning and swelling. He initially described it in an 1872 article, then expanded on it in 1878, and wrote on it intermittently throughout his career. A notable fact is that erythromelalgia was not perceived as arising secondary to nerve trauma, as it has been noted in the case of causalgia [19].

Mitchell's work began gaining influence in Europe, when in 1874 the French translation of *Injuries of Nerves and Their Consequences* by M. Dastre was published. Prefaced by a 48-page introduction by the famed French neurologist Alfred Vulpian, the book was echoed in the subsequent work of physicians who focused on peripheral nerve lesions that were the result of World War I. Both sides of the conflict were tasked with treating tens of thousands of combat victims. France, where Mitchell's monograph had the most significant impact, was the channel through which his ideas began to be disseminated through Europe [20].

Mitchell was extensively referenced around the time of WWI by the two prominent French physicians, Jules Tinel and Chiriachitza Athanassio-Bénisty. In his 1916 *Les Blessures des nerfs* [Nerve Injuries], Tinel wrote extensively on symptoms of causalgia, distinguishing it from non-traumatically acquired neuritis that could at times be cured with nerve resection. Like many of his contemporaries, he felt that causalgia symptoms stemmed from reflex sympathetic irritation, a term that took into account the paroxysmal nature, vasomotor characteristics, emotional influence, and symptom radiation. While Tinel did not find that resection and suture was curative, as the pain returned within a few weeks of the nerve section, he did report significant success with periarterial sympathetectomy in refractory cases in the upper extremity, proposing a similar treatment for the lower extremity. Tinel also found that radiotherapy to the nerve roots was more effective in causalgia than in neuritis, and while it did not eliminate the pain, it did diminish its paroxysmal nature [20, 21].

The French vascular surgeon, Rene Leriche (1879-1955), established the connection between the sympathetic nervous system and causalgia from his observation and treatment of injured soldiers during World War I. In 1916, he proposed that a peripheral and central nervous systems shared a feedback loop, a "viscious circle," as he called it, in which the sympathetic nervous system served as the efferent limb. Noting similarity between extremities affected by ischemia and those affected by causalgia, he applied the existing treatment of the ischemic limbs, periarterial nerve stripping, to causalgic limbs.

The resulting sympathetectomy was successful in relieving pain. Leriche's report and subsequent reproduction of his method by others gave credence to the sympathetic origins of the disorder [22]. This directed research and clinical efforts for decades to come [23-25].

Chiriachitza Athanassio-Bénisty published her works towards the end of WWI and immediately after the war. In 1918, *Formes cliniques des lésions des nerfs* [Clinical Forms of Nerve Lesions] was published in Paris, and in 1919, *Les lésions des nerfs: traitement et restauration* [Treatment and Repair of Nerve Lesions] appeared in Paris as well [26, 27]. With both works, which cited Mitchell prominently, her goal was to not only present the cases but also to aid in improving peripheral nerve lesion examination by less experienced physicians, focusing on distinguishing causalgia from other neurological disorders in order to effect more appropriate treatment. In her works, she noted fine intention tremor in cases of median and some sciatic nerve injuries and proposed irritation of the sympathetic nerves as the cause. Complex anastomoses of the sympathetic fibers were thought to be able to most likely explain why nerve lesions could cause sympathetic irritation beyond their area of distribution. This was a likely explanation for the fact that she did not see Leriche's periarterial sympathetic stripping produce successful relief in her own patients.

In the United Kingdom, in 1905, H. Head and J. Sherren published an article, *The consequences of injury to the peripheral nerves in man,* where they referenced Mitchell and used the term causalgia. The paper dealt with both civilian and military injuries due to Boer War. Eleven years later, James Purves-Stewart, a consulting physician to Her Majesty's forces, along with Arthur Henry Evans, a surgeon at the 4th London General Hospital published *Nerve Injuries and their Treatment* in 1916, a practical clinical text. Instead of causalgia, the authors advocated the use of the word *thermalgia*. Hartley Sidney Carter, a physician at the 2nd Northern General Hospital reviewed over 1,000 cases of post-WWI peripheral nerve injuries, publishing his observations in 1922 as *On Causalgia and Allied Painful Conditions Due to Lesions of Peripheral Nerves.*

In 1900, the German physician, Paul Sudeck (1866-1945) discovered a localized bone atrophy he termed "*Knochenatropie.*" He observed it in the setting of acute, focal extremity disorders and fractures, and reported his findings during the German Society of Surgery's 24th meeting. This "acute inflammatory bone atrophy," as he termed it, later became known as "Sudeck's Dystrophy." He also posited an inflammatory ctiology (*entzündliche*) for causalgia [24, 28-30].

By the time WWI had begun, a number of treatments became available, offering hope outside of the standard approach that consisted of morphine injections or blister application to areas affected by pain. In 1916, Jean A. Sicard was the first physician to suggest alcohol injection into the trunk of the nerve as a treatment modality for causalgia. His idea was based on his previous work in treating facial spasms and tics with alcohol injections [31]. Lewis Yealland reported in 1916 a single case in which a successful intraoperative alcohol injection was performed. It, however, worked only on the second attempt which was carried out 8 months after the initial injection [32]. That same year, E. Farquhad Buzzard along with Sicard advocated the use of alcohol injections into the affected nerve, citing their good results [33, 34]. Dean Lewis and Wesley Gatewood also reported 3 successful cases in 1919, while also that year, Sicard and Dambrin presented 47 cases of which 27 were deemed "cured" [35]. Ultimately, the results were deemed to be inconsistent, with significant interoperator variability, and the injections fell out of favor [18]. Resection of the affected part of the nerve constituted another approach which was favored by Carter, who felt that the resection and suture should be carried out in all cases of causalgia. Although good results were reported, the fact that minimal neurological deficits were often present in a setting of incomplete nerve injury presented a source of hesitation in performing an essentially destructive procedure. Other approaches that were sometimes successful included Tinel's arterial sympathectomy, arterial ligation distal to site of injury, and dorsal nerve root resection [18].

In 1930, James C. White demonstrated the application of a diagnostic sympathetic block with procaine, in a procedure designed to test the efficacy of sympathetic ganglionectomy. This approach was based on the work of prior investigators in which the excision of upper dorsal or lower lumbar sympathetic ganglia resulted in vasomotor paralysis of the ipsilateral limb, anhydrosis, and a relief from a number of painful conditions transmitted over the sympathetic fibers. Citing Leriche's past work on sympathetically-mediated pain transmission, White predicted the procedure's utility in treating causalgia [36]. At the same time, Spurling published a report of a causalgia case subsequent to a gunshot wound of the brachial plexus [37]. Several procedures were already tried, including periarterial sympathectomy, but without success. After the cervicothoracic sympathetic ganglionectomy was performed, a complete cure was effected. Five years later, Kwan suggested that causalgia was a result of sensory hypertony that arose from sympathetic modulation of non-sympathetic nerves, and in 1935 he reported a successful treatment of a case of causalgia with thoracic sympathetic gangilonectomy [38]. Livingston and Homans followed up in 1938 and 1940, respectively, their excellent results demonstrating both diagnostic and therapeutic applicability [39, 40].

In 1937, De Tákats applied the term "Reflex Dystrophy" postulating an activation of the preganglionic nerves of the sympathetic system by nociceptive stimuli, leading to the formation of a somatic-sympathetic reflex arc that may intensify significantly in the absence or decrease of inhibition from the higher centers. Such reflexes were then known to exist acutely in the setting of diseased or thrombosed blood vessels, contributing to a vasospasm. In the 5 cases presented by DeTákats, a slow afferent outflow was noted, with either vasoconstricting or vasodilatory effects, suggesting a variability in the level of control of the higher centers [41]. In the same article, De Tákats described the progression of the reflex dystrophy in three broad phases, anticipating Bonica's proposal of three stages of reflex sympathetic dystrophy by 16 years [41, 42].

Livingston in 1943 posited his explanation for the pathophysiology of the disease. It was known as the theory of reverberating circuits in the spinal cord. Such circuits form under the influence of intensely painful stimuli in the internuncial pools of neurons. Once formed, these circuits also respond to seemingly innocuous stimuli which will be received as pain [43]. A year later, Granit et al. proposed that an injured nerve in causalgia can act as an artificial synapse, causing signals from the ventral root to be transmitted via the sensory fibers to the dorsal root. Thus a shunt is created that can induce the sensation of pain [44]. The same year, Doupe theorized that sympathetic efferents may be responsible for activation of sensory fibers in causalgia [45].

As World War II raged, physicians were caring for increasingly larger numbers of the war wounded. Once again, high-velocity bullet injuries brought attention to causalgia. Attention was at this point shifting away from distal sympathectomies as a viable treatment option, with James White's pioneering work setting the stage for interrupting the sympathetic efferents at the ganglion. By the end of WWII, a standard approach to treatment of soldiers affected by causalgia resulting from combat injuries was a diagnostic block at a sympathetic ganglion involved with the injured limb, followed by surgical excision if the block failed to achieve a therapeutic effect. Spiegel and Milowsky, in 1945, reported a series of 9 cases that were successfully treated by sympathectomy at the sympathetic ganglion. Of the 9, every patient responded to a local anesthetic block of the sympathetic ganglion. Permanent and complete pain relief with surgery was obtained by 7 patients. Of the remaining 2 patients, one's condition resolved with just the diagnostic block, and the other, who for technical reasons could not undergo surgical sympathectomy, was treated with an alcohol block of the affected sympathetics [46].

In 1947, Evans introduced the term "Reflex Sympathetic Dystrophy" in order to differentiate causalgic symptoms that were present in the setting of minor injury where no evident physical nerve damage was present [47]. In 1948, Steinbrocher discussed the shoulder hand syndrome which he saw as a subclassification of the RSD [48]. More name changes appeared in 1949 when Echlin, Owens, and Warner extended the concept originally discussed by Homans in 1940. Homans introduced the term "minor causalgia" with the intent for it to include only painful osteoporosis, Sudeck's atrophy, and a few others in which hyperesthesia was the overriding complaint. Echlin et al. proposed a delineation of the disorder into "minor" and "major" causalgia, although they did not wish to suggest that two distinct forms of the disorder exist, merely highlighting the variation in severity. In a fully manifested "major causalgia," the extremity would be affected by a constant and diffuse burning pain that is perceived deep in the tissue and it spreads beyond the area supplied by the affected nerve [49].

Attempts at delineating the pathophysiology between RSD and causalgia continued after WWII. Nathan, in 1947, noted in patients with partial nerve injury the existence of abnormal stimulation of somatic sensory axons in the area of the nerve. Postganglionic sympathetic efferents were responsible, and he also proposed the existence of an artificial synapse that would allow for this form of crosstalk [50]. In 1959, Drucker's observation that relatively minor soft-tissue injuries can result in the same RSD symptoms as nerve injury led him to propose that artificial synapses can form among the tiny peripheral nerve endings, in a manner similar to larger nerves [51]. In 1965, Melzack & Wall proposed the *gate-control theory of pain*, which in part was designed to explain causalgia [52]. They theorized that modulation of sensory input takes place in the substantia gelatinosa where second-order neurons act as gates in transmission of sensation by inhibiting incoming signals. Later on, in 1971, Melzack posited that a potential central biasing mechanism exists, which may decrease its tonic inhibitory effect once a nerve is injured [53].

In 1981, Kozin compared radiography and scintigraphy in terms of sensitivity and specificity. While scintigraphy was more specific, radiography was more sensitive [54]. However, the diagnostic ganglion block continued to be the favored diagnostic method.

Roberts, in 1986, proposed the concept of *sympathetically maintained pain* (SMP) to describe the pathology of RSD, which was based on the observation that a blockade of the sympathetic nervous system frequently resulted in the relief of symptoms of RSD, and sometimes even remission [55]. In many cases, however, sympatholysis did not produce the expected relief, even in cases when the patients had most of the symptoms of RSD. The explanation came in the form of *sympathetically independent pain* (SIP), a term coined by Campbell in 1992 [56].

By the early 1990's, the term RSD was losing its usefulness as a clinical name. Its application to cases that were both sympathetically mediated and to those where such relationship was unclear, created an unwelcome challenge in utilizing it as a precise descriptor. In the absence of standardized diagnostic criteria, Gibbons and Wilson in 1992 proposed a scoring system designed to aid in the diagnosis of RSD. They found it had good clinical correlation, proposing its application to research settings as well [57]. Still, a definitive decision was made a year later, as researchers and clinicians moved to revise the taxonomy of the disorders grouped under the RSD and causalgia umbrella. In 1993, a Special Consensus Workshop was held in Orlando, Florida between 31st of October and 3rd of November, with specific goals to examine the four terms in greatest use (RSD, causalgia, SMP, and SIP) and to determine the need for taxonomic revision of the International Association for the Study of Pain (IASP) conventions. As the direct result of the workshop, Stanton-Hicks et al. published a revised taxonomic system, originating the term Complex Regional Pain Syndrome, CRPS, with defined classification into two subtypes along with diagnostic criteria. The 1995 paper proposed that CRPS I would encompass what was previously termed RSD, allowing for the clinical variability that was heretofore observed. It postulated a presence of an inciting noxious event without clear evidence of nerve injury. CRPS II would be reserved for the cases reflecting the classical definition of causalgia, in which the inciting event is clearly associated with nerve injury. Under these IASP criteria, the diagnosis of CRPS took into account only elements of history, symptoms, and clinical findings. SMP, which was also present in other disorders such as phantom pain, herpes zoster, neuralgias, and metabolic neuropathies, was not a key component of the CRPS diagnosis. As it may or may not be present through omission from diagnostic criteria, utilization of a diagnostic sympathetic block was not required for diagnosis of CRPS henceforth. Furthermore, eliminating the focus on the sympathetic nature of the pain clarified the diagnostic approach [58].

Since their introduction, the CRPS diagnostic criteria have been subject to much concern from both clinicians and investigators. It was felt that the chief limitation was the lack of specificity in spite of excellent sensitivity. A negative impact on diagnostic accuracy was seen due to the sole reliance on subjective symptoms and signs that can also be subject to clinicians' interpretations along with significantly permissive diagnostic rules. Such limitations carry a risk of non-CRPS patients being over-diagnosed as suffering from CRPS [59]. In 1999, Bruehl et al. proposed empirically-derived research diagnostic criteria which were designed to address the concerns over the lack of specificity [60]. These "Bruehl criteria" underwent small changes at an international consensus meeting that was held in Budapest, Hungary in August of 2003 [61-63]. A modification utilizing statistically-derived diagnostic criteria was proposed, with aim to replace the original IASP criteria proposed in Orlando. The "Budapest criteria" consisted of both clinical and, somewhat more stringent, research diagnostic criteria. Clinical diagnostic criteria incorporated 4 symptom and 4 sign categories, with clinical diagnosis being made if at least one symptom in 3 out of 4 symptom categories was present and at least one sign in 2 out of 4 sign categories was positive. Research criteria required at least one symptom present in all 4 symptom categories. A recent validation of the clinical Budapest criteria noted the retention of excellent sensitivity as compared to the original criteria while producing a significant improvement in specificity [64].

While the Budapest criteria offer a significant improvement in terms of clinical utility and specificity, and clarity of the diagnosis, the objective criteria are still lacking, and investigational work continues. With the 2013 publication of the CRPS Practical Diagnostic and Treatment Guidelines, the Committee for Classification of Chronic Pain of the IASP has accepted and codified the Budapest criteria for clinical and research diagnoses. A third diagnostic subtype was also introduced to encompass about 15% of patients who were originally diagnosed with CRPS, but would not meet the new clinical criteria. It is called CRPS-not, and allows the inclusion of patients whose signs and symptoms do not offer any other diagnosis. It is considered a compromise subtype and is not seen as a permanent feature, with hopes that future research provides more clarification [10].

SUMMARY

- The first documented reports of CRPS were likely from the 16th century
- Denmark was credited with the first description of CRPS II

- Bernard was first to note sympathetic involvement in pain
- Mitchell coined "causalgia"
- Leriche established sympathetic involvement and utilized sympathetectomy in treatment
- Evans coined "RSD" in 1947
- Bonica elucidated the three stages of RSD in 1953
- Orlando Criteria in 1993
- Budapest Criteria in 2007

CRPS EPIDEMIOLOGY

Epidemiologic and outcome study data involving CRPS are sparse and stem from the difficulty in unequivocal classification of CRPS, both historically and in recent years.

The changes in diagnostic criteria since the introduction of the Orlando criteria in 1994 and subsequent modifications that emerged as the Budapest criteria in 2003 along with researchers' own alterations have created an environment in which a single set of mutually-agreed-upon standards is difficult to achieve. This presents a diagnostic challenge that results in a significant hardship in attempting to study CRPS on a broader population level. At this point, true incidence and prevalence of CRPS are not known and can be only estimated. Nevertheless, two recent publications that focused on the epidemiological aspects of the disease in specific geographic areas have yielded results that reveal the incidence to be between 5.46 and 26.6 per 100,000 person-years at risk [65, 66]. For the United States, this predicts over 16,000 - 80,000 new cases of CRPS type I per year if applying this incidence to the US population of 300 million people in the year 2000 [67]. Globally, this can be extrapolated to 380,000 to 1.8 million new cases annually, assuming a global population of 7 billion people.

Women are more frequently affected than men, with a female to male ratio ranging from 2.3:1 to 4:1, although Choi et al. have observed a ratio slightly directed towards higher frequency among men (0.8:1 male to female). As Choi's study was done in Korean population, it remains uncertain whether cultural, societal, or other factors played a role in this finding [68]. In all other studies, the majority of the affected individuals were Caucasian (79-100%). This may, however, be only the reflection of the population being serviced by the pain centers performing the epidemiological studies. Older individuals are more likely to present with CRPS symptoms, with peak age of incidence falling between 50 and 70 years old [65, 66, 69]. Depending on the study, age of affected persons could range from 2.5 to 85 years old, with a mean age at diagnosis being 41.8 − 52.7 years. Patients' sex had no impact on the mean age at diagnosis.

Upper extremities were affected more commonly, almost 1.5-2 times as often as the lower extremities, although at least one older study (Allen et al.) noted a slight preference (48% vs 44%) of the lower limb versus the upper limb [66, 70-72]. A small percentage of bilateral involvement has also been noted. Left and right sides were distributed equally, without preference for sex or extremity. Most commonly observed precipitating events include fractures (16-46%), sprains (12-29%), and surgery (12.2-24%), although up to 11% of cases cannot be correlated with any inciting injury.

Prior to being referred to the specialty pain centers, a patient typically sees an average of 4.8-5 physicians. The average time to presentation in the pain center was 11.6-30 months, which is concerning for the lack of recognition of CRPS among non-specialist physicians [68, 70]. Most of the injuries were work-related. From 56% to 75.6% of the affected individuals were injured while performing their job. Permanent disability occurred in 11% to 68.1% cases; however, it is often difficult to determine whether the disability occurred directly because of CRPS or if it was already present. Workers' compensation was being received by 33% to 54% of the individuals, suggesting a significant financial impact for the individual [70, 72].

Epidemiological data have been acquired over the years from single-center studies that have provided crucial information, but have not been amenable towards generalization to a broader section of the population. In 2003 and 2007, two population studies were published that attempted to address this issue. While Sandroni et al., in their 2003 work, focused their efforts on a single county in the United States, de Mos et al. expanded their efforts to the entire country of Netherlands in 2007 by sampling a 600,000 patient database in the Integrated Primary Care Information project (IPCI).

POPULATION STUDY: OLMSTED COUNTY, MINNESOTA

By 2003, very little was known about the broader societal burden of CRPS. This first population study was conducted by Sandroni et al., who investigated incidence, prevalence, and the natural history and response to treatment. The 1994, IASP [73] diagnostic criteria were used for inclusion criteria in this retrospective study, covering the 11-year time period from 1989 to 1999 and encompassing the population of Olmsted county, Minnesota. In 1990, the population of Olmsted county numbered in 106,470. The population under investigation reflected the surroundings of the Mayo Clinic and all affiliated medical systems. It consisted of approximately 95% Caucasians and bore a demographically close resemblance to that of broader Caucasian population in the United States. A comprehensive data system encompassed all residents who sought care within the county, making for a pool of reliable records available for research. Results encompassed the following 6 categories: demographics, clinical characteristics, signs and symptoms, laboratory indices, treatments, and predictors of outcomes. A total of 74 cases of CRPS I were recognized. The resulting incidence rate was calculated to be 5.46 per 100,000 person years at risk. Prevalence was determined for the year 1999, with 25 cases noted at that time, giving 20.57 per 100,000 person years at risk. CRPS I appeared to affect women at a significantly higher ratio of 4:1, resulting in per-100,000 person year incidence rates of 8.57 for females and 2.16 for males. Prevalence among women was 35.33 and 5.06 among men. Mean age of onset was 46.9 years (46.5 years in men and 47.7 years in women), with the range being 15 to 86 years. With the exception of a single Asian patient, all individuals affected were Caucasian. Peak age of incidence was 50-59 years old. Little difference was noted between women and men in terms of the age of onset. In terms of affected sites, upper extremities were recognized to be two times as frequently affected as lower extremities. All cases reported an initiating event, with fractures predominating at 46%, followed by sprains at 12%. Resolution was seen in 74% of the cases, with a mean symptom duration of 11.6 months, and no sex-related differences.

Symptoms and signs shared similar frequencies, with swelling, and the presence of color and temperature changes being the most common. Further characteristics of pain, such as type and severity could not be analyzed due to lack of consistency in the charts. In 85% of the cases in which the three-phase bone scan was performed, a pattern reflecting CRPS I was observed. Asymmetry in autonomic testing was seen in 80% of the patients.

Treatment arms were divided into three categories: physical therapy, sympathetic block, and prescription medication. In each treatment modality, a very significant majority reported beneficial effect. Physical therapy was utilized in 93% of the patients, with 87% improvement. Sympathetic blocks were performed on 45% patients, of whom 79% noted positive effect. Prescription medications were used in 49% cases, with 80% positive outcomes. Symptom resolution was used to assess outcomes ("good" vs. "poor" based on symptom resolution) when analyzing putative predictors. Sex, age, and affected site did not exhibit close association with outcomes. Injury types, however, offered predictive possibility. Greatest possibility of resolution was observed with fractures (91%) and sprains (78%). Symptoms with predictive value were limited to presence of swelling and absence of sensory deficits. It is known that work-related injuries are most commonly involved in being the cause of CRPS. Of the 55 cases considered for evaluation of disability, 2 had complete disability due to CRPS, 4 had partial disability, and 11 were disabled for reasons unrelated to CRPS.

While the study focused primarily on CRPS I, cases of CRPS II were taken into consideration. Over the period of the entire study, 11 cases of CRPS II have been noted, resulting in incidence of 0.82 per 100,000 person years at risk, while reflecting prevalence of 4.2 per 100,000. In terms of demographics, no sex differentiation was seen. Upper extremity prevalence was seen (82% vs. 18%). Due to the scarcity of cases available for analysis, no further investigation was performed.

Sandroni et al. found a surprising number of patients with resolution of CRPS-related signs and symptoms, along with a paucity of severe disability directly resultant from CRPS. Also impressive was the number of cases with good outcomes utilizing physical therapy alone, suggesting a possible treatment avenue other than an initially aggressive or interventional approach. Incidence following injury, in the light of past lack of standardization of diagnostic criteria, remained difficult to determine.

Furthermore, there was a large divergence in incidence between this study and Veldman et al. in 1993, where the incidence of RSD was reported to be 1-2% [74]. The reason for upper extremity frequency being twice that of the lower extremity was unknown as well. The female to male ratio (3:1) in the Sandroni et al. investigation was similar to Veldman et al. Vasomotor symptoms were present more often than sudomotor changes, possibly reflecting easier clinical detection at the time of this study compared to Veldman's. A similar high rate of resolution was also seen by A. Zyluk, who noted a large percentage of resolution for patients with post-traumatic RSD of the hand where no intervention was made [75].

Weaknesses of the Sandroni et al. study included the fact that the diagnostic criteria likely varied between clinicians due to lack of unified rules in the period encompassing the duration of this study. There was also close temporal clustering of symptoms; in clinical settings, symptoms and signs can be temporally separated [66].

POPULATION STUDY: NETHERLANDS

Little data on incidence of CRPS existed prior the 2007 article by de Mos. The most thorough analysis available was based on a single county in the United States, and no appreciation of CRPS in general population was available. This did not give a concrete understanding or appreciation of the societal or medical burden of CRPS. Hence, the de Mos retrospective cohort study analyzed electronic records of more than 600,000 patients in the Netherlands, within the timeframe of 1996 to 2005 with the intent of obtaining population-based data.

Because case diagnoses were not always apparent in the record and needed to be elucidated in the analysis, a sensitive search algorithm was utilized with implementation of synonyms and abbreviations for CRPS. Further record review and correspondence with the diagnosticians validated the cases thus filtered, obtaining a more reliable sample. The overall incidence rate was 26.2 per 100,000 person-years and the incidence rate was not seen to change significantly over the time of the study. Female predominance was noted with a 3.4:1 ratio over males. Highest incidence was in females in their sixth decade of life. In terms of sites affected, upper extremity was affected with a higher frequency, while fractures were the most common precipitating event. The study noted a fourfold higher incidence than the prior Olmsted County study from 2003.

Mean age at diagnosis was 52.7, with individuals' ages ranging from 7 to 90 years old. The male mean age was 51.1 years and the female mean age was 53.0 years. Peak incidence occurred at age 61-70. The most common precipitating events were fractures (44.1%), sprains or strains (17.6%), and "none identified" (10.8%). The distribution of limb involvement was 59.2% for upper extremity and 39.1% for lower extremity; left and right side were affected with similar frequency.

Unfortunately, the broad symptomatology and complexity of CRPS ensured it was treated by a range of clinicians with disparate backgrounds, including anesthesiologists, orthopedic surgeons, neurologists, rheumatologists, and physiatrists.

This likely made a concrete diagnosis more difficult to attain, posing a significant challenge to this and any other study attempting to characterize the general population. De Mos ultimately conducted an analysis on a total sample of individuals consisting of 61 patients diagnosed by a general practitioner and 177 patients diagnosed by a specialist [65].

INCIDENCE FOLLOWING SURGICAL PROCEDURES

Surgery is one of the iatrogenic risk factors for CRPS. Characterization of incidence and prevalence of CRPS following surgery has yet to be fully investigated; however, multiple studies have addressed post-surgical incidence of the syndrome in a variety of contexts. Reported incidence following upper extremity surgery after fasciectomy for Dupuytern contracture was 4.5% to 40%, after carpal tunnel surgery 2% to 5%, and after distal radius fracture 22% to 39% [25, 76]. Lower extremity surgery encompassing the foot and the ankle produced a range from 4.4% to 9.6% [77, 78]. Anesthetic technique did not correlate with the incidence of postoperative CRPS [79, 80].

PEDIATRIC EPIDEMIOLOGY

Within the pediatric population, CRPS is still considered to be in the early stages of investigation. This applies to diagnosis and treatment as much as it does to epidemiology. Clinicians are still unclear how to apply the diagnostic criteria and treatment modalities developed for adults in the pediatric realm – a concern that is becoming an increased focus in research. The current epidemiological data is also the reflection of this present state of uncertainty, with no uniform pediatric diagnostic criteria being applied across studies [81, 82]. Most of the data concerns CRPS type I, which has been subject of recent attention.

True incidence and prevalence in the pediatric cohort is unknown. For the population 16 years old or younger, the gender ratio has been reported as 1:6 – 1:9 male to female, suggesting that adolescent girls are the pediatric group with the highest incidence of CRPS type I. While the youngest child reported was 2.5 years old, the median age is 11.8 to 13 years. Lower extremities were more frequently affected (72.6-85%) than upper extremities (15.0-23.3%), while both extremities were involved 4.1% of the time. This of course contrasts with the adult population data, in which the involvement of the upper extremity predominates.

The inciting factor was usually a mild injury such as contusion, strain, or sprain, seen in 62.5-80% cases, with ankle sprains contributing 45% of the cases, while a severe injury such as fracture or surgery was noted in 29.2% cases. No known initiating event was present in 8.3-20% cases. The pediatric population was also noted to be affected by CRPS I more frequently in the winter time, a situation not observed in adults. Mean time from injurious event to diagnosis was reported as 11.9 to 13.6 weeks. Recurrence rate was reported to be 20-33% [82, 83].

For CRPS type II, less data is available, and no studies targeting the disorder specifically in the pediatric population have been performed. The youngest individual reported was 3 years old [84].

QUALITY OF LIFE

A protracted course of the disease or incomplete recovery can result in significant consequences for the patient. Long term impact on quality of life can be profound, with levels of disability pronouncedly interfering with daily life, and pain and decrease in mobility resulting in further problems for affected individuals. Previous quality of life studies have noted the above concerns with focus on the long-term effects on patients' lives, generally limited by relatively small sample sizes.

In 2014, however, the first study reporting a large sample of CRPS patients was published, describing long-term morbidity and quality of life for CRPS patients with the specific aim of generalizability of findings. This study analyzed 975 Dutch patients from a time span covering 10 years, encompassing 5 CRPS clinics and 1 neurology department of a university hospital, focusing on the quality of life associations with gender, affected limb location, duration of disease, and pain perception [85].

The Medical Outcomes Study 36-Item Short-Form Health Survey (SF-36) translated to Dutch was used. The chief determinant of the quality of life of CRPS patients was their degree of physical disability, with much less being attributed to the impact of their mental condition. Low scores were notable in the physical domains of the SF-36 scoring instrument, especially in the categories of Role Physical (males 16.34, females 18.48) and Bodily Pain (males 28.27, females 27.36).

There were no gender disparities noted in quality of life, and pain scores differed little between male and female cases, as noted previously. CRPS Severity Score did not significantly change among the three age groups (<40 years, 40.1-55.0 years, and >55.1 years). Lower quality of life scores were noted for younger patients, however, suggesting that CRPS prevents full participation in the potentially demanding work and family schedules of such individuals, whereas an older patient may not find the limitations imposed by CRPS as restrictive. Physical Health Summary (PHS) scores were higher in individuals with affected lower extremity than in those with upper extremity deficits.

There was a moderate association of pain intensity with the PHS and Mental Health Summary (MHS) scores, yet symptom severity correlated poorly with quality of life in terms of PHS, and not at all for MHS. CRPS patients scored low in Physical Functioning and Role Physical categories. Their scores were lower than in other musculoskeletal or neuropathic pain conditions, such as rheumatoid arthritis, neuralgic amyotrophy, and lower limb amputees with or without phantom limb pain [86]. Quality of life was explained by the effect that CRPS had on the patient's physical health. Of note was the fact that patients diagnosed using the Budapest criteria had worse quality of life than those diagnosed using the older Orlando criteria for CRPS. All studied patients fulfilled the Orlando criteria, while 71% met the Budapest clinical criteria. Because the Budapest criteria include motor signs and symptoms, lower PHS scores and, consequently, lower quality of life scores were not surprising [87, 88].

SUMMARY

- On an international scale, limited population-based data is available regarding the incidence and prevalence of CRPS.
- The Olmsted County study was the first in 2003 and found the incidence to be 5.46 per 100,000 person-years.
- The Netherlands study followed in 2007 and found an incidence of 26.6 per 100,000 person years.
- Each of these studies' populations was primarily Caucasian in a developed country, limiting generalizability of data internationally.
- Pediatric incidence of CRPS I or II is not yet clear.

REFERENCES

[1] Perez, R.S., et al., Evidence based guidelines for complex regional pain syndrome type 1. BMC *Neurol.*, 2010. 10: p. 20.

[2] Woodhouse, A., Phantom limb sensation. *Clin. Exp. Pharmacol. Physiol.*, 2005. 32(1-2): p. 132-4.

[3] Dommerholt, J., Complex regional pain syndrome—1: history, diagnostic criteria and etiology. *Journal of Bodywork and Movement Therapies*, 2004. 8: p. 167-177.

[4]   Hernigou, P., Ambroise Pare's life (1510-1590): part I. *Int. Orthop.*, 2013. 37(3): p. 543-7.

[5]   Webb, E.M. and E.W. Davis, Causalgia; a review. *Calif. Med.*, 1948. 69(6): p. 412-7.

[6]   Woodhall, B.B., G.W., Peripheral Nerve Regeneration: A Follow-up Study of 3,656 World War II Injuries, ed. B.B. Woodhall, G.W. 1956, Washington, D.C.: United States Government Printing Office.

[7]   Denmark, A., An example of symptoms resembling Tic Douloureux produced by a wound in the Radial Nerve. *Medico-Chirurgical Transactions, 1813*. 4: p. 48-52.

[8]   Duttagupta, S., Causalgia: An Historical Perspective. *The History of Anaesthesia Society Proceedings*, 2010. 42: p. 76-87.

[9]   Hamilton, J., On some effects resulting from Wounds of Nerves. *Dublin Journal of Medical Science*, 1838. 13: p. 38-57.

[10]   Harden, R.N., et al., Complex regional pain syndrome: practical diagnostic and treatment guidelines, 4th edition. *Pain Med.*, 2013. 14(2): p. 180-229.

[11]   Hooshmand, H., Chronic Pain: Reflex Sympathetic Dystrophy, Prevention, and Management. 1993: CRC Press.

[12]   Paget, J., Clinical lecture on some cases of local paralysis. *Medical Times and Gazette*, 1864. 26(1): p. 331-332.

[13]   Freemon, F.R., The first neurological research center: Turner's Lane Hospital during the American Civil War. *J. Hist Neurosci.*, 1993. 2(2): p. 135-42.

[14]   Coupland, W., Notes, Short Comments, and Answers to Correspondents. *Lancet*, 1918. 191(4936): p. 520.

[15]   Ross, J., Surgery of the Sympathetic Nervous System. 3 ed. 1958, London: Balliere, Tindall & Cox.

[16]   Richards, R.L., The term 'causalgia.' Med Hist, 1967. 11(1): p. 97-9.

[17]   Dunglison, R., *A Dictionary of Medical Science*. 1874, London: J. & A. Churchill.

[18]   Richards, R.L., Causalgia. A centennial review. *Arch. Neurol.*, 1967. 16(4): p. 339-50.

[19]   Olson, W.L., Historical differentiation between erythromelalgia and causalgia. *J. Am. Acad. Dermatol.*, 1991. 24(1): p. 153-4.

[20]   Koehler, P.J. and D.J. Lanska, Mitchell's influence on European studies of peripheral nerve injuries during World War I. *J. Hist Neurosci.*, 2004. 13(4): p. 326-35.

[21]   Tinel, J., Les Blessures des Nerfs. 1916, Paris: Masson.

[22]   Turco, A., A Case of Causalgia Treated by Decortication of the Artery. Surgery, Gynecology, and Obstetrics, 1921. 33: p. 126.

[23]   Harden, R., Stanton-Hicks, M, Diagnosis of CRPS: Summary. Progress in Pain Research and Management, ed. R. Harden, Baron R, Janig, W. 2001: IASP Press.

[24]   Schott, G.D., Complex? Regional? Pain? Syndrome? *Pract. Neurol.*, 2007. 7(3): p. 145-57.

[25]   Sebastin, S.J., Complex regional pain syndrome. *Indian J. Plast. Surg.*, 2011. 44(2): p. 298-307.

[26]   Athanassio-Benisty, C., *Formes cliniques des lesions des nerfs*. 2 ed. 1918, Paris: Masson.

[27]   Athanassio-Benisty, C., *Les lesions des nerfs: traitement et restauration*. 1919, Paris: Masson.

[28]   Sudeck, P., Über die akute entzündliche Knochenatrophie. *Archiv für klinische Chirurgie*, 1900. 62: p. 147-56.

[29] Maihofner, C., F. Seifert, and K. Markovic, Complex regional pain syndromes: new pathophysiological concepts and therapies. *Eur. J. Neurol.*, 2010. 17(5): p. 649-60.

[30] Gay, A.M., N. Bereni, and R. Legre, Type I complex regional pain syndrome. *Chir. Main,* 2013. 32(5): p. 269-80.

[31] Stookey, B.P., Surgical and Mechanical Treatment of Peripheral Nerves. 1922, Philadelphia: W.B. Saunders Company.

[32] Yealland, L., Median Nerve Injury; Causalgia; Alcohol Injections. *Proceedings of the Royal Society of Medicine,* 1916. 9: p. 61-62.

[33] Buzzard; Farquhad, E., Transactions of the Medical Society of London, 1916. 39: p. 79.

[34] Sicard, J.A., Traitement des nevrites douloureuses de guerre causalgies par l'alcoolisation nerveuse locale. La Presse Medicale, 1916.

[35] Spiller, W.G., Diseases of the Nervious System. Progressive Medicine, ed. H.A. Hare. 1920, Philadelphia and New York: Lea & Febiger.

[36] White, J.C., Diagnostic blocking of sympathetic nerves to extremities with procaine: test to evaluate the benefit of sympathetic ganglionectomy JAMA, 1930. 94(18): p. 1382-1388.

[37] Spurling, R.G., Causalgia of the Upper Extremity: Treatment by Dorsal Sympathetic Ganglionectomy. *Archives of Neurology & Psychiatry,* 1930. 23: p. 784-788.

[38] Kwan, S.T., The Treatment of Causalgia by Thoracic Sympathetic Ganglionectomy. *Ann. Surg.,* 1935. 101(1): p. 222-7.

[39] Homans, J., Minor Causalgia: A Hyperesthetic Hemovascular Syndrome. *New England Journal of Medicine,* 1940. 222: p. 870-874.

[40] Livingston, W.K., Fantom limb pain: A report of ten cases in which it was treated by injections of procaine hydrochloride near the thoracic sympathetic ganglions. *Archives of Surgery,* 1938. 37(3): p. 353-370.

[41] De Takats, G., Reflex dystrophy of the extremities. *Archives of Surgery,* 1937. 34(5): p. 939-956.

[42] Bonica, J., The Management of Pain. 1953, New York: Lea and Febiger.

[43] Livingston, W.K., Pain Mechanisms. 1943, New York: Macmillan Publishing Co, Inc.

[44] Granit, R. and C.R. Skoglund, Facilitation, inhibition and depression at the ;artificial synapse' formed by the cut end of a mammalian nerve. *J. Physiol.,* 1945. 103(4): p. 435-48.

[45] Doupe, J., C.H. Cullen, and G.Q. Chance, Post-Traumatic Pain and the Causalgic Syndrome. *J. Neurol. Psychiatry,* 1944. 7(1-2): p. 33-48.

[46] Spiegel, I.M., JL, Causalgia: a preliminary report of nine cases successfully treated by surgical and chemical interruption of the sympathetic pathways. *JAMA,* 1945. 127(1): p. 9-15.

[47] Evans, J.A., Reflex sympathetic dystrophy; report on 57 cases. *Ann. Intern. Med., 1947.* 26(3): p. 417-26.

[48] Friedman, H.H., T.G. Argyros, and O. Steinbrocker, Neurovascular syndromes of the shoulder girdle and upper extremity: the compression disorders and the shoulder-hand syndrome. *Postgrad. Med. J.,* 1959. 35: p. 397-404.

[49] Echlin, F., F.M. Owens, Jr., and W.L. Wells, Observations on major and minor causalgia. *Arch. Neurol. Psychiatry,* 1949. 62(2): p. 183-203.

[50] Nathan, P.W., On the pathogenesis of causalgia in peripheral nerve injuries. *Brain,* 1947. 70(Pt 2): p. 145-70.

[51] Drucker, W.R., et al., Pathogenesis of post-traumatic sympathetic dystrophy. *Am. J. Surg.*, 1959. 97(4): p. 454-65.

[52] Melzack, R. and P.D. Wall, Pain mechanisms: a new theory. Science, 1965. 150(3699): p. 971-9.

[53] Melzack, R., Phantom limb pain: implications for treatment of pathologic pain. *Anesthesiology*, 1971. 35(4): p. 409-19.

[54] Kozin, F., et al., The reflex sympathetic dystrophy syndrome (RSDS). III. Scintigraphic studies, further evidence for the therapeutic efficacy of systemic corticosteroids, and proposed diagnostic criteria. *Am. J. Med.*, 1981. 70(1): p. 23-30.

[55] Roberts, W.J., A hypothesis on the physiological basis for causalgia and related pains. *Pain*, 1986. 24(3): p. 297-311.

[56] Campbell, J.M., RA; Raja, SN, Is nociceptor activation by alpha-1 adrenoreceptors the culprit in sympathetically maintained pain? *APS Journal*, 1992. 1(1): p. 3-11.

[57] Gibbons, J.J. and P.R. Wilson, RSD score: criteria for the diagnosis of reflex sympathetic dystrophy and causalgia. *Clin. J. Pain*, 1992. 8(3): p. 260-3.

[58] Stanton-Hicks, M., et al., Reflex sympathetic dystrophy: changing concepts and taxonomy. *Pain*, 1995. 63(1). p. 127-33.

[59] Harden, R.N., Objectification of the diagnostic criteria for CRPS. *Pain Med.*, 2010. 11(8): p. 1212-5.

[60] Bruehl, S., et al., External validation of IASP diagnostic criteria for Complex Regional Pain Syndrome and proposed research diagnostic criteria. International Association for the Study of Pain. *Pain*, 1999. 81(1-2): p. 147-54.

[61] Harden, R.N., et al., Proposed new diagnostic criteria for complex regional pain syndrome. *Pain Med.*, 2007. 8(4): p. 326-31.

[62] Harden, R.N. and S.P. Bruehl, Diagnosis of complex regional pain syndrome: signs, symptoms, and new empirically derived diagnostic criteria. *Clin. J. Pain*, 2006. 22(5): p. 415-9.

[63] Wilson, P.S.-H.M., Harden, RN, CRPS: Current Diagnosis and Therapy. 2005, Seattle, WA: IASP Press.

[64] Harden, R.N., et al., Validation of proposed diagnostic criteria (the "Budapest Criteria") for Complex Regional Pain Syndrome. *Pain*, 2010. 150(2): p. 268-74.

[65] de Mos, M., et al., The incidence of complex regional pain syndrome: a population-based study. *Pain*, 2007. 129(1-2): p. 12-20.

[66] Sandroni, P., et al., Complex regional pain syndrome type I: incidence and prevalence in Olmsted county, a population-based study. *Pain*, 2003. 103(1-2): p. 199-207.

[67] Bruehl, S. and O.Y. Chung, How common is complex regional pain syndrome-Type I? *Pain*, 2007. 129(1-2): p. 1-2.

[68] Choi, Y.S., et al., Epidemiology of complex regional pain syndrome: a retrospective chart review of 150 Korean patients. *J. Korean Med. Sci.*, 2008. 23(5): p. 772-5.

[69] Raja, S.N. and T.S. Grabow, Complex regional pain syndrome I (reflex sympathetic dystrophy). *Anesthesiology*, 2002. 96(5): p. 1254-60.

[70] Allen, G., B.S. Galer, and L. Schwartz, Epidemiology of complex regional pain syndrome: a retrospective chart review of 134 patients. *Pain*, 1999. 80(3): p. 539-44.

[71] Duman, I., et al., Reflex sympathetic dystrophy: a retrospective epidemiological study of 168 patients. *Clin. Rheumatol.*, 2007. 26(9): p. 1433-7.

[72] Sharma, A., et al., A web-based cross-sectional epidemiological survey of complex regional pain syndrome. *Reg. Anesth Pain Med.*, 2009. 34(2): p. 110-5.

[73] Der Sarkissian, C., et al., Ancient genomics. *Philos Trans R Soc. Lond B Biol. Sci.*, 2015. 370(1660).

[74] Veldman, P.H., et al., Signs and symptoms of reflex sympathetic dystrophy: prospective study of 829 patients. *Lancet,* 1993. 342(8878): p. 1012-6.

[75] Zyluk, A., The natural history of post-traumatic reflex sympathetic dystrophy. *J. Hand Surg. Br.,* 1998. 23(1): p. 20-3.

[76] Li, Z., et al., Complex regional pain syndrome after hand surgery. *Hand Clin.,* 2010. 26(2): p. 281-9.

[77] Besse, J.L., et al., Effect of vitamin C on prevention of complex regional pain syndrome type I in foot and ankle surgery. *Foot Ankle Surg.,* 2009. 15(4): p. 179-82.

[78] Rewhorn, M.J., et al., Incidence of complex regional pain syndrome after foot and ankle surgery. *J. Foot Ankle Surg.,* 2014. 53(3): p. 256-8.

[79] da Costa, V.V., et al., Incidence of regional pain syndrome after carpal tunnel release. Is there a correlation with the anesthetic technique? *Rev. Bras. Anestesiol., 2011.* 61(4): p. 425-33.

[80] Zyluk, A., Complex regional pain syndrome type I. Risk factors, prevention and risk of recurrence. *J. Hand Surg. Br.,* 2004. 29(4): p. 334-7.

[81] Katholi, B.R., et al., Noninvasive treatments for pediatric complex regional pain syndrome: a focused review. PM R, 2014. 6(10): p. 926-33.

[82] Tan, E.C., et al., Complex regional pain syndrome type I in children. *Acta Paediatr.,* 2008. 97(7): p. 875-9.

[83] Low, A.K., K. Ward, and A.P. Wines, Pediatric complex regional pain syndrome. *J. Pediatr. Orthop.,* 2007. 27(5): p. 567-72.

[84] Wilder, R.T., Management of pediatric patients with complex regional pain syndrome. *Clin. J. Pain,* 2006. 22(5): p. 443-8.

[85] van Velzen, G.A., et al., Health-related quality of life in 975 patients with complex regional pain syndrome type 1. *Pain,* 2014. 155(3): p. 629-34.

[86] Kemler, M.A. and H.C. de Vet, Health-related quality of life in chronic refractory reflex sympathetic dystrophy (complex regional pain syndrome type I). *J. Pain Symptom Manage,* 2000. 20(1): p. 68-76.

[87] Galer, B.S., et al., Course of symptoms and quality of life measurement in Complex Regional Pain Syndrome: a pilot survey. *J. Pain Symptom Manage,* 2000. 20(4): p. 286-92.

[88] Tan, E.C., et al., Quality of life in adults with childhood-onset of Complex Regional Pain Syndrome type I. *Injury,* 2009. 40(8): p. 901-4.

In: Complex Regional Pain Syndrome
Editors: Nader D. Nader and Ognjen Visnjevac

ISBN: 978-1-63483-130-7
© 2015 Nova Science Publishers, Inc.

Chapter 2

PATHOPHYSIOLOGY AND RELATED MECHANISMS

Nader D. Nader[1,], MD, PhD, FACC, FCCP*
and Harsha Nair[2], MD
[1]Departments of Anesthesiology and Surgery,
University at Buffalo, Buffalo, NY, US
[2]School of Medicine and Biomedical Sciences,
University at Buffalo, Buffalo, NY, US

INTRODUCTION

Complex Regional Pain Syndrome (CRPS) is a chronic neuropathic pain disorder that involves one or more extremity with dystrophic changes of skin, muscle, and bone. CRPS is characterized by constant regional neuropathic pain that does not follow the usual dermatomal distribution or nerve territory. In addition to neuropathic pain patients suffer from sensory loss, autonomic dysfunction, vasculature changes and motor dysfunction in the region affected. [1, 2] As a debilitating disease with an unclear pathophysiology, patients suffering from this disorder often do not get the adequate level of care or treatment. Until recently, many clinicians believed CRPS was a purely psychiatric ailment and was lumped together with conditions such as conversion disorder. Recent strides in the understanding of both the nervous system's and body's responses to trauma has allowed both researchers and clinicians to elucidate possible pathophysiology components for this disorder, as well as to better understand the CRPS patient. Currently, CRPS is viewed to be a multiple component disorder activated by the dysfunction of multiple systems. This includes local injury response, inflammatory response, central and peripheral nervous sensitization, abnormal vasculature changes and psychiatric components.

Claude Bernard, a French physiologist credited with proposing what is now known as homeostasis in the 1800's is credited with first theorizing the link between the sympathetic nervous system and pain. One of his students was Silas Weir-Mitchell, a surgeon during the American Civil War. As a field surgeon, Weir-Mitchell was responsible for many surgical treatment and follow up care for his patients. He noted that about 10% of his patients who had

---

[*] E-mail: nnader@buffalo.edu.

trauma to peripheral nerves in limbs began to express unusual symptomology. [3, 4] These symptoms included a basal level of a burning pain sensation that was easily aggravated by minor touch, and movement. Within these injured limbs, he also noted considerable swelling of the limb, excessive sweating, and inappropriate hair loss with smoothing of the skin. He noted that these injuries never fully transected the peripheral nerve, leading him to believe that the damaged nerve in addition to skin pathology was the cause of these symptoms. He termed this condition "causalgia". [3, 5, 6] One of the first instances of formal documentation of CRPS dates back to the twentieth century when German surgeon Paul Sudeck first published a paper describing posttraumatic pain syndrome with edema and trophic changes in posttraumatic bone dystrophy patients. [7, 8] Sudeck noted that these patients exhibited the classic CRPS symptomology in patients who had not undergone any discernable nerve injury. His findings contributed to the hypothesis that postulated what was initially termed Reflex Sympathetic Dystrophy (also known as Sudeck's Atrophy after Sudeck). Since 1900, debate over the pathophysiology has been an important point of discussion and debate. In 1993, the International Association for the Study of Pain (IASP) selected the name CRPS in order to clarify and provide more uniformity for diagnosis.

CRPS has a variety of presentations that vary greatly between patients and even within individuals over time. The pain itself is generally characterized as neuropathic-described as burning, stinging, tingling, stabbing or shock like sensation. This differs from nociceptive pain, which is typically described as sharp, aching and throbbing type pain. Edema, body temperature dysfunction, paresthesia and even paralysis are often seen in the affected limb. This presentation makes CRPS a disorder that is a mixture of positive symptoms and negative symptoms. Positive symptoms are behaviors or sensations that are absent in the normal patient. Examples of this in CRPS are pain, hyperesthesia, allodynia, edema, and paresthesia. Negative symptoms are functions that are normally found in normal patients, but are diminished or not present in affected persons. Negative symptoms include paralysis, and sensory loss. [5, 9, 10]

The IASP divides CRPS into two subtypes based on the presence of an identifiable nerve lesion post injury. CRPS Type I (CRPS I) makes up 90% of cases. It generally begins with a noxious event much like CRPS Type II (CRPS II), but differs in that no neural lesion can be confirmed with testing or imaging post injury. CRPS I was formerly known as Reflex Sympathetic Dystrophy, Sudeck's atrophy, algoneurodystrophy, and shoulder-hand syndrome. These previous names are indicative of the possible pathologies that have been explored to explain the condition. CRPS II, formerly known as causalgia consists of CRPS symptoms with evidence of nerve lesions. The majority of CRPS instances are linked with a causative trauma or insult. Still, there are cases of CRPS developing with no discernable insult or trauma. These spontaneous cases make up about 10% of total cases. [11-13]

Another important stride in the understanding and care for patients with CRPS came with the formation of commonly accepted set of diagnostic criteria for CRPS. These criteria were created in 2003 through an invitation-only workshop held in Budapest, Hungary for IASP members from around the world.

Together, these members created the consensus statement commonly known as the Budapest Criteria, named so after the location where they met. These criteria soon became a useful diagnostic tool in identifying patients with CRPS. These criteria (Table 1) have two separate versions: one for clinical criteria and another for research criteria.

Table 1. Budapest Clinical and Research diagnostic criteria for CRPS [14]

Patient must report at least one symptom in three out of the four categories	
Sensory	Hyperalgesia and/or allodynia
Vasomotor:	Skin color change/asymmetry, temperature changes/asymmetry
Sudomotor/Edema:	Swelling or sweating changes/asymmetry
Motor/Trophic:	Weakness, tremor, dystonia, decreased range of motion, trophic changes/asymmetry involving nails, skin and or/ hair
Patients must display at least one symptom at the time of assessment in two or more of the four aforementioned categories.	
Sensory	Evidence of hyperalgesia (to pinprick) and/or allodynia (to a light touch) and/or deep somatic pain for joint movement.
Vasomotor:	Skin color change/asymmetry, temperature changes/asymmetry
Sudomotor/Edema:	Evidence for a decreased range of motion and/or motor dysfunction (weakness, tremor or dystonia) and/or trophic changes involving nails, skin or hair
Patient must report continuing pain that is disproportionate in duration and degree to the usual course of pain after any trauma or noxious event.	
Research Version	
Research Criteria in an effort to balance sensitivity and specificity differs only in the second requirement of the Clinical Criteria. Instead, the Research Criteria requires at least one symptom for all four categories mentioned in the second requirement.	

Since it has recently established for the first time, the validity of the Budapest Criteria has been questioned at times. Harden et al. boast that the Budapest Criteria have a high sensitivity of 92% in diagnosing CRPS, but there is room for improvement with regards to its 36% specificity. [14] Hence, the Clinical Criteria maximizes sensitivity, while the Research Criteria serves to maximize specificity (70% sensitivity and 94% specificity). [9, 15] Still, any added criterion that would be able to maximize both the sensitivity and the specificity would be beneficial in assessment and diagnosis. One step towards this would be developing a greater understanding of the pathophysiology of CRPS.

Recent epidemiologic studies exploring CRPS incidence and prevalence utilized the diagnoses made by general practitioners in 2007 to estimate the number of cases in the general population.

This has yielded the figure of 26.2 patients per 100,000 with 16,000-80,000 new cases yearly in the United States. [10] Using more specific IASP criteria to diagnose, this number is lowered to 16.8 per 100,000. There has been an increase in diagnoses from 5.4 per 100,000 in studies from 1999. [16] Studies show that CRPS 1 occurs in 10% of various fractures, and 7-

35% of Colles' fractures of the wrist. [2] CRPS has a large variation in its presentation; the patient course of the syndrome is also highly variable. A Dutch study looking at patients at a mean of 5.8 years after a triggering injury shows 30% of patients consider themselves completely recovered from their condition. 16% report severe progressive disease, and 54% report stability of the disease. [9] In terms of anatomical distribution the arm is affected 60% of patients vs. 40% in the leg. [10]

Genetically, Human leukocyte antigen class I and II (HLA-I, HLA-II) factors have become an area of study to discern a genetic predisposition to developing CRPS. [17] Evidence for genetic predisposition is still weak for CRPS. Class I and Class II major HLA typing was done in 52 CRPS patients by Kemler et al. in 1999. The frequency of HLA DQ1 was higher among the patients with CRPS. HLA DR13 positive patients tend to manifest CRPS symptoms over multiple sites and develop generalized tonic dystonia. [18] Moreover, a different centromeric locus on HLA class I has been described an association with spontaneous development of CRPS. [19]

The general timeline for CRPS presentation starts with a patient presenting within nine weeks after a minor or moderate injury such as a small fracture or crush injury. [20] Initially, the injured limb is warm, painful and red – also known as warm CRPS. During this time the patient may start experiencing the classical limb-confined symptomology of allodynia, hyperalgesia, inappropriate sweating, blunted hair growth, blunted nail growth, and muscle weakness. Mechanical and thermal dysregulation is the most prominent in acute CRPS. [10] As the disease progresses, pain does not subside but spreads to distributions that are outside of a specific nerve or nerve root distributions.

In 2000, a study analyzed the course of the spread of CRPS within a patient. In this study, Maleki et al. discerned three types of spread: contiguous, independent, and mirror image. CRPS spread can present as all three of these patterns, or just remain in the isolated region it initially presents at. Contiguous spread is seen when you have proximal and distal expansion of symptoms from the initial symptomatic region. [21] Theories regarding the mechanism of contiguous spread range from an abnormal inflammatory process to therapeutic interventions such as splints or cast triggering exacerbations. Independent spread occurs when a new localization of symptoms is found in an area distant and non-contiguous with the initial CRPS site (e.g., initial site being the right foot, the independent spread site being the left shoulder or arm). Similarly, theories regarding this mechanism stem from new trauma, such as misuse of crutches causing brachial plexus injury, or as sequelae to an ill placed nerve block. In fact, Maleki et al. state there was an association of a causative event with independent spread in a majority of cases. [21] Mirror image spread consists of CRPS appearing on the opposite side of an initial site (e.g., left foot, then right foot.) The onset of this spread is proposed to stem from compensatory movement in the opposite limb, causing trauma in an already susceptible CRPS patient. [21] Maleki et al. were unable to definitively link secondary trauma or overuse to any of these spreads patterns. It was suggested the variable latency of onset of these patterns (two days to 13 months for contiguous, 1 month to 12 years for independent, and 1 month to 7.6 years for mirror image made an exaggerated abnormal inflammatory response unlikely to be a source of CRPS spread. Van Rijn et al. also studied spread in their 2011 study at a tertiary center, examining patients with multiple limbs expressing CRPS on presentation, termed Multiple-CRPS. They found a significant difference in age, with multiple-CRPS patients being significantly younger at onset than single-CRPS patients. This was thought to be suggestive of a genetic component that makes some patients experience more severe and prolific disease than others. [17]

As the syndrome progresses from "warm" or acute (4 months) CRPS to the chronic phase or "cold" CRPS (18 months), the limb may appear bluish in color and rapid hair growth and skin changes are often visible. A third phase of progression can be discerned with further advancing of symptoms with dystrophic changes continuing coupled with new-onset dystonia. [22] Patients can complain of myoclonus, dystonia as well as movement induced worsening of pain. While the general progression of CRPS usually begins with warm CRPS, patients can experience any three of these phases at any time. Symptoms tend to worsen proximally rather than distally though patients may start having symptoms in other limbs as well. Patients without resolution of CRPS for more than 5 years can express more advanced neurological symptoms such as syncope, and urological dysfunction. Cognitive impairment is another advanced symptom associated with long term CRPS, though this has not been seen often and is credited to other possible etiology. [10] Like other neuropathic pain disorders, CRPS also affects quality of life beyond physical symptoms. It has been documented that patients who suffer from CRPS often suffer economic and personal life problems. Disabling pain can lead to loss of working days or even loss of employment depending on job requirements. Furthermore treating chronic pain can be very expensive leading to increased health care costs. Aside from financial difficulty, patients often find their condition takes a toll on their married, social, and sexual life, leading to social isolation. [22]

With an unclear pathophysiology, the treatment for CRPS is another source of discussion and debate. Recent systematic reviews on interventions have shown that there is a low quality evidence base for most CRPS treatments. [23] This is particularly regarding the variety of block therapies that have been the staple first line treatment for CRPS. Like opioid administration during pain breakthrough and crisis, blocks provide pain free periods, but do not provide long lasting therapy. [3] Glucocorticoids are the only oral therapy that has demonstrated significant efficacy in some clinical trials. [24] Patient management is clinician-dependent with a variety of treatments utilized to manage symptomology. Currently, it is recommended that patients with moderate to severe CRPS be treated and assessed by a pain specialist who has experience treating other forms of neuropathic pain. These providers have experience in integrated interdisciplinary pain care while additionally providing the opportunity for more advanced, invasive procedures for patients with severe refractory pain. [9] Physical therapy and gradual desensitization to sensory stimuli performed by occupational therapists in the United States are important components of restoring functionality to patients. [3] Some physical therapy pain modulation techniques used are hot and cold packs, ultrasound, short-wave diathermy, transcutaneous electrical nerve stimulation (TENS), high voltage galvanic stimulation, and deep brain stimulation. Another route of treatment focuses on the possible psychiatric and neurologic links to CRPS. Tricyclic antidepressants (TCAs), serotonin-norepinephrine reuptake inhibitors (SNRIs) and anticonvulsants such gabapentin and pregablin have also been used to some limited success. With a high incidence of anxiety and depression linked with CRPS, psychological intervention such as cognitive based therapy (CBT) has been shown to be a possible non-pharmacologic pain modulation tool. There has been some success utilizing CBT in patients with anxiety and depression associated CRPS. [3] Links to osteoporosis coupled with some clinical trial data has shown benefit of bisphosphonate treatment for patients, though this is a pharmacological treatment with many unanswered questions. [5, 9]

CRPS Type I

The more common of the two subsets of CRPS, type I's key characteristic is the absence of an associated nerve lesion. This distinction has come under criticism recently. With trauma that does not cause an obvious nerve lesion, there is still peripheral damage. These post-fracture and post-surgical cases are placed into the CRPS I category. Placzek et al. argue that an immediate evaluation for peripheral nerve compression should be sought in all post-surgical cases of CRPS. [10, 25] More recent studies have noted that while patients with CRPS I do not have obvious nerve lesions, there is a change in the nerve densities of the affected limbs, suggesting pathology linked to the maintenance of nerve integrity. [26, 27] The unclear pathophysiology and multi-faceted nature of CRPS I have made it an increasingly popular subject of interest for pain research.

Currently CRPS I has been characterized by the following: spontaneous pain, allodynia, or hyperalgesia not localized purely to a single peripheral nerve, tending to have a disproportionate regionalization with disproportionate intensity of symptoms. Edema, disturbed blood flow, local temperature dysfunction and abnormal activity of the sweat glands are found in the affected limb. It is a diagnosis of exclusion; no other conditions can be attributed to the pathophysiology. [2, 16]

CRPS Type II

As mentioned above, CRPS II is distinguished from type 1 by the presence of a confirmed peripheral nerve lesion. This identification can be done by imaging or electrophysiological studies. As mentioned above, some experts argue that this distinction is merely a distinction of semantics based purely on imaging and lesion verification. With the presence of a lesion, the argument for intervention is stronger. Nerve decompression is one procedure that can provide rapid improvement in symptoms if a nerve in distress can be identified. [25]

Pathophysiology

The pathophysiology of CRPS remains unclear though in the past two decades insight into the mechanism has gradually increased with current avenues of exploration, which consist of the following: abnormal tissue response to injury, peripheral and central nervous sensitization and inflammation, vasomotor dysfunction, endothelial dysfunction, neurogenic inflammation, supraspinal reorganization or maladaptation, disturbed sympathetic-afferent coupling, hyperalgesic priming, and autoimmunity. [1, 3, 9, 10]

This combination of possible causes led researchers to propose peripheral afferent, efferent and central mechanisms to explain CRPS, making it a unique cause of holistic neuropathic pain.

The previous names used to describe CRPS, particularly Reflex Sympathetic Dystrophy point to the sympathetic-afferent coupling dysfunction that many believe to be the largest component of CRPS.

ABNORMAL TISSUE RESPONSE TO INJURY

The majority of CRPS incidents occur after some type of noxious event. The most common documented source of this injury is a fracture, specifically wrist fracture. Additionally, other forms of trauma such as stroke, crush injuries and even long term immobility have been linked to CRPS. There are three major phases of response to soft tissue damage. These include an inflammatory phase, a proliferative phase and remodeling phase. [28] The inflammatory phase is responsible for hemostasis, removal of dead tissue, and prevention of infection from possible pathogens. The proliferative phase is a time of growth, reconstruction and revascularization. The remodeling phase is a time of restoration and reconfiguration of the temporary measures made by the previous two phases. [28] Much like CRPS, wound healing, particularly the remodeling phase, is not a completely understood process. While the aforementioned phases described have been shown to occur in chronological order, there is a fluidity to which phase of healing a patient may be in. This fluidity and variation in time is the product of a plethora of molecular signaling and changing chemical concentrations that trigger more molecular signaling. In fact, the remodeling phase is reported to take between 21 days to an entire year. This leaves ample time and opportunity for complication.

All three of these phases are driven by molecular messengers that activate potent biochemical cascades. These signals in turn serve to bring a variety of different cell types responsible for immunity, debris clearing, and repair. White blood cells such as monocytes and macrophages, and neutrophils arrive for the immune defense and clearance of damaged tissue. Platelets, keratinocytes fibroblasts and endothelial cells play important roles in clotting, damage control and revascularization. [28] Studies have shown that CRPS patients tend to have normal white blood cell counts compared to controls. Being that an elevated white blood cell count has been the first indication of infection and pan-inflammation, these studies suggest a local inflammation process during the initial phase of CRPS I. [29] While this acute phase is a beneficial and essential part of the healing process, it is important to keep it in check. Recent studies exploring the venous blood of patients with suction blisters in acute CRPS patients (4 months of symptomology) have shown elevation of pro-inflammatory cytokines, specifically interleukin 6 (IL-6), interleukin 8 (IL-8), interleukin 1β (IL-1β), macrophage inflammatory protein-1 β (MIP-1 β), and Tumor Necrosis Factor α (TNF-α) in blister fluid. [2] Complementing these findings, a reduction in the concentration of a number of anti-inflammatory agents such as interlukin-1 receptor antagonist (IL-1RA) has also been shown. [30] TNF-α and MIP-1 β in CRPS I patients have been shown to be significantly elevated when compared to patients with other pain syndromes suggesting inflammation plays a key role in CRPS I. It is of note that TNF-α represents an acute phase marker of inflammation while IL-6 is a late phase marker leading researchers to believe it plays a role in late phase healing during the proliferative and remodeling phase. [31] TNF-α has shown an increase in serum levels within 3 days of a fracture in humans. [7] CRPS patients with inciting traumas occurring months to years prior to testing have higher levels of TNF-α protein in affected limbs compared to both osteoarthritic patients and acute trauma. Patients with elevated serum TNF-α levels show weak correlations to classic inflammation signs such as pain and elevated skin temperature in some CRPS patient groups. This is suggestive of multiple mechanisms for TNF-α regulation. [7] Until recently, many studies had shown that there was an elevation of these cytokines in the affected limb of patients while, more recent studies have shown that there is an elevation in unaffected CRPS limbs as well. These levels were elevated in samples from both affected and unaffected limbs, suggesting more than a localized response. [30]

While measurement of cytokines has been shown to be indicative of a possible inflammation trigger, it is important to note that changes in cytokine levels in CRPS patients have not been found to correlate to clinical outcomes. [30] Table 2 tabulates the role of various cytokines; growth factors and neuropeptides involved in inflammation and injury responses leading to the development of CRPS.

Aside from the cytokines, elevated concentrations neuropeptides such as neuropeptide Y (NPY), substance P [29], endothelin-1 (ET-1), and calcitonin gene-related peptide (CGRP), also lend credence to an initial localized insult causing uninhibited activation of a multiple factor mediated response. [32]

Table 2. Inflammatory mediators role in development of CRPS

Mediator	Abbr	Source	Description
Transforming Growth factor β	TGF-β	Platelets, macrophages, T and B cells, hepatocytes	Angiogenesis, chemo-attraction, induces adhesion molecule expression, pro-inflammatory [28]
Tumor necrosis factor α	TNF-α	Macrophages, T and B cells, fibroblasts natural killer (NK) cells	Induces collagen synthesis in wounds, regulates immune cells, pyrogenic, pro inflammatory, activation of NF-κB [37]
Macrophage Inflammatory protein-1β	MIP -1β	Macrophages	Activate immune cells (granulocytes), induce synthesis of other pro-inflammatory cytokines [38]
Interleukin 1	IL-1β	Macrophages, fibroblasts, dendrite ells, epithelial cells	Pyrogen, proinflammatory, hyperalgesia, vasodilation, hypotension [39]
Interleukin 1 receptor antagonist	IL- 1RA	Epithelial cells, keratinocytes, immune cells	Anti-inflammatory, inhibit IL-1β, IL-6 [40]
Neuropeptide Y	NPY	Neurons	Stress, food intake, anti-anxiolytic, analgesia, circadian rhythm control, immune mediation [41]
Substance P	SP	Neurons, macrophages, eosinophils, lymphocytes, dendritic cells	Pain perception and transmission, mood disorder, neurogenic inflammation, nociception, extravasation of plasma proteins [36, 42]
Endothelin-1	ET-1	Endothelial cells	Vasoconstriction [32]
Calcitonin gene related peptide	CGRP	Neurons, Keratinocytes	Vasodilatation, pain transmission [43]

Neurons are ectodermal tissue in origin and produce and store many neuromodulators such as CGRP. Likewise, keratinocytes are the predominant cell in the epidermis, are also of ectodermal origin, and produce CGRP as well.

Recent studies propose CGRP production in keratinocytes could play a role in initiating more central sensitization and neuropathic pain after an injury or insult. [33] In addition to this change in molecular chemistry and signaling in CRPS patients, studies looking at sectioned muscle tissue and peripheral nerve tissue from CRPS effected limbs have shown evidence of pathologic changes in the innervation and vasculature of these limbs.

With regards to this musculature change, a study performed by Van er Laan et al. showed muscle change consistent with ischemic microangiopathy. The authors of this study describe capillaries in the tissue specimens as having thickened basal membranes and showed improved oxygen consumption when treated with free radical scavenger dimethylsulfoxide (DMSO). These tissue changes combined with the improvement of oxygen utilization with DMSO led the authors to propose oxygen-derived free radicals are involved in the pathophysiology of CRPS. [26] Coderre et al. proposed a model of chronic post ischemic pain (CPIP), which entailed a tourniquet inducing ischemia and reperfusion injury in a rat. Their model focuses on this ischemia leading to deep tissue injury secondary to acute inflammation causing a compartment syndrome-like injury (Figure 2.1). This micro compartment syndrome leads to microvascular ischemia reperfusion injury, which in turn leads to vasospasm and alteration of blood flow dynamics. These alterations in blood flow and vessel patency cause deep tissue ischemia.

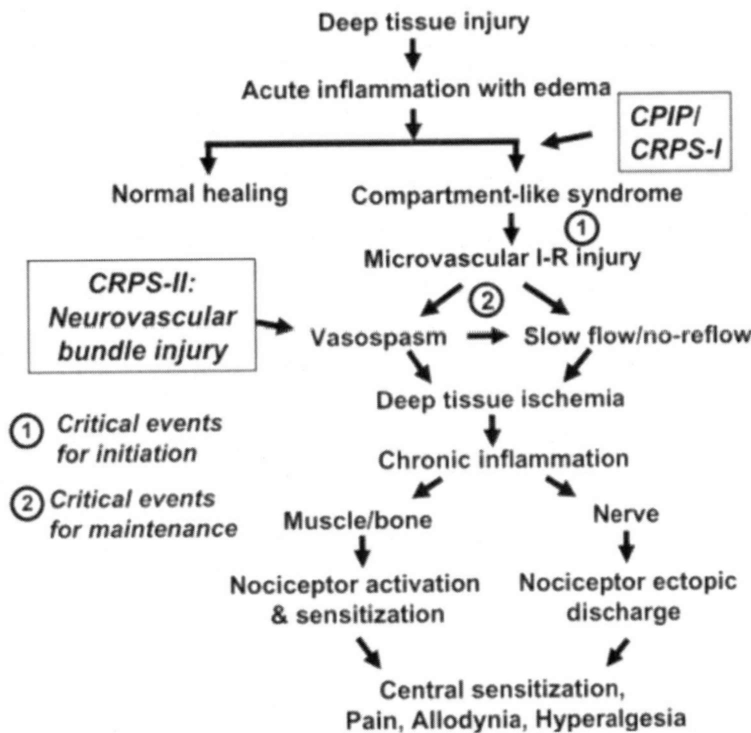

Figure 2.1. A mechanistic model that was proposed by Coderre and Bennett (Adopted with permission).

Deep tissue ischemia serves as a nidus for chronic inflammation that in turn causes the sensitization and activation of muscle and bone tissue nociceptors as well as adrenoreceptors. Additionally, chronic inflammation triggers the pain nerve fibers in the area to ectopically fire, initiating signal cascades, leading to central nervous system sensitization. [34] Tissue has been shown to have high level of oxidative enzymes post ischemia. When reperfusion occurs, these enzymes are privy to oxygen rich blood leading to oxidative reactions and free radical formation. These free radicals cause damage to the vascular endothelial and smooth muscle cells. This same study also argues that the pain felt by CRPS patients is very similar to muscle inflammatory pain. The authors cite a correlation regarding muscle lactate, a marker of muscle ischemia, with the level of symptomology in CRPS patient. The importance of the initial insult or injury, and the body's inappropriate or skewed reaction to it is an essential component of CRPS.

PERIPHERAL NERVOUS SYSTEM INJURY AND SENSITIZATION

The perception of noxious stimuli by free end pain receptors is known as nociception. It falls to the peripheral nervous system (PNS) to relay this information to the central nervous system in order to process and react to these signals. These free endings are known as nociceptors and can be triggered by stimuli of different modalities. These modalities consist of mechanical (pinches, crush injury), thermal, and chemical (capsaicin, acetic acid, and melatin). [35] There are two types of major nociceptor classes: the Aδ fibers and the C fibers. These primary afferents have the unique property of being pseudo-unipolar. [36] Pseudo-unipolar neurons consist of a centrally positioned soma with two large axons terminating in the periphery as free nerve endings associated with nociceptors, and synapses on the spinal cord. With a centrally located cell body, stimuli from both the peripheral and central synapses can be relayed throughout the nerve. Proteins synthesized in a soma housed in the DRG or trigeminal nuclei can be distributed to both terminal sites. With the same proteins available at each terminal, the nerve endings attain biochemical equivalency. [36] Combining this synapse equivalency with a pseudo unipolar structure, primary afferents are able to convey signals bi-directionally. Additionally, this leads to central terminal receptor ligand interactions exerting local changes at the peripheral endings and vice versa (Figure 2.2). [36]

These bi-directional effects of the PNS primary afferents give credence to an inflammatory trigger for initiating CRPS. Whether it is an inflammatory response to injury acting on peripheral afferents to generate changes at the afferent spinal cord synapse, or neurogenic inflammation at the spinal cord acting on central afferents to affect the peripheral synapses, inflammation at either end may play a role in sensitizing the entire neuron (Figure 2.2).

If this inflammation causes signals to be relayed from central synapses of the primary afferent, it is then possible for the peripheral synapse to release CGRP or SP causing vasodilation and plasma extravasation – hallmarks of CRPS. [36] In addition to factor release, the nerves of the peripheral nervous system may undergo a phenotypic switch when injured. Genes are upregulated and downregulated, causing alterations in excitability, transduction and transmission. Rapidly, fibers that were expressing nociceptors for mechanical stimulation are now expressing receptors that respond to CRGP or SP. [44]

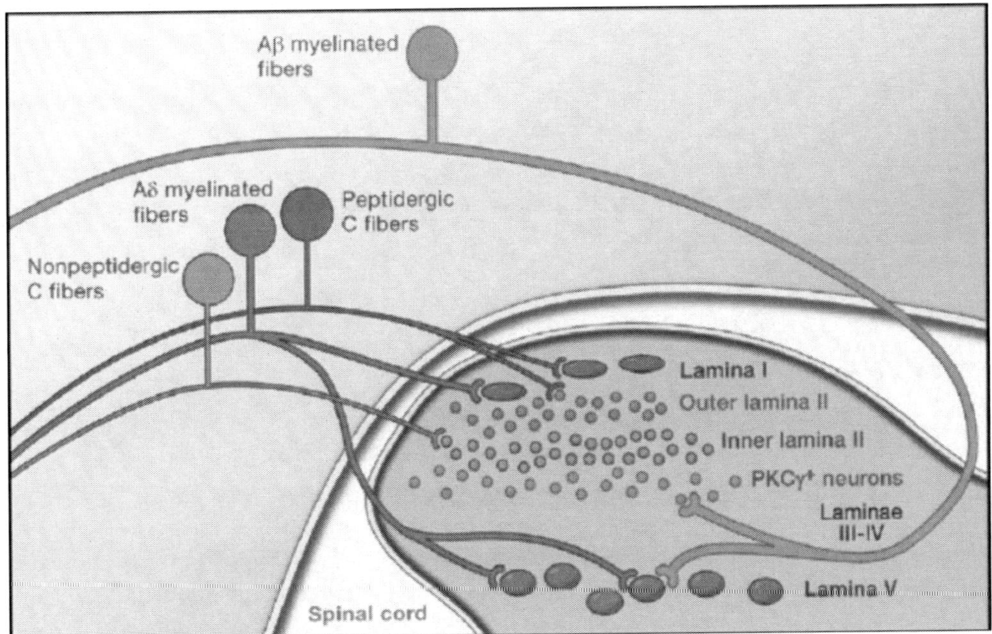

Figure 2.2. The mechanistic model of neuronal centralization and sensitization adopted from "Cellular and molecular mechanism of pain" by Basbaum et al. [36]

This change in fiber gene expression is another avenue that lends credence to the idea that CRPS is a multi-system disorder based on chronic changes of the nervous system.

These chronic peripheral changes are also key components of initiating central nervous sensitization. Damage to peripheral afferents have been shown to cause changes to central axons (due to the pseudo unipolar biochemical equivalency), as well as post synaptic neurons in the dorsal horn and higher level central nervous structures (Figure 2.3). Furthermore this damage and the aforementioned inflammatory response has been shown to trigger microglia and astrocytes of the CNS. [4]

Aβ Fibers

Aβ fibers are responsible for the conduction of light touch. Of the afferent nerve fibers, they are the largest and have the fastest conduction times. These large caliber fibers are associated with low thresholds with high conduction rates receptors such as Merkel cells, Pacinian corpuscles, and hair follicles. These endings transduce mechanical stimulation, specifically pressure, texture and vibration. [36]

Aδ Fibers

The Aδ afferent group consists of medium diameter myelinated (2 to 5 micrometers) fibers with medium conduction velocity. Nerve signals generally travel 2 to 30 meters per second.

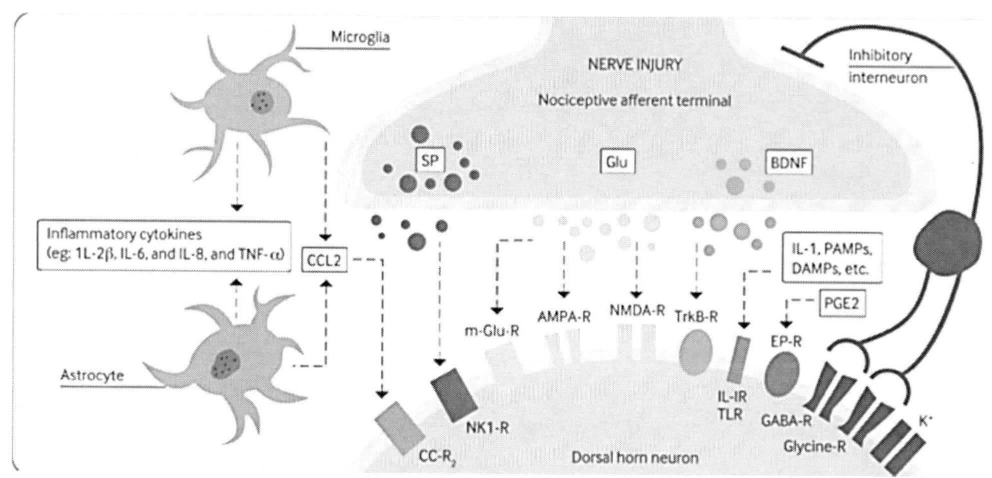

Figure 2.3. The mechanistic model of neuropathic pain adopted from "Neuropathic pain: mechanisms and their clinical implications" by S P Cohen. [44]

These nerve fibers differ from the Aβ fibers which possess larger diameters and faster conduction velocities.

Aδ fibers are further broken down into two sub categories. [36] Type 1 Aδ consist of high-threshold mechanical nociceptors which respond to mechanical and chemical stimuli, but require an intense (> 50°C) or long acting thermal stimuli to trigger firing. These fibers are responsible for the rapid response to pinprick pain.

It is important to note that Type 1 Aδ fibers sensitize to both mechanical and heat stimuli in the presence of injury. [36] This is especially important in CRPS, a condition where allodynia and hyperalgesia occur to disproportionate stimuli. Type 2 Aδ fibers are the inverse of type 1 Aδ fibers in that these nociceptors have low heat threshold and very high mechanical stimuli threshold.

As the type 1 Aδ fiber is responsible for the rapid first response to pinprick, the type 2 Aδ fibers are responsible for the first response to severe thermal stimuli. [36]

These fibers have endings in the epidermis, tunica adventitia of blood vessels, and around hair follicles of free nerve endings. [45] Being that these are primary afferent fibers of the peripheral nervous system, where they synapse within the spinal cord is important. The Aδ axons have synapses in both Lamina I of the spinal cord, as well as Lamina V. [36]

C FIBERS

C fibers are unmyelinated afferents that are thinner than their Aδ counterparts. C fibers range between 0.2-1.5 micrometers with a conduction velocity less than 2 meters per second. They too are subdivided into subgroups with one population that is more responsive to thermal stimuli, and another that is more responsive to mechanical stimuli. Of these populations, there is a subgroup of C fibers that are at baseline mechanical insensitive that become mechanical sensitive in the presence of injury. These nociceptors are termed silent or sleeping nociceptors. [36] These silent nociceptors are generally more sensitive to chemical stimuli, in the form of capsaicin or histamine. These nociceptors are especially important in the context of CRPS due to the possibility of being sensitized to mechanical stimulation after being immersed in the chemical mediators of the inflammatory or injury state. Being that these fibers are more responsive to chemical stimulation, it is possible that this exposure awakens mechanical sensitization in these sleeping nociceptors. Another subsets of C fibers are responsible for itch reactions in the presence of pruritogens.

Finally, not all C fibers are nociceptors, with some of these unmyelinated fibers responsible for producing a pleasant sensation to light stroking. [36] Another quality of C fibers that distinguish between populations is the peptidergic versus non-peptidergic populations. These peptidergic C fibers release SP and CRGP at synapses. Additionally, they express a nerve growth factor (NGF) receptor. These qualities of C fibers serve to further provide evidence for a multiple faceted CRPS pathophysiology model. Like Aδ fibers, C fibers have peripheral terminal endings located in the epidermis, around blood vessels, and as free nerve endings with hair follicles. [45] Peptidergic C fibers synapse in Lamina I and outer Lamina II, while non-peptidergic C fibers send axons to the inner Lamina II. [36] With regards to CRPS, deep-tissue C-fibers that are exposed to the inflammatory milieu post injury have been theorized to ectopically fire and cause central sensitization of peripheral nerves and the central nervous system. Venules are also innervated by C fibers. Damage to C Fibers can lead to de-innervated venules that are no longer able to maintain their integrity. This may lead to fluid extravasation and neurogenic edema. [4] A number of studies have shown a correlation of decreased C fiber density in the epidermis of patients with CRPS. Recent studies looking at amputated limbs of CRPS patient also demonstrated a significant loss of C fibers in the sural nerve. [4] With neuron loss, collateral sprouting may occur. With this sprouting, incorrect matching between fiber and ending can lead to sensitization, excessive activation, sensory loss or constant stimulation. [44]

Aδ and C Fiber Damage

A number of neuropathies are linked to small Aδ and C Fiber damage. Diabetes, shingles, and certain forms of chemotherapy have been noted to cause neuropathic pain through small fiber injury. [4] While neuron loss and damage is a key part of these neuropathies, it is important to note that fiber loss does not correlate with positive symptoms such as pain. Rather, it is the sequelae of regeneration and re-innervation that is responsible for the pain associated with pain syndromes. [4] When a nerve is damaged, cascades are triggered that induce growth factors and generation of new stalks from healthy nerve tissue. Additionally, Wallerian degeneration and programmed atrophy of damaged nerves occurs. Both of these changes may cause maladaptive innervation, leading to neuropathic pain.

Thermal Nociceptors

Thermal nociceptors have the ability to transduce temperatures that reach levels of injury into a noxious signal. This threshold, per Basbaum et al, is 43°C. This temperature serves as a parallel to the heat sensitivity of the aforementioned thermal sensitive C fibers and type 2 Aδ nociceptors. Heat sensation has some cross over with chemical nociception as demonstrated by the ability of capsaicin to activate a vanilloid receptor in populations of C and Aδ nociceptors. This receptor is named TRPV1, representing a group of transient receptor potential (TRP) ion channel receptors. [36] This seemingly misplaced receptor allows for sensations classically paired with thermal stimuli to be triggered by chemical stimuli. Basbaum et al. refer to TRPV1 as the "molecular integrator of thermal and chemical stimuli." [36] Further proof of this comes in the form of capsaicin and thermal evoked stimuli eliciting similar current patterns. An important factor to consider regarding TRPV1 is that its evoked responses are potentiated by pro-inflammatory and painful stimuli. These stimuli include protons, bradykinin and neurotrophins. Inflammation has been demonstrated to potentiate thermal nociception. In times of injury, the TRPV1 channel is exposed to the many chemical agents of inflammation, collectively known as "inflammatory soup." These agents can have an allosteric modulation effect on the TRP channel, or potentiate the downstream cascade. [36] Aside from direct involvement with nerves, TRPV1 channels found in abundance within keratinocytes also suggests a dermal-nervous component to thermal nociception. [33] While the role of TRPV1 has been shown to be significant in inflammation disorders such as sunburn, infection, and inflammatory bowel disease, the possibility of a link to CRPS is a promising area of exploration. In fact, tissue samples taken from patients with CRPS by Albrecht et al. noted that many CGRP positive fibers in deep nerves of CRPS patients co-expressed TRPV1 receptors. When compared to controls, an association with TRPV1 is not typically noted. [45]

MECHANICAL NOCICEPTOR

Mechanical nociceptors are responsible for a large variety of stimulation. This ranges from light touch on hair follicles, to noxious intense pressure stimulation. Within the nociceptor fiber families, Aδ and C fibers both have subpopulations dedicated to both high and low threshold mechanoreceptor endings. These stimulation thresholds can vary in speed, intensity and frequency. To allay these varied stimuli into a common signaling pathway, it requires a receptor system capable of subtle signaling. Acid sensing ion channels or ASICs are one subgroup of mechanical transduction channels responsible for nociception. Found on both high threshold and low threshold neurons, these channels respond to tissue acidosis and ischemia. This quality makes these receptors candidates for nerve sensitization in response to inflammation and tissue damage. TRPV2 is a protein related to the aforementioned TRPV1 and is also responsible for nociception. TRPV2 serves as a both a noxious heat receptor and an osmotic stretch receptor. It is found in vascular smooth muscles have been shown to be triggered by direct suction and osmotic pressure changes. [36] TRPV2 is a prominently expressed ion channel in medium and large diameter Aδ fibers responsible for mechanical and thermal stimuli. Additionally, the TRPV4 and TRPA1 are members of the TRP family that have been singled out for their role in nociception. [36] While neither of these two channel types has been shown to be responsible for primary mechanical stimuli transduction, research points towards possible roles in CRPS. TRPV4 has been linked with injury-evoked pain hypersensitivity. Likewise, TRPA1 studies have provided evidence of its involvement in modulating the excitability of mechanosensitive afferents, particularly post injury and inflammation. [36] TRPA1 channels are activated via chemical interactions between the cysteine residues found on the channel. During oxidative processes, like that of the inflammatory response, electrophilic reactants are formed that bind to those cysteine residues. [36] Additionally, TRPA1 can be indirectly modulated via second messenger cascades triggered by the interaction of pro-inflammatory factors with their own receptors located on afferent fibers. These include pro-inflammatory agents such as bradykinin.

Outside of the TRP family, the role of two pore potassium channels (KCNK) have been identified as other possible mechanical trasnducers with crossover chemical stimulation. KCNK18 a receptor expressed on a peptidergic population of C fibers and low mechanical threshold Aβ fibers has been shown to react with hydroxyl-α-sanshool, an ingredient in Szechuan peppercorns. Studies have shown that exposure to this ingredient can cause a numbing paresthesia-like sensation. This has led researchers to speculate a mechanical-chemical nociception crossover. [36] CRPS has been shown to follow a variety of insults and injuries. One unique trigger noted in a case study was a patient who developed CRPS after receiving a tetanus vaccination. [24] Vaccinations trigger local inflammatory responses. Chemical sensitization of the mechanoreceptor is a property that allows a connection to be made between a toxoid injection and CRPS.

CHEMICAL NOCICEPTOR

Chemo-nociception plays the important role of providing the body with an ability to respond to chemical irritants in the environment, as well as to physiologic stress. As mentioned above, TRP channels play a very prominent role in chemo-transduction. TRPA1 is a particularly important member of this family due to fact that it responds to compounds that form covalent adducts with thiol groups. This allows TRPA1 to be activated by a variety of different chemical triggers. Intriguingly, isofluorane and some other general anesthetics as well as chemotherapy metabolites of drugs like cyclophosphamide have shown to trigger TRPA1 embedded fibers. Side effects of these drugs include acute pain and neuroinflammation. [36] Especially relevant to TRPA1's potential role in CRPS is its activation by factors released due to tissue damage or oxidative stress. This activation can lead to sensitization, with lower thresholds causing patients more pain symptoms.

ION CHANNELS

The factors and signals that activate the nerve fibers make up the primary afferents of the PNS open a variety of ion channels, serving as the medium by which chemical signals are transduced to electric potential signals. Sodium channels in particular are known targets of anesthetics. One of these channels singled out as being overly expressed in patients with pain symptoms due to inflammation is Nav1.7. [46] This channel has been shown to be overly expressed in both paroxysmal extreme pain disorder and erythromelalgia – both disorders that share symptoms such as burning pain with CRPS. Erythromelalgia has been linked to mutation of SCN9A, a gene that codes for Nav1.7. [47] It has been postulated that Nav1.7 is responsible for mechanical and thermal hypersensitivity. Surprisingly, there has been no evidence of overexpression of these channels in patients with evident nerve damage. [36]

Calcium channels are some of the most common players in human biology. From neuronal synapses to muscle contraction, it is no surprise that calcium channels have been shown to play a role in nociception. Cav2.2 and Cav2.3 are calcium channels that have been shown to play a role in sensitization to mechanical and thermal stimuli. [48] Further evidence of calcium channel involvement in hypersensitivity lies in the upregulation of particular subunits. C fiber nociceptors have a dramatically upregulated α2δ subunit population after nerve injury. These subunits are current modulators responsible for current activation and inactivation within the channel. [36] Researchers have shown that increased α2δ subunit populations are found to be associated with allodynia in rats, and lower in populations of rats recovering from tactile allodynia. [49] Gabapentin, a drug often used to treat neuropathic pain has been shown to target this subunit, providing further evidence of an extensive roll in neuropathic pain. Furthermore, its role in the up regulation post nerve injury makes it an area of interest for CRPS.

PERIPHERAL INFLAMMATION

As mentioned above, inflammation is a response to tissue damage. This response is facilitated the release of numerous biological signals (e.g., TNF-α, IL-1ß, IL-6) and mediators that act on multiple systems to initiate immunity and repair. A side effect of this activation is that these systems can have excessive stimulation, which increases the likelihood that sensitization will occur due to excessive activation. Endogenous factors accumulate and activate nociceptors of the PNS triggering signal cascades and total system modulation. These factors consist of neurotransmitters, peptides (SP, CGRP, bradykinin), cytokines, chemokines, prostaglandins and extracellular proteins collectively referred to as the "inflammatory soup." [36] One of the systems greatly affected by the inflammatory soup is the PNS. Nociceptors populate the primary afferent fibers and respond to multiple factors released during the inflammatory response. This property makes nociceptors prime targets for inflammation-induced sensitization, particularly the nociceptors responsible for transduction of noxious temperature and touch stimuli. [36]

Nerve growth factor (NGF) is one specific growth factor noted to be increased in the inflammatory state. In the normal state, NGF is a neurotrophic factor required for the growth and development of neurons during neurogenesis. In the injury and inflammatory state NGF plays a role in growth and repair. As a component of the inflammatory soup, NGF has been found to have interactions with nociceptors on peptidergic C-Fibers. [36] There are two arms of the NGF effect on nociception. The first is a local cascade driven pathway, while the second is a more global factor synthesis and transcription-based pathway. The first of these aforementioned arms begins with nociceptors on C-fibers causing local chemical ion changes. C-Fibers that respond to NGF possess high affinity receptors such as the tyrosine kinase TrkA and low affinity p75 receptor. [36] NGF interaction with these receptors leads to activation of the second messenger cascade via proteins such as phospholipase c (PLC), mitogen-activated protein kinase (MAPK), and phosphoionositide 3-kinase (PI3K). A channel of specific interest is the aforementioned TRPV1. This channel has allosteric modification sites that inflammatory agents can bind to in order to increase the channels activity. Furthermore, components of the inflammatory soup such as NGF, bradykinin and ATP can act on their own receptors to trigger downstream TRPV1 modulation through second messengers. [36] These modulations to TRPV1 facilitate a rapid sensitization to heat stimuli by lowering the thermal activation threshold. The second way NGF promotes sensitization and increased pain is by triggering increased transcription of genes encoding pro-inflammatory and pro-nociceptive proteins. This is done via retrograde migration of NGF to the nucleus of the neuron and action on receptors there. Activation of nuclear receptors leads to the increased production of agents such as SP, TRPV1, Nav1.8. [36] Thus, this local and global activation by NGF causes both immediate and sustained sensitization in the nociceptor.

In the normal state, the peripheral nerve relies on the interaction and action of glial cells in maintaining functionality through immune surveillance and ion channel clearance for synaptic transmission. [50] Schwann cells are the glial cells of the PNS. They are responsible for the myelination of nerves as well as for phagocytic clearance for growth and repair. With injury, glial cells as well as macrophages, neutrophils and other cells responsible for maintenance of local environments became activated. They began to release factors that induce an inflammatory response. Additionally there is migration between systems. For example, macrophages and neutrophils in the vicinity of a peripheral nerve injury began migrating into the DRG. [51] Pro-inflammatory agents such as IL-1β, NADPH oxidase 2 (Nox2) and Toll-like receptor 4 (TLR4) are also increased in this activated state. This occurs through gene upregulation, leading to increased inflammatory and oxidative state. [50] TLR4 has emerged as a particular pathological target in recent years. Toll-like receptors are responsible for recognizing pathogen associated molecular patterns, making them important agents in detecting infectious agents and triggering an immune response. [51]

While the increase in production of these factors is one important factor about glial activation, the activated glial cells are also less capable of performing their normal functions. This includes serving as buffers for the excitatory transmitters released by the neurons they police. Altered expression or function of astroglia glutamate transporters GLAST and GLT-1 has been shown in activated astroglia. Conversely, neuropathic pain studies have shown microglia increase the synthesis of glutamate transporters. [50] This leads to pain synapses having greater levels of excitation and stimulation, providing another potential cause of hypersensitivity and pain. Furthermore, glutamate exerts both a synaptic and paracrine signal on the neurons and local tissue around the neuron. Evidence of the involvement of glutamate receptors in CRPS pain, specifically NMDA Receptors (NMDARs), can be seen by the therapeutic combination of ketamine and low dose naltrexone. [15] Both microglia and astroglia have been shown to be key players in the onset and sustainment of allodynia and hyperalgesia after peripheral nerve injury. [50]

TOLL LIKE RECEPTORS

Toll Like receptors (TLR) are a family of receptors that are responsible for the maintenance of innate and adaptive immunity. As receptors that react with ligands associated with various pathogens, they are the key in the maintenance of a first line of defense against many bacteria, fungi and viruses. At the same time the ability of TLRs to react to patterns without the vetting of an adaptive immune process means that many self-associated ligands can trigger responses at the receptor. [52] Research has shown that the peripheral immune system plays an important part in the initiation and maintenance of chronic pain. Recent studies have also shown that TLRs and their associated cascades play a role in pain hypersensitivity. TLRs are found in both the CNS and PNS. This property has led to the hypothesis that TLRs serve as a link between the nervous systems. Neurogenic inflammation is induced by the activity of non-neuronal cells like microglia, astrocytes, oligodendrocytes and Schwann Cells. [52] TLRs are found in high density on these cells. Furthermore, these receptors have shown expression levels that correlate both to intensity of pain sensation and inflammation signs, providing evidence for TLRs to serve as potential quantifiable pain biomarkers. Clinical evidence has demonstrated that TLRs (TLR4 and TLR2 specifically) found in peripheral blood and spinal column may serve as system biomarkers for the chronic pain state. [53] TLR4 agonist LPS and TLR4 agonist PolyI:C administration causes pain like behavior in rodents, while the blockade of these receptors can subdue the pain response.

TLRs function as pattern recognition receptors (PRR) that form complexes with pathogen associated molecular patterns (PAMP). [54] These interactions initiate cascades to fight potential immune threats. PAMPs can come in the form proteins, double stranded DNA, and single stranded DNA. [55] Sources of these ligands can be viruses, fungi, bacteria or even native proteins found in the body's natural environment. Another source of these ligand triggers are the components of the aforementioned inflammatory soup. In addition to initiating cascades, these ligands upregulate the receptors they act on by triggering parallel cascades to increase production of the TLR molecules. Cytokines and cascade byproducts of inflammation have been shown to form complexes with TLRs the same way the aforementioned pathogen molecules do. TLRs share the same intracellular structure to interleukin-1 receptors (IL-1R), and thus have the ability to trigger similar cascades triggered by Il-1R. Some components of these cascades include IL-1R associated kinases (IRAKs), transforming growth factor-β activated kinase (TAK1), tumor-necrosis-factor-receptor associated factor 6 (TRAF6), MAPK and nuclear factor −κβ (NF- κβ). [56] Peripheral nerve damage products and inflammatory soup products have both been demonstrated to form complexes with TLRs. These complexes in turn have been speculated to lead to CNS sensitization and glial activation. Strong evidence for TLRs triggering glial activation in the CNS post peripheral nerve injury provides further evidence for an inflammation-sensitization linkage. [57] This linkage is an important concept with regards to the pathology of CRPS being a multisystem disorder. Furthermore, TLRs are currently being explored as possible therapeutic targets for chronic pain disorders. [57] A study by Christianson et al. explored the role TLRs played in arthritic pain. They hypothesized that there is a transition from slow resolving inflammatory state to a neuropathic pain phenotype. They then showed that the activation of TLR4 located in the spinal cord play is an important contributor to chronic mechanical hypersensitivity. [57]

Found in the outer membrane as surface expressing receptors (TLR 1,2,3,4,5,6,7,10) and intracellularly (TLR 3,7,8,9), a total of 12 mammalian-type TLRs have been identified by researchers thus far. Most TLRs can be found in homodimer form, but non-covalent dimers and heterodimers are also seen. [52] The distribution of TLRs, particularly in nervous tissue suggests TLRs may play an important role in nociceptive processing. Of these subtypes, TLR1, TLR2, and TLR4 have been linked with host origin triggering ligands. TLR 4,7,8,9 all correspond to microglia and are thought to be contributors to microglial-mediated neurotoxicity. [52]. TLR1,2,3,4,5,7,9 can all be found in astrocytes. TLR2 and TLR3 both see upregulation in astrocytes in response to pro-inflammatory cytokine triggers. TLR3 is especially interesting in the astrocyte since studies have shown its activation triggers the release of factors responsible for cellular growth, differentiation, and migration. [52] Outside of the CNS, TLRs can be found in primary afferent fibers, DRG and trigeminal ganglion. Liu et al. theorized that the primary afferent triggered by endogenous or exogenous TLR ligands may send a transduced signal to the brain. TRPV1, an aforementioned vanilloid receptor shown to be up regulated and stimulated by chemokines, is known to have an increase in expression and activity during times of inflammation. TLR7 has been linked to the up regulation of TRPV1 expressing nociceptors and gastrin-releasing peptide (GRP) causing pruritus in some patients. [52] Additionally, Kwok et al. demonstrated TRPV1 expression and gene transcription rises with TLR stimulation. [55] CRGP, PGE2 and IL-1β also have up regulation within DRG neurons activated by ligand interactions with TLR3, TLR7 and TLR9.

A subgroup of TLRs recognizes endogenous molecules released from damaged tissue and cells. This leads researchers to postulate the role of TLRs in the body's monitoring of internal damage. TLR2, TLR3, and TLR4 have been linked to this latter role. [58] Current models focus on the interaction between endogenous ligands originating from damaged peripheral neurons and TLR to induce macrophage activation and infiltration into nerves. These endogenous molecules include heat shock proteins, hyaluronic acid and high-mobility group protein B1 – all chemokines and markers of inflammation. [51] Additionally, these receptors play an important role in Wallerian degeneration. [58] Of these TLRs, TLR2 and TLR4 have been the most promising targets to explore with regards to pain-mediation and pro-inflammatory gene expression, particularly in the DRG (TLR3 has been demonstrated to bind necrotic nuclei mRNA). [51, 59] Knockout mice studies have shown that TLR2 knockouts have attenuated pain responses after nerve injury compared to controls. [51] A study by Kim et al. explored the role of TLR2 in chemokine release. The authors found markedly increased DRG levels of MCP-1 and MIP-1α mRNA expression in mice with peripheral nerve induced injury. Conversely, TLR2 knockout mice showed a reduced macrophage infiltration and chemokine production.

TLR4 activation leads to cascades of pro-nociceptive cytokines and spinal sensitization. [57] Ligands such as heat shock proteins, hyaluronic acid, fibrinogen, fibronectin, and lipopolysaccharide (LPS) are known to activate the receptor. TLR4 is found on both microglia and astrocytes. Animal studies with TLR4 deletions demonstrated a subdued spinal astrocyte and microglia immunoreactivty. [57] Furthermore, pharmacological studies have shown that antagonism of TLR4 suppresses allodynia secondary to bone cancers. [15] The aforementioned NF-κB also is linked to TLR4 activation via two distinct pathways. The first pathway involves TLR4 activation inducing expression of myeloid differentiation primary response gene 88 (MyD88). This leads to cascade that activates NF-κB. [57] Additionally, this cascade is also responsible for upregulation of inflammatory soup components like TNF, IL-18, COX-2, p38 and C-Jun-N terminal kinases (JNK). The second route of NF-κB stimulation is a slower pathway that is triggered by TLR4's activation of TIR-domain containing adapter-inducing interferon β (TRIF). Additionally, morphine binds to TLR4 accessory proteins and causes TLR4 oligomerization and spinal inflammation. [60]

As mentioned above, TLRs are located in the spinal column, brain stem, and DRG – three sites that correspond to chronic pain sensitization. The activation of TLRs within microglia facilitates microglia-neuron interactions that lead to chronic pain symptoms. [52] Spinal cord microglia see a rise in activity post nerve trauma, and opioid exposure. This activity results in production and release of pro-inflammatory products such as TNF-α, IL-1β and brain derived neurotrophic factor BDNF. [52] In addition to microglia and astrocytes, TLRs can be found in different dermal type tissue. Keratinocytes, Langerhans cells, macrophages, dendritic cells, T and B Cells, as well as mast cells all bear TLRs. While the role of TLRs in pain has been established, a link to itch sensation is another area of study that has grown recently. A link to pruritic conditions such as psoriasis, and atopic dermatitis has been deemed a point of further study by researchers. [52] Such markers include ionized-calcium binding adaptor molecule 1 (Iba1), and Glial fibrillary acidic protein (GFAP) [50]. Iba1 and GFAP correspond respectively to microglia and astroglia. Since CRPS is a pain condition of inappropriate response to seemingly innocuous stimuli, over sensitization is a process, which hypothetically makes sense in explaining at least part of CRPS' unique pathology. After, the vast majority of CRPS cases are triggered by some type of injury or inflammation causing insult.

NEUROCUTANEOUS ROLE

Most of the small fibers responsible for nociception have nerve endings that interact with the dermis. Interestingly, patients with the polyneuropathy show either high or low cutaneous neurite densities when compared against controls. This variation in neurite density did not show any correlation to symptom severity. [4, 5] It has been demonstrated that disease of the skin such as psoriasis, atopic dermatitis, and palmoplantar psoriasis have an increased level of morphologic contact between primary afferent sensory nerves and tryptase-positive mast cells housed in the dermis. [61] CRPS patients have been noted to possess elevated tryptase levels in the skin of affected limbs, suggesting an increased mast cell activation degranulation process. [4, 5] Cutaneous mast cells are important players in providing the first line of defense of the body, housing granules filled with many preformed inflammatory mediators. [62] These pro-inflammatory agents include histamines, cytokines, prostaglandin D2, and proteases. It has been shown that this connection between the primary afferent neurons and cutaneous mast cells is mediated by N-Cahderins. [62] N-cadherins are adhesion molecules responsible for connecting the biochemical environments of neighboring cells. [62] These molecules allow for the formation of "synapse-like" interaction between mast cells and neurons. Animal studies using a tibia fracture in the rat as model for CRPS have shown cutaneous nerves can induce mast cell degranulation through the actions of neurotransmitters. Li et al. demonstrated mast cell degranulation secondary to SP release by nerves. Their experiments verified an increase in SP firing and NK-1 receptor expression in neurons and epidermal keratinocytes. [61] The authors also found intraplantar SP injection induced degranulation, providing more evidence for mast cell response to SP. Further evidence lies in the use of NK-1 receptor antagonist to attenuate the nociceptive sensitization in the injured hind paws.

CNS SENSITIZATION AND INFLAMMATION

Another important component of CRPS lies in the central nervous system. There are a number of central pain syndromes where the CSF shows an increase in pro-inflammatory cytokines. These syndromes include multiple sclerosis, stroke, post herpetic neuralgia and

AIDS. While inflammation is believed to be an initial trigger for CRPS, its chronic duration and effect on multiple systems makes a central component very likely. Symptoms such as allodynia, hyperhidrosis, motor dysfunction and sensory loss are all controlled by different circuits within the nervous system. It is believed that for all these circuits to be affected, a central process must be involved. [31]

Hyperexcitability is another component of CRPS that has central nervous system origins. The root pathology of this dysfunction stems from inappropriate and exaggerated response to stimuli. While there is a peripheral component to this symptom, central sensitization plays a vital role in its pathology. Central sensitization is defined as nociceptive messaging triggering out of proportion to pain reactions. Basbaum et al. focused on three mechanisms in their 2009 publication in *Cell* (Figure 2.4). These mechanisms include: alteration in glutamatergic neurotransmission and NMDA receptor mediated hypersensitivity, loss of disinhibition, and glial-neuronal interaction. [36]

GLUTAMATE AND NMDA RECEPTOR-MEDIATED SENSITIZATION

Like all transduced signaling, pain as a sensation is dependent on the release of neurotransmitters initiating excitatory currents. Glutamate is a key neurotransmitter in this process. Glutamate is released from the central terminal of nociceptors, triggering excitatory postsynaptic currents (EPSC) in second order dorsal horn neurons. [36] Transduction of chemical signaling to excitatory currents is enabled by glutamate binding postsynaptic α-amino-3-hydroxy-5-methyl-4-isoxazolepropionic acid receptors (AMPA), kainite, and NMDA channels. These channels are all ionotropic glutamate receptors. [36] The NMDA channel is an essential component of synaptic plasticity. NMDA receptors have been proven to be essential for both memory and learning, and possess unique voltage gated properties.

While still an area of study, the NMDA receptor is composed of hetero tetramers – two NR1 subunits, and two NR2 or NR3 subunits.

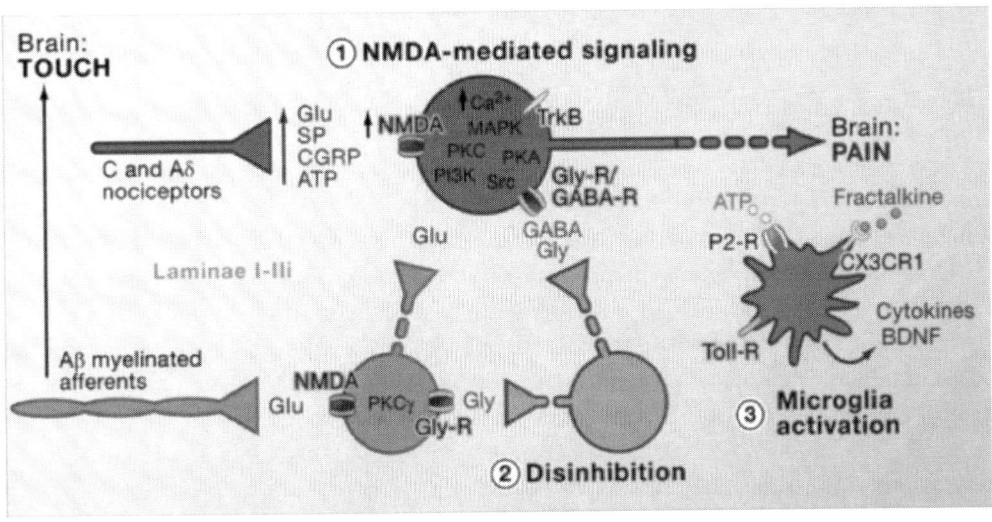

Figure 2.4. The molecular mechanisms pain centralization and sensitization adopted from "Cellular and molecular mechanism of pain" by Basbaum et al. [36]

Different combinations of these subunits form different isoforms with unique functions. This is especially seen in different brain distributions where specific NMDA receptor subunits give rise to unique functions. In the non-injury or chronic pain states, the NMDA glutamate channel is quiescent. When injury occurs, downhill primary nociceptive neurons are activated and a greater amount of glutamate is released by these presynaptic neurons. Glutamate, in turn, triggers the opening of its receptor-associated channels causing an influx of depolarizing calcium. These currents depolarize the postsynaptic NMDA receptors and activate them. This allows for even greater calcium influx, perpetuating the activated state.

Additionally, the calcium influx promotes an increase in the number of synaptic connections between the primary nociceptor and dorsal horn pain neurons. This increase in synapses leads to greater neurotransmitter induced EPSPs, thereby causing sensitization. Subsequently, noxious stimuli that once initiated appropriate pain responses now cause hyperalgesia. In addition to the activity of glutamate neurons, other ligands such as substance P also cause rises in cytosolic calcium levels via receptor ligand interactions. This increase of calcium in the cell does not remit and induces changes that cause long-term potentiation. Long-term potentiation in turn leads to plastic changes and permanent alterations in multiple synapse pathways, including the nociceptive pathways.

NMDA receptor function is also modulated by the actions of second messengers from inflammatory soup triggers. These include kinases such as MAPK, PKA, PKC, PI3K, and Src. [36] Spinal injections of Src peptide fragments disrupt the NMDA receptor interaction with Src and blunt the hypersensitivity caused by peripheral injury. Interestingly, these injections do not alter acute pain sensations. While glutamate alterations play a role in the nociceptor to second order neuron sensitization (primary hyperalgesia), there is also evidence of changes in higher level neurons causing secondary hyperalgesia. These higher level neurons form multiple synapse processes, and are responsible for the alteration and modulation of input response. As mentioned above, Aβ afferents are responsible for rapid light touch response. After central sensitization, some of these Aβ afferents now transmit nociceptive signals and cause severe mechanical allodynia – a typical finding in CRPS. Additionally, suppression of Aβ conduction with compression blocks can terminate the nociceptive signaling, giving additional credence to this mechanism.

DISINHIBITION

Reduced activity of inhibitory interneurons in the dorsal horn appears particularly important in triggering the abnormal firing of central pain neurons that coalesce into the final common pathway of neuropathic pain. [4] GABAergic and glycinergic interneurons and their interactions with other neurons are responsible for the inhibitory inputs of the CNS. Densely distributed in the superficial dorsal horn, these neurons are key players in pain sensation. Loss of these inhibitory neurons leads to greater excitatory signaling down the pain pathway and greater pain sensation. [36] When spinal treatments of bicuculline, a GABA receptor antagonist, are administered, pain symptomology like that secondary to peripheral nerve injury occurs. [36] Similar consequences occur with spinal treatments of strychnine glycine receptor antagonists. In peripheral nerve injury, a loss of inhibitory post synaptic tone in superficial dorsal horn neurons occurs, whether this change is purely from the death of inhibitory interneurons or other mechanisms. [36] The loss of inhibitory input leaves unopposed excitatory inputs to enhanced depolarization and excitement of projection neurons. Uninhibited NMDA receptor sensitization also leads to enhanced spinal cord output due to injury-induced mechanical hypersensitivity. [36] Glycinergic signaling also has its role in inhibition of pathways in the injury state. When injury occurs, spinal receptors are activated by prostaglandin PGE_2. This prostaglandin acts on EP2 receptors found on excitatory interneurons and superficial dorsal horn projection neurons. Once activated, these receptors induce a cAMP-PKA cascade that in turn phosphorylates glycine receptor units GlyRα3. This renders the receptor unresponsive to glycine, thus eliminating the inhibitory effects of glycine. This has been verified in knockout mice studies. Mice without the GlyRα3 gene show decreased thermal and mechanical hypersensitivity in the setting of injury. [36]

The gamma isotype of protein kinase C (PKCγ) is a kinase activated by calcium and diacylglycerol- members of the inflammatory cascade. Uniquely, PKCγ is expressed solely in neurons of the spinal cord and brain sections such as the hippocampus, cerebral cortex and cerebellum. PKCγ is an essential component in long-term potentiation and depression of neurons. [55, 63] Located in the second lamina of the spinal cord, PKCγ neurons are especially prone to increased excitatory tonc hypersensitivity secondary to disinhibition. One result of this aforementioned change is allodynia. Another component of disinhibition that leads to symptoms such as allodynia and hypersensitivity is the alteration of potassium chlorine co-transporters (KCC2) found in lamina I of the spinal cord. [63] Peripheral nerve injury has been linked to down regulation of KCC2 expression. Normally, GABA-A receptors normally initiate hyperpolarizing currents when activated. When KCC2 is down-regulated, a change in the chloride gradient occurs. This change in the chloride gradient subsequently causes GABA-A receptor activation to initiate depolarization currents rather than inhibitory hyperpolarizing ones. This change in GABA-A receptor function thus leads to increase in pain transmission. In-vivo studies have reproduced this relationship by causing mechanical allodynia in the rat via the administration of siRNA or pharmacological inhibitor of KCC2. [36]

GLIAL-NEURONAL INTERACTIONS

Glial neuronal interactions serve as the link between inflammation and central nervous sensitization. As the macrophages of the central nervous system, microglia are distributed throughout the gray matter of the spinal cord patrolling for infection and injury. During times of peripheral nerve injury, these microglia migrate to the superficial dorsal horn within the termination zone of the injured nerve. Here, they begin inducing a number of signaling cascades including release of inflammatory cytokines including TNF α, IL- 1β and IL-6. These signals induce neuronal sensitization and persistent allodynia. [36] Further evidence of microglia involvement in the CRPS was demonstrated by rat studies in which researchers injected activated CNS microglia into the CSF at the level of the spinal cord. [64] These treatments induced behavioral changes in subjects most consistent with post nerve injury. Based on these important experiments, researchers believe microglia hold a vital component in both the initiation and maintenance of chronic pain conditions like CRPS. The activation of microglia is another important topic of study in understanding CRPS. The primary afferent's extent of injury is not the most predominant factor determining microglia activation. Rather, the amount of ATP reacted with P2-type purinergic receptors has a greater influence. Of these receptors, the $P2X_4$, $P2X_7$, and $P2Y_{12}$ subtypes have become especially interesting to pain researchers. [64] These ionotropic ATP receptors, when activated, have been shown to trigger allodynia-like pain in rats. Coull et al. specifically demonstrated that ATP-activated $P2X_4$ receptors lead to the release of BDNF from microglia. BDNF is a ligand for tropomyosin receptor kinase B (TrkB) located on lamina I projection neurons. With TrkB is activated, a change in the Cl-gradient occurs and GABA receptor's hyperpolarizing actions become depolarizing. [65] The complete mechanism for this process is not yet fully understood, but the net result is a sensitization of the lamina I neurons. These post-sensitization neurons show enhanced response to both direct and indirect nociceptor input. [36] Both genetic and pharmacologic blockade of these purinergic receptors' function prevents and reverses the mechanical-induced allodynia seen in rats with post nerve injury. [64] Chemokines, cytokines, neurotransmitters also play an important role in the activation of microglia. [66] Even neuromodulators such as nitric oxide have an effect on the neuro-immune system. The neuromodulator, fractalkine, has been identified as a link specific to the neuronal glial interaction. [36, 66] Fractalkine has only been isolated in sensory afferent and dorsal horn neurons, while the corresponding fractalkine receptor CXCR31 has only been found on microglia. [36, 66] In the normal state, fractalkine is located on the exterior of the neuron surface in an inactive unfractionated form. When fractalkine release is triggered post injury, the inactive state is cleaved by the protein cathepsin S, and becomes a soluble signaling molecule, free to interact with receptors on microglia. Injury also induces increased expression of the fractalkine receptor CXCR31. [36] Spinal administration of fractalkine has been shown to cause and enhance neuropathic pain. Wild-type mice treated with cathepsin S also express neuropathic pain symptomology. Conversely, the administration of fractalkine receptor antagonists as well as antibodies against CXCR31 cause delay in pain onset and a reduction of severity. CXCR31 knockout mice do not show pain symptomology when administered spinal injections of cathepsin S. Further research regarding purinergic receptors will lead to possible avenues for better understanding and treatment of CRPS. Both the role of signaling via ATP and neuromodulation via fractalkine and other cytokines lend credence to CRPS having multiple components to explain its pathology.

NEUROGENIC INFLAMMATION

Aδ and C fibers innervate multiple organ systems. In addition to having nociceptor free endings in soft tissue, Aδ and C fibers innervate vascular beds. When neurons degenerate or begin ectopically releasing modulators, an inflammatory like response can be seen in the blood vessels innervated by these nerves. It is important to note that there may not be any cause of direct injury or insult within these blood vessels. Rather their changes have been brought about by the alterations in their innervation. Extravasation secondary to the loss of fluid from the vascular beds that may be innervated by small fiber nerves can also serve as a nidus for unwanted aggregates. Plasma extravasation leads to an increase in the hemoconcentrate within the vasculature. This triggers migration of white blood cells, and propagates inflammation. [4, 5] Post-mortem studies of patients with CRPS have shown evidence of active ischemia-evoked inflammation. This includes liposfuscin deposits, atrophic fibers and extreme hypertrophy of capillary basal membranes in muscle and subcutaneous tissue.

AUTOIMMUNITY

Recent avenues into the study of CRPS have focused on an autoimmune component to CRPS pathophysiology. The root of this possible pathology focuses on anti-autonomic autoantibodies. [67] Tekus et al. studied this through a series of experiments in which they treated naïve mice with IgG from subjects suffering longstanding CRPS. In these studies, the authors discovered behavioral changes, with reduced exploratory behavior, but did not see any allodynia or edema-like swelling classically seen in CRPS patients. They theorized that for CRPS to manifest, an environment had to be ready for an inciting event in order to manifest symptomology. To test this hypothesis, the team designed an experiment in which the environment would be set by anti-autonomic autoantibodies by passively treating mice with IgG before administering the inciting event in the form of a nerve injury surgery. [67] In this scenario, mice began to express the classic persistent mechanical allodynia and edema seen in CPRS.

An interesting point raised by the study showed a greater occurrence in cold-induced allodynia versus mechanical allodynia. This area of study regarding CRPS is still in its infancy, though the interconnectedness of the syndrome makes an autoimmune component a highly pertinent area of study.

SYMPATHETIC AFFERENT COUPLING ISSUES

Treatment of CRPS by sympathetic blockade suggests a pivotal role of the autonomic nervous system in the pathophysiology of CRPS. Particularly in CRPS I, a significant component of the pain is sympathetically maintained. Primary afferents are influenced by both circulating cathecolamines and by adrenergic sympathetic nerve endings. Sympathetically maintained pain not only is relieved by sympathetic blocks, it also can be experimentally induced by sympathetic activation maneuvers such as cooling. [68] It is important to note that the sympathetic neurons couple with both nociceptive afferent neurons and non-nociceptive ones, such as thermal and mechanosensitive neurons. Sympathetic activation excites already hyperexcitable central neurons and thereby evokes severe states of hyperalgesia and allodynia. Although there is sympathetic afferent coupling in both types of CRPS, the coupling tends to involve deeper tissues such as vascular beds in CRPS I, more so than in CRPS II, the type that is commonly seen following trauma. [69] Coupling of the sympathetic with the primary afferent may also occur through inflammatory mediators such as bradykinin and neuronal growth factors. [70, 71] Lastly, adrenal medulla plays a significant role in coupling with primary afferent of patents with CRPS. In animal models of pain, preganglionic stimulation of adrenal medulla results in release of adrenaline which in turn sensitizes nociceptors for mechanical stimulation and cause hyperalgesia-like symptoms in rats. [72, 73]

ARCHIDONIC ACID METABOLISM

Ramsden et al. described elevated levels of omega 6 highly unsaturated fatty acids in 20 patients diagnosed with CRPS compared to 15 pain-free patients, noting that there was no difference in serum concentrations of omega 3 fatty acids. [74] Although the number of patients was too low to draw definitive conclusions from this study, the data imply a role for polyunsaturated fatty acids and inflammation in pathophysiology of CRPS. Additionally, Kalita et al. demonstrated that oral administration of prednisolone reduced CRPS and related pain scores by more than 2 in 60 patients who developed CRPS following a cerebrovascular event. [75] Fischer et al. was unable to detect any difference in the serum concentrations of malone dialdehyde, F2 isoprostanes, or 8-hydroxy-2-deoxyguanosine from among 9 patients with CRPS I and 9 matched controls, but this study was too underpowered to detect such a change in this patient population. The effectiveness of steroids in reducing CRPS pain is commonly believed to be mediated through its inhibitory effect on phospholipase A and the metabolism of arachidonic acid. This polyunsaturated eicosanoid fatty acid is the substrate for synthesis of prostaglandins (Cyclo-oxygenase pathway; COX) and leukotrienes (Lipo-oxygenase pathway; LOX) in the body. Inhibition of COX-2 either with non-selective or selective COX-2 inhibitors is a common therapeutic tool in treating inflammatory pain. Non-steroidal anti-inflammatory drugs (NSAID) work to inhibit the production of such prostaglandin and are used in treatment of CRPS, albeit without strong evidence of effectiveness.

WORKING PAIN MODEL

The pathophysiology of pain and trophic changes in CRPS is fairly complex. We tried to shed some light into this complex interaction between the inflammatory process and neurogenic mechanisms involving both sympathetic and somatic sensory nervous systems and affecting sudomotor pathology. There is ample evidence that CRPS is a disease of central nervous system, including changes in regulation of sympathetic, sensory and somatic motor components.

However, the presence of peripheral changes like sympathetic afferent coupling, local inflammation, edema and trophic changes indicate that the disease process may initially start peripherally and it then centralized later into a full-blown clinical disease at the time of presentation.

SUMMARY

We conclude that future studies still should aim toward identifying the underlying mechanisms and the pathophysiology of this pain syndrome. By doing this, new therapeutic modalities will evolve to be more effective in treating CRPS pain, improving not only quality of life but also adding to each patient's productive time, helping to return them to baseline function and reducing the days of work lost among this often highly morbid patient population.

REFERENCES

[1] de Mos M., Huygen F. J., Dieleman J. P., Koopman J. S., Stricker B. H., Sturkenboom M. C. Medical history and the onset of complex regional pain syndrome (CRPS). *Pain,* 2008; 139(2):458-66.

[2] Huygen F. J., De Bruijn A. G., De Bruin M. T., Groeneweg J. G., Klein J., Zijlstra F. J. Evidence for local inflammation in complex regional pain syndrome type 1. *Mediators Inflamm.,* 2002; 11(1):47-51.

[3] Harden R. N. Complex regional pain syndrome. *Br. J. Anaesth.,* 2001; 87(1):99-106.

[4] Oaklander A. L., Fields H. L. Is reflex sympathetic dystrophy/complex regional pain syndrome type I a small-fiber neuropathy? *Ann. Neurol.,* 2009; 65(6):629-38.

[5] Bruehl S. An update on the pathophysiology of complex regional pain syndrome. *Anesthesiology,* 2010; 113(3):713-25.

[6] McMahon S. B. Wall and Melzack's textbook of pain. Philadelphia, PA: Elsevier/Saunders,; 2013. Available from: ClinicalKey http:// www.clinicalkey.com/ dura/browse/bookChapter/3-s2.0-C20090526712.

[7] Kramer H. H., Eberle T., Uceyler N., Wagner I., Klonschinsky T., Muller L. P., et al. TNF-alpha in CRPS and 'normal' trauma--significant differences between tissue and serum. *Pain,* 2011; 152(2):285-90.

[8] Sudeck P. On acute inflammatory bone atrophy. *Journal of hand surgery,* 2005; 30(5):477-81.

[9] Fukushima F. B., Bezerra D. M., Villas Boas P. J., Valle A. P., Vidal E. I. Complex regional pain syndrome. *BMJ,* 2014; 348:g3683.

[10] Marinus J., Moseley G. L., Birklein F., Baron R., Maihofner C., Kingery W. S., et al. Clinical features and pathophysiology of complex regional pain syndrome. *Lancet Neurol.,* 2011; 10(7):637-48.

[11] Allen G., Galer B. S., Schwartz L. Epidemiology of complex regional pain syndrome: a retrospective chart review of 134 patients. *Pain,* 1999; 80(3):539-44.

[12] Sandroni P., Benrud-Larson L. M., McClelland R. L., Low P. A. Complex regional pain syndrome type I: incidence and prevalence in Olmsted county, a population-based study. *Pain,* 2003; 103(1-2):199-207.

[13] Sharma A., Agarwal S., Broatch J., Raja S. N. A web-based cross-sectional epidemiological survey of complex regional pain syndrome. *Regional anesthesia and pain medicine,* 2009; 34(2):110-5.

[14] Harden R. N., Bruehl S., Stanton-Hicks M., Wilson P. R. Proposed new diagnostic criteria for complex regional pain syndrome. *Pain medicine,* 2007; 8(4):326-31.

[15] Chopra P., Cooper M. S. Treatment of Complex Regional Pain Syndrome (CRPS) using low dose naltrexone (LDN). *J. Neuroimmune Pharmacol.,* 2013; 8(3):470-6.

[16] Bruehl S., Chung O. Y. How common is complex regional pain syndrome-Type I? *Pain,* 2007; 129(1-2):1-2.

[17] van Rijn M. A., Marinus J., Putter H., Bosselaar S. R., Moseley G. L., van Hilten J. J. Spreading of complex regional pain syndrome: not a random process. *J. Neural. Transm.,* 2011; 118(9):1301-9.

[18] van Hilten J. J., van de Beek W. J., Roep B. O. Multifocal or generalized tonic dystonia of complex regional pain syndrome: a distinct clinical entity associated with HLA-DR13. *Annals of neurology,* 2000; 48(1): 113-6.

[19] van de Beek W. J., Roep B. O., van der Slik A. R., Giphart M. J., van Hilten B. J. Susceptibility loci for complex regional pain syndrome. *Pain,* 2003; 103(1-2):93-7.

[20] Quisel A., Gill J. M., Witherell P. Complex regional pain syndrome underdiagnosed. *J. Fam. Pract.,* 2005; 54(6):524-32.

[21] Maleki J., LeBel A. A., Bennett G. J., Schwartzman R. J. Patterns of spread in complex regional pain syndrome, type I (reflex sympathetic dystrophy). *Pain,* 2000; 88(3): 259-66.

[22] Akyuz G., Kenis O. Physical therapy modalities and rehabilitation techniques in the management of neuropathic pain. *Am. J. Phys. Med. Rehabil.,* 2014; 93(3):253-9.

[23] O'Connell N. E., Wand B. M., McAuley J., Marston L., Moseley G. L. Interventions for treating pain and disability in adults with complex regional pain syndrome. *The Cochrane database of systematic reviews,* 2013; 4:CD009416.

[24] Al-Nesf M. A., Abdulaziz H. M. Complex regional pain syndrome type I following tetanus toxoid injection. *J. Clin. Rheumatol.,* 2014; 20(1): 49-50.

[25] Placzek J. D., Boyer M. I., Gelberman R. H., Sopp B., Goldfarb C. A. Nerve decompression for complex regional pain syndrome type II following upper extremity surgery. *The Journal of hand surgery,* 2005; 30(1): 69-74.

[26] van der Laan L., ter Laak H. J., Gabreels-Festen A., Gabreels F., Goris R. J. Complex regional pain syndrome type I (RSD): pathology of skeletal muscle and peripheral nerve. *Neurology,* 1998; 51(1):20-5.

[27] Oaklander A. L., Rissmiller J. G., Gelman L. B., Zheng L., Chang Y., Gott R. Evidence of focal small-fiber axonal degeneration in complex regional pain syndrome-I (reflex sympathetic dystrophy). *Pain,* 2006; 120(3):235-43.

[28] Thorne C., Grabb W. C., Smith J. W. Grabb and Smith's plastic surgery. 6th ed. Philadelphia: Wolters Kluwer Health/Lippincott Williams & Wilkins,; 2007.

[29] Schinkel C., Gaertner A., Zaspel J., Zedler S., Faist E., Schuermann M. Inflammatory mediators are altered in the acute phase of posttraumatic complex regional pain syndrome. *The Clinical journal of pain,* 2006; 22(3): 235-9.

[30] Lenz M., Uceyler N., Frettloh J., Hoffken O., Krumova E. K., Lissek S., et al. Local cytokine changes in complex regional pain syndrome type I (CRPS I) resolve after 6 months. *Pain,* 2013; 154(10):2142-9.

[31] Alexander G. M., van Rijn M. A., van Hilten J. J., Perreault M. J., Schwartzman R. J. Changes in cerebrospinal fluid levels of pro-inflammatory cytokines in CRPS. *Pain,* 2005; 116(3):213-9.

[32] Parkitny L., McAuley J. H., Di Pietro F., Stanton T. R., O'Connell N. E., Marinus J., et al. Inflammation in complex regional pain syndrome: a systematic review and meta-analysis. *Neurology,* 2013; 80(1):106-17.

[33] Hou Q., Barr T., Gee L., Vickers J., Wymer J., Borsani E., et al. Keratinocyte expression of calcitonin gene-related peptide beta: implications for neuropathic and inflammatory pain mechanisms. *Pain,* 2011; 152(9):2036-51.

[34] Coderre T. J., Bennett G. J. A hypothesis for the cause of complex regional pain syndrome-type I (reflex sympathetic dystrophy): pain due to deep-tissue microvascular pathology. *Pain medicine,* 2010; 11(8): 1224-38.

[35] Nair H. K., Hain H., Quock R. M., Philip V. M., Chesler E. J., Belknap J. K., et al. Genomic loci and candidate genes underlying inflammatory nociception. *Pain*, 2011; 152(3):599-606.

[36] Basbaum A. I., Bautista D. M., Scherrer G., Julius D. Cellular and molecular mechanisms of pain. *Cell*, 2009; 139(2):267-84.

[37] Gaur U., Aggarwal B. B. Regulation of proliferation, survival and apoptosis by members of the TNF superfamily. *Biochem. Pharmacol.*, 2003; 66(8):1403-8.

[38] Maurer M., von Stebut E. Macrophage inflammatory protein-1. *Int. J. Biochem. Cell. Biol.*, 2004; 36(10):1882-6.

[39] Contassot E., Beer H. D., French L. E. Interleukin-1, inflammasomes, autoinflammation and the skin. *Swiss Med. Wkly*, 2012; 142:w13590.

[40] Perrier S., Darakhshan F., Hajduch E. IL-1 receptor antagonist in metabolic diseases: Dr Jekyll or Mr Hyde? *FEBS Lett.*, 2006; 580 (27):6289-94.

[41] Farzi A., Reichmann F., Holzer P. The homeostatic role of neuropeptide Y in immune function and its impact on mood and behaviour. *Acta Physiol. (Oxf.)*, 2014.

[42] O'Connor T. M., O'Connell J., O'Brien D. I., Goode T., Bredin C. P., Shanahan F. The role of substance P in inflammatory disease. *J. Cell. Physiol.*, 2004; 201(2):167-80.

[43] Ma H. Calcitonin gene-related peptide (CGRP). *Nat. Sci.*, 2004; 2:41-7.

[44] Cohen S. P., Mao J. Neuropathic pain: mechanisms and their clinical implications. *BMJ*, 2014; 348:f7656.

[45] Albrecht P. J., Hines S., Eisenberg E., Pud D., Finlay D. R., Connolly M. K., et al. Pathologic alterations of cutaneous innervation and vasculature in affected limbs from patients with complex regional pain syndrome. *Pain*, 2006; 120(3):244-66.

[46] De Rooij A., Gosso M., Alsina- Sanchis E., Marinus J., Van Hilten J., Van Den Maagdenberg A. No mutations in the voltage- gated NaV1. 7 sodium channel α1 subunit gene SCN9A in familial complex regional pain syndrome. *European Journal of Neurology*, 2010; 17(6):808-14.

[47] Drenth J. P., te Morsche R. H., Guillet G., Taieb A., Kirby R. L., Jansen J. B. SCN9A mutations define primary erythermalgia as a neuropathic disorder of voltage gated sodium channels. *J. Invest. Dermatol.*, 2005; 124(6):1333-8.

[48] Tedford H. W., Zamponi G. W. Direct G protein modulation of Cav2 calcium channels. *Pharmacol. Rev.*, 2006; 58(4):837 62.

[49] Luo Z. D., Chaplan S. R., Higuera E. S., Sorkin L. S., Stauderman K. A., Williams M. E., et al. Upregulation of dorsal root ganglion (alpha)2(delta) calcium channel subunit and its correlation with allodynia in spinal nerve-injured rats. *J. Neurosci.*, 2001; 21(6):1868-75.

[50] Berger J. V., Deumens R., Goursaud S., Schafer S., Lavand'homme P., Joosten E. A., et al. Enhanced neuroinflammation and pain hypersensitivity after peripheral nerve injury in rats expressing mutated superoxide dismutase 1. *J. Neuroinflammation*, 2011; 8:33.

[51] Kim D., You B., Lim H., Lee S. J. Toll-like receptor 2 contributes to chemokine gene expression and macrophage infiltration in the dorsal root ganglia after peripheral nerve injury. *Mol. Pain*, 2011; 7:74.

[52] Liu T., Gao Y. J., Ji R. R. Emerging role of Toll-like receptors in the control of pain and itch. *Neurosci. Bull.*, 2012; 28(2):131-44.

[53] Kwok Y. H., Tuke J., Nicotra L. L., Grace P. M., Rolan P. E., Hutchinson M. R. TLR 2 and 4 responsiveness from isolated peripheral blood mononuclear cells from rats and humans as potential chronic pain biomarkers. *PLoS One*, 2013; 8(10):e77799.

[54] Iwasaki A., Medzhitov R. Toll-like receptor control of the adaptive immune responses. *Nat. Immunol.*, 2004; 5(10):987-95.

[55] Qi J., Buzas K., Fan H., Cohen J. I., Wang K., Mont E., et al. Painful pathways induced by TLR stimulation of dorsal root ganglion neurons. *J. Immunol.*, 2011; 186(11): 6417-26.

[56] Akira S., Takeda K. Toll-like receptor signalling. *Nat. Rev. Immunol.*, 2004; 4(7):499-511.

[57] Christianson C. A., Dumlao D. S., Stokes J. A., Dennis E. A., Svensson C. I., Corr M., et al. Spinal TLR4 mediates the transition to a persistent mechanical hypersensitivity after the resolution of inflammation in serum-transferred arthritis. *Pain*, 2011; 152(12):2881-91.

[58] Boivin A., Pineau I., Barrette B., Filali M., Vallieres N., Rivest S., et al. Toll-like receptor signaling is critical for Wallerian degeneration and functional recovery after peripheral nerve injury. *J. Neurosci.*, 2007; 27(46):12565-76.

[59] . !!! INVALID CITATION !!! { }.

[60] Sauer R. S., Hackel D., Morschel L., Sahlbach H., Wang Y., Mousa S. A., et al. Toll like receptor (TLR)-4 as a regulator of peripheral endogenous opioid-mediated analgesia in inflammation. *Mol. Pain*, 2014; 10:10.

[61] Li W., Shi X., Wang L., Guo T., Wei T., Cheng K., et al. Epidermal adrenergic signaling contributes to inflammation and pain sensitization in a rat model of complex regional pain syndrome. *Pain*, 2013; 154(8): 1224-36.

[62] Li W. W., Guo T. Z., Liang D. Y., Sun Y., Kingery W. S., Clark J. D. Substance P signaling controls mast cell activation, degranulation, and nociceptive sensitization in a rat fracture model of complex regional pain syndrome. *Anesthesiology*, 2012; 116(4):882-95.

[63] Saito N., Shirai Y. Protein kinase C gamma (PKC gamma): function of neuron specific isotype. *J. Biochem.*, 2002; 132(5):683-7.

[64] Tsuda M., Shigemoto-Mogami Y., Koizumi S., Mizokoshi A., Kohsaka S., Salter M. W., et al. P2X4 receptors induced in spinal microglia gate tactile allodynia after nerve injury. *Nature*, 2003; 424(6950):778-83.

[65] Coull J. A., Beggs S., Boudreau D., Boivin D., Tsuda M., Inoue K., et al. BDNF from microglia causes the shift in neuronal anion gradient underlying neuropathic pain. *Nature*, 2005; 438(7070):1017-21.

[66] Watkins L. R., Maier S. F. The pain of being sick: implications of immune-to-brain communication for understanding pain. *Annual review of psychology*, 2000; 51:29-57.

[67] Tekus V., Hajna Z., Borbely E., Markovics A., Bagoly T., Szolcsanyi J., et al. A CRPS-IgG-transfer-trauma model reproducing inflammatory and positive sensory signs associated with complex regional pain syndrome. *Pain*, 2014; 155(2):299-308.

[68] Janig W., Levine J. D., Michaelis M. Interactions of sympathetic and primary afferent neurons following nerve injury and tissue trauma. *Progress in brain research*, 1996; 113:161-84.

[69] Janig W., Baron R. Complex regional pain syndrome: mystery explained? *The Lancet Neurology*, 2003; 2(11):687-97.

[70]   McMahon S. B. NGF as a mediator of inflammatory pain. Philosophical transactions of the Royal Society of London Series B, *Biological sciences,* 1996; 351(1338):431-40.

[71]   Woolf C. J., Ma Q. P., Allchorne A., Poole S. Peripheral cell types contributing to the hyperalgesic action of nerve growth factor in inflammation. *The Journal of neuroscience: the official journal of the Society for Neuroscience,* 1996; 16(8): 2716-23.

[72]   Khasar S. G., McCarter G., Levine J. D. Epinephrine produces a beta-adrenergic receptor-mediated mechanical hyperalgesia and in vitro sensitization of rat nociceptors. *Journal of neurophysiology,* 1999; 81(3): 1104-12.

[73]   Khasar S. G., Miao F. J., Gear R. W., Green P. G., Isenberg W. M., Levine J. D. Sympathetic-independent bradykinin mechanical hyperalgesia induced by subdiaphragmatic vagotomy in the rat. *The journal of pain: official journal of the American Pain Society,* 2002; 3(5):369-76.

[74]   Ramsden C., Gagnon C., Graciosa J., Faurot K., David R., Bralley J. A., et al. Do omega-6 and trans fatty acids play a role in complex regional pain syndrome? A pilot study. *Pain medicine,* 2010; 11(7):1115-25.

[75]   Kalita J., Vajpayee A., Misra U. K. Comparison of prednisolone with piroxicam in complex regional pain syndrome following stroke: a randomized controlled trial. *Qjm,* 2006; 99(2):89-95.

Chapter 3

MOLECULAR PATHOPHYSIOLOGY AND THE ROLE OF TNF IN THE NEURO-INFLAMMATORY REFLEX

Tracey A. Ignatowski[1,*], PhD, Shabnam Samankan[1], MD and Robert N. Spengler[2], PhD

[1]Department of Pathology and Anatomical Sciences,
University at Buffalo, Buffalo, NY, US
[2]NanoAxis, LLC, Clarence, NY, US

INTRODUCTION

It is well known that unresolved chronic pain results in decreased quality of life, inability to interact with others, and an overall patient disability, even to the point of not being able to perform one's activities of daily living. Complex regional pain syndrome (CRPS) constitutes chronic pain with a neuroinflammatory component that culminates in disabilities and impairment, as well as comorbid disease onset. CRPS often affects a limb following a trauma (sprain, strain and fracture) to the limb or immobilization (i.e., casting). [1] There are two diagnostic categories for CRPS: CRPS-1 occurs in the absence of an identifiable nerve lesion, and CRPS-2 arises in the presence of an identifiable nerve injury. Both CRPS-1 and -2 display similar symptoms, but only the latter type meets the formal classification of neuropathic pain. The CRPS-1 subtype distinction is less thoroughly described in the literature, because the microscopic nerve damage would be hard to detect clinically. [2] In addition to pain out of proportion to the initial injury, other CRPS symptoms due to damage to nerves controlling temperature and blood flow frequently do not appear until much after the injury, and therefore, patients often experience a delay in diagnosis. [3, 4] Unfortunately, delayed diagnosis may translate to ineffective treatment, because early initiation of treatment

---

[*] Research Associate Professor in the Department of Pathology and Anatomical Sciences, University at Buffalo, Buffalo, NY tail@buffalo.edu.

is important to prevent a vicious cycle of ongoing, chronic pain that becomes even more difficult to treat medically.

A neuro-immunologic approach to understanding the pathogenesis of CRPS has gained popularity over the past several years, because of the realization that injury and inflammation trigger bidirectional communication between the nervous system (neurons) and immune system. [5, 6] The balanced release of pro- and anti-inflammatory cytokine proteins, as well as neurotransmitters such as norepinephrine, orchestrates the ensuing inflammatory response, which normally proceeds to injury resolution that is actively mediated by lipid-based immuno-resolvants. [7] If this active process fails, the pro-inflammatory state persists, or an exaggerated post-traumatic inflammatory response occurs, then chronic inflammation often ensues. The resultant shift that favors a pro-inflammatory profile over an anti-inflammatory profile signifies loss of physiological homeostasis and is a harbinger of disease onset, including the chronic pain of CRPS.

A comprehensive understanding of the etiologic and pathophysiologic mechanisms contributing to the incidence of CRPS is key to the development of an efficacious treatment. This chapter is a review of the determinants of CRPS, including the neuromodulator and inflammatory mediator, tumor necrosis factor-α (TNFα), various neurotransmitters, particularly norepinephrine, and neuroanatomical pathways and structures, including higher cortical brain regions. The role of elevated levels of TNFα that is associated with CRPS is our major focus. We hypothesize that TNFα overexpression locally in the afflicted extremity and in the brain serves as a therapeutic target for the management of CRPS.

CRPS PATHOGENESIS

CRPS is generally considered a neuroinflammatory disorder that is initiated by a peripheral injury that includes damage to a nerve. How inflammatory mediators direct the onset and development of CRPS is controversial. Inflammation and altered autonomic function are well-recognized symptoms of CRPS. Interestingly, detection of autoantibodies suggests an immunologic component. [8, 9] Therefore, three hypotheses predominate for the causative mechanisms driving the development of CRPS: trauma or stress as an initiating event, inflammation, and autoimmunity.

TRAUMA OR STRESS

After injury or trauma to a limb, CRPS may develop resulting in impaired or loss of limb function and chronic pain that is disproportionate to the insult. In greater than 90% of cases, there is a clear history of an injury that precipitates development of CRPS. [10] Some common triggers include bone fractures, sprains, strains, minor tissue injury (burn or cut), surgical procedures, routine medical procedures such as injections, and limb confinement in a cast. Even when normal healing of the inciting injury occurs, excruciating and overwhelming pain may continue to be perceived due to the development of CRPS. The question arises: why do some people develop CRPS while others do not? The answer lies in the multiple underlying mechanisms that contribute to CRPS development, such as genetic and environmental factors (stress).

CRPS usually affects the afflicted limb, but the pain can often be perceived in other parts of the body. This perceived spread of pain to non-injured areas reflects the involvement of the nervous system and the release of cellular protein mediators, such as cytokines, that transmit information throughout the body. It is well-accepted that stress is associated with activation of the immune system and release of pro-inflammatory cytokines, such as tumor necrosis factor-alpha (TNFα), interleukin-1 (IL-1), and IL-6. [11, 12] Therefore, individuals with CRPS who experience flare-ups, or worsening of the pain, that last days to weeks at a time, may be suffering from stress. Enhanced pro-inflammatory cytokine production would be expected to contribute to the ongoing dysfunction of the inflammatory process associated with the immune and nervous systems and perpetuate pathophysiologic changes that underlie the development of chronic pain.

PRO-INFLAMMATORY CYTOKINES

The inflammatory response is a common feature to injury, trauma, and stress, which are all noted precipitating factors for the induction of CRPS. Activation of the inflammatory response initiates increased production of TNFα, the first cytokine to appear in the pro-inflammatory cytokine cascade. [13] TNFα is a key mediator involved in neuropathic pain. Experimentally, TNFα increases locally and centrally following peripheral nerve injury. [14-19] Sciatic nerve chronic constriction injury (CCI) is associated with increased infiltration of macrophages to the site of nerve injury with concomitant dysregulation of TNFα production by the peripheral macrophages. [19-21] Pain and hyperalgesia result, at least in part, from pro-inflammatory cytokine-induced sensitization of peripheral nociceptors. An increase in brain-TNFα also contributes to peripheral hypersensitivity. Microinfusion of rat recombinant TNFα (rrTNF) into the cerebral ventricle of naive rats induces thermal hyperalgesia (increased sensitivity to a painful stimulus) and enhances hyperalgesia that is induced by CCI. [22] Stereotactic injection of TNFα expression plasmid directly into hippocampi of naive rats induces peripheral hypersensitivity that mimics clinical neuropathic pain behaviors. [23] Treatment of CCI rats with drugs that inhibit TNFα decreases hyperalgesia. [21, 22]

Similar to other neuropathic pain states, CRPS has been shown to be associated with elevated cytokine levels, particularly TNFα. Experimentally, it was shown that pro-inflammatory TNFα upregulation occurs after bone fracture and with immobolization by cast. [24] Using a CRPS-1 tibia fracture model, protein levels of TNFα were determined to be increased in the fractured ipsilateral hindpaw skin and sciatic nerve as compared to non-fractured controls, and in the fractured ipsilateral hindpaw skin, sciatic nerve, and tibia bone as compared to the contralateral side. The development of mechanical allodynia associated with this CRPS model was prevented when rats were treated with soluble TNF receptor-1 (sTNF-R1) for four weeks following the fracture in order to block TNFα signaling. [24] The increase in ipsilateral hindpaw edema and temperature that was induced by tibial fracture were unaffected by the prophylactic sTNF-R1 administration regimen, indicating that local TNFα signaling may not be required for the development of vascular abnormalities after fracture. Similarly, anti-TNFα alleviation of CCI-induced hyperalgesia and allodynia was associated with lack of effect on CCI-induced vascular abnormality. [21, 25]

Elevated levels of TNFα were demonstrated in fluid from artifically-induced suction blisters on affected CRPS patient extremities. [26] Similarly, blister fluid of CRPS patients showed increased pro-inflammatory cytokines TNFα and macrophage inflammatory protein-1β and decreased anti-inflammatory cytokine IL-1 receptor antagonist, which occurred bilaterally, when compared to non-CRPS patients. [27] Mechanical hyperalgesia in patients with CRPS was associated with increased plasma levels of soluble TNF receptor 1 (sTNF-R1) and TNFα. [28] Another study reported that patients with CRPS had higher blood pro-inflammatory TNF and IL-2 mRNA levels and lower IL-8 mRNA levels when compared to controls. [6] In this study, TNF mRNA levels were increased while TNFα protein levels were not, but the authors cite the low stability of the TNF protein for this discrepancy. Likewise, in the early stages of CRPS, IL-8 and sTNF-R1 and -R2 levels were elevated in serum from both arms of patients, when compared with healthy control subjects. [29] TNFα was shown to be increased in the skin of the affected limb of CRPS patients, when compared to patients with an acute fracture trauma and subjects with osteoarthritis. [30] Taken together, the majority of clinical and experimental evidence supports a predominant pro-inflammatory cytokine profile during CRPS, indicating that these mediators, especially TNFα which is the proximal cytokine that initiates activation of the pro-inflammatory cytokine cascade, may contribute to the induction and maintanence of neuropathic pain. In fact, a 2013 systematic review and meta-analysis of the literature determined that CRPS is associated with a predominant pro-inflammatory cytokine profile in the blood (serum and plasma), blister fluid (affected appendage), and cerebrospinal fluid (CSF) of patients. [31]

Inflammation not only induces neuropathic pain (hyperalgesia and allodynia), but can also lead to ischemia, resulting in microvascular changes that are observed during CRPS. Many CRPS patients experience changes in skin color, temperature, and swelling of the affected limb. This occurs, in part, because inflammation-mediated damage to nerves that regulate temperature and blood flow results in abnormal microcirculation in the affected limb. Small nerve fibers (sympathetic phenotype) that innervate blood vessels control dilatation and constriction in the affected limb, both of which can occur during CRPS, but the former of which contributes to edema. [10] Tissue underlying the injury may become ischemic, which in turn, causes activation of the afferent nociceptive nerve fibers. Using an animal model whereby rats experience a prolonged hind paw ischemia and reperfusion injury, called chronic post-ischemia pain (CPIP), it was shown that the ischemic hind paw developed hyperemia and edema, as well as long-lasting (at least 4 weeks post-reperfusion) hyperalgesia and allodynia, symptomology similar to CRPS. [32] Ischemia-induced inflammation and reperfusion-induced edema leading to increased tissue pressure may compromise blood flow thereby causing more tissue damage. This persistent state of ischemia may contribute to the activation of afferent nociceptive nerve fibers resulting in sensitization and persistent pain. The injured nerve fibers also secrete neuropeptides that contribute to the ongoing inflammatory process and circulatory problems, resulting in a viscous cycle of chronic, excruciating pain that is characteristic of CRPS. [32] One such neuropeptide is substance P (SP) that is released from sensory nerve fiber terminals and transmits pain information to the CNS. [33] This release of SP is involved in neurogenic inflammation, which is the local inflammation characteristic of CRPS, that contributes to both the vascular and nociceptive consequences. [34] In addition to nerves, SP is also produced by and released from inflammatory cells. [35] In turn, SP stimulates the production and release of TNFα, IL-1β, and IL-6 from monocytes and macrophages, IL-1β and TNFα from neutrophils, and TNFα from mast cells. [35]Thus, trauma-induced SP release could stimulate the release of TNFα from resident and infiltrating immune cells, thereby contributing to over-expression of TNFα and the development of chronic pain during CRPS. [24] Another neuropeptide released from nociceptive nerve fibers is calcitonin gene related peptide (CGRP). This neuropeptide causes vasodilatation and is associated with transmission of pain signals. [36] Cytokines not only activate and sensitize primary afferents, but also increase the neuropeptide content of primary afferent neurons. [37] Neurogenic inflammation, characterized by the release of neuropeptides from nociceptors, is linked with nociceptor activation. Thus, a feed-forward cycle is perpetuated whereby chronic production and release of pro-inflammatory cytokines and neuropeptides in the afflicted limb may underlie the chronic pain and vascular dysfunction typical of CRPS. [5, 28, 29]

IMMUNE DYSFUNCTION - AUTOANTIBODIES

The signs and symptoms in the affected limbs of CRPS patients meet the classic definition of inflammation: dolor (pain), calor (heat), rubor (redness), tumor (swollen), and loss of function. Due to the presence of an exaggerated inflammatory reaction, recent research into the involvement of the immune system identified autoantibodies in many CRPS patients. Initially, serum obtained from 12 CRPS patients that was used for immunohistochemical staining of rat myenteric plexus nerve fibers and sympathetic ganglia showed autoantibody reactivity to autonomic nervous system structures in 5 of 12 patients (41.6%). [38] In this same study, Western blot analysis using SKN-SH neuroblastoma cells as antigen determined autoantibody neuronal reactivity in 11 of 12 patients (91.6%). However, the specific autoantibody neuronal target(s) remained unidentified. Flow cytometric analysis of serum from subjects (30 CRPS, 20 neuropathy, and 30 healthy controls) that was added to autonomic neuron primary cultures and differentiated neuroblastoma cells revealed 43.3% (CRPS), 5% (neuropathy), and 0% (controls) specific surface binding to autonomic neurons. [39] Differentiation of neurons to a cholinergic phenotype induced expression of a surface antigen that was recognized by 60% of the CRPS sera, but not by control sera, whereas differentiation to a catecholaminergic phenotype decreased surface binding of CRPS sera. [39] These results suggested a predominant cholinergic neuronal antigen may be the target for autoantibody formation during CRPS. Autoantibodies to the autonomic G-protein-coupled neurotransmitter receptors, the β$_2$-adrenergic receptors and muscarinic-2-acetylcholine (m$_2$Ach) receptors were subsequently identified and functionally characterized. [9] The production of autoantibodies by B-cells implies a breakdown of immunologic self-tolerance. Cytokine-induced activation of the immune system may be at fault. Importantly, TNFα plays a role in B-cell activation and proliferation. [40] Nerve injury that leads to excessive cytokine production, disturbances in the microcirculation, and tissue damage would be expected to produces deficits in the affected limb vasculature, allowing for autoantibodies to gain access to the neural antigens in these patients, which may explain the distinctive pattern of spread (i.e., spontaneous, contralateral) throughout the body. [41] Autoantibody reaction against both β$_2$-adrenergic receptors and m$_2$Ach receptors could help explain the autonomic disturbances and chronic pain that is characteristic of CRPS. For example, in the absence of functional m_2Ach receptors on peripheral nociceptors, which when activated under physiological conditions interferes with nerve excitability, neurogenic inflammation would proceed unhindered, contributing to the abnormal vascular and nociceptive symptoms. [42] Similarly, in the absence of functional β_2-adrenergic receptors on immune cells, the normal inhibition of TNFα production by catecholamines would be compromised, supporting a pro-inflammatory environment. [43] A major source of TNF is the macrophage; these immune effector cells possess norepinephrine-sensitive α_2- and β_2-adrenergic receptors that regulate TNF production. [43-45] Depending on its concentration, norepinephrine has either immune-enhancing (α_2-adrenergic receptor) or –suppressive effects (β_2-adrenergic receptor), resulting in tight control of TNF production by macrophages. [46] Thus, in the absence of functional β_2-adrenergic receptors on macrophages, the normal inhibition of TNF production would be absent, resulting in unobstructed TNF production. In fact, abnormal cytokine production by macrophages is implicated during neuropathy and is associated with dysregulated sympathetic activity. [47-51]

The question remains as to the importance of neuron receptor autoantibodies in the pathogenesis of CRPS, since not all patients demonstrate their presence. It may be that the methods used for detection of these autoantibodies were not sensitive enough for all patient autoantibody levels, or it may reflect the presence of inhibitory factors that mask the ability to detect the autoantibodies in certain assays. For instance, non-specific serum immunoglobulin background staining (immunohistochemical procedures) and unspecific background binding of sera from controls and patients to neuronal cells (flow cytometry) may limit specificity and sensitivity of these methods. It is noteworthy that as the stringency of the methods was improved, for example by affinity purification of the IgG fraction from serum samples prior to testing for the presence of autoantibodies and preabsorbing IgGs prior to flow cytometry analysis to avoid unspecific binding, as well as by use of functional bioassays and ELISA assays, the detection of autoantibodies increased (to 90%) in CRPS patients, with the concomitant presence of both receptor autoantibodies detected in 55% of CRPS subjects. [9] It has also been suggested that patients expressing autoantibodies may represent a special pathophysiological CRPS subtype. [39] Due to the variation in clinical presentation amongst CRPS patients (i.e., differences in the temperature or sensory impairment of the affected limb), subtypes of this condition may materialize.

MOLECULAR PATHOPHYSIOLOGY

Neuroinflammatory spread along the neuroaxis (peripheral nervous system (PNS) to central nervous system (CNS)) is postulated to occur during CRPS pathogenesis and pathophysiology, which may explain the chronicity and spread of symptoms in these patients. [52] This transfer of pain to sites distant to that of the initial site of injury may exist as a result of transport of cytokines, such as TNFα, IL-1β, and IL-6, as well as by microglial and astrocytic activation. Furthermore, evidence for aberrant neurophysiology along the neuroaxis during chronic pain in response to a peripheral nerve injury confirms neuroplasticity at both the cellular and molecular levels. Figure 1 provides a schematic diagram illustrating these proposed changes during development of neuropathic pain.

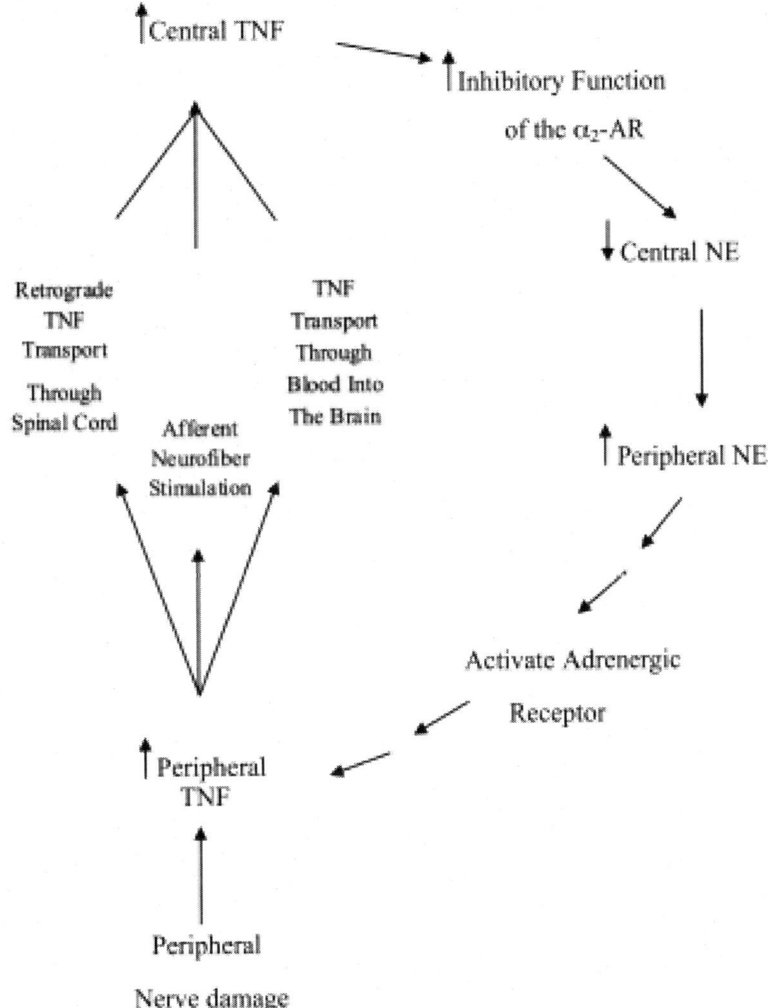

Figure 1. Proposed schematic diagram of TNFα function in neuropathic pain. Injury with nerve damage induces TNFα production from both neurons and inflammatory cells. The localized peripheral increase in TNFα may be transmitted to the CNS by several means including: transport of TNFα along the injured axon to the DRG and spinal cord;[83, 84] as a hormonal or endocrine transportation of TNFα through the systemic circulation to the brain (actively transported across the blood-brain barrier (BBB) via receptor-mediated mechanism, entry at circumventricular sites lacking functional BBB, or signal transduction across the BBB imparted by generation of diffusible second messenger mediators within the brain following TNF binding to its receptor on the BBB); direct stimulation of afferent (sympathetic and/or vagal) nerve fibers that transmits noxious information to the CNS. [104, 141] This spread of neuroinflammation along the neuroaxis induces an increase in TNFα at higher brain regions involved in pain processing and perception. [15, 21, 25] TNFα induces an increase in Gαi-protein expression that allows for enhanced α₂-adrenergic receptor-second messenger coupling and functioning that results in decreased norepinephrine release, as demonstrated in the hippocampus. [14, 15, 111, 142] The enhanced inhibition of central norepinephrine release would fail to engage the descending inhibitory pain pathway (loss of sensory gating), thereby contributing to pain facilitation. Also, an enhanced sympathetic outflow with the exception of the afflicted extremity in CRPS neuropathic pain would ensue, and thereby stimulate adrenergic receptors present on inflammatory cells that regulate TNFα production. These events would invoke a cycle of ongoing pain, as stimulation of the α₂-adrenergic receptor increases TNFα production.

NEUROINFLAMMATION

Peripheral nerve injury has been shown to induce neuroinflammation at sites distant from the site of injury. This spread of neuroinflammation was demonstrated in the thalamus following peripheral nerve injury using radiolabeled PK11195, a ligand for the peripheral benzodiazepine binding site that is absent in normal brain parenchyma but strongly expressed by activated microglia in the vicinity of injured neurons, for imaging of activated microglia and brain macrophages. [53] Seven patients with peripheral nerve injury or spinal root lesions underwent [^{11}C](R)-PK11195 PET imaging. All patients showed increased binding of [^{11}C](R)-PK11195 in the thalamus contralateral to the side of injury. Interestingly, this contralateral, thalamic microglial activation was evident up to 20 years after the injury, indicating persistence in the targeted migration of neuroinflammation from the site of peripheral nerve injury. This trafficking of inflammation progresses from the injured neurons to the first order synapse that is located in the spinal cord and continues progressing trans-synaptically to the second order synapse located in the brain. [53] Activated microglia participate in synapse removal from injured neurons, the persistence of which may contribute to pathologic neuroplasticity and central sensitization during neuropathic pain. [54] In fact, during CRPS, resultant microglial activation in the spinal cord is proposed to drive the spread of neuroinflammation to supraspinal sites. [41, 55]

Release of signaling molecules such as cytokines including TNFα and IL-1β and chemokines, for example monocyte chemoattractant protein (MCP) 1 that is also known as cysteine-cysteine chemokine ligand 21 (CCL21), from first order nociceptive neuron terminals initiates neuroinflammation at secondary sites (for example, at the spinal level) due to stimulation of respective receptors on immune cells, thereby triggering their activation and migration. [56, 57] Neuroimmune activation via neuronal projections to second order synapses where these neurons terminate in the thalamus may account for the spread of glial activation at supraspinal sites. [52] The spread of neuroinflammatory signals was also demonstrated by showing that a unilateral, peripheral nerve chronic constriction injury increased levels of TNFα in the contralateral hippocampus, which was associated with the development of hyperalgesia and allodynia. [25] Whether distinct peripheral nerve injuries lead to discrete persistent sites or patterns of spinal and supraspinal neuroinflammation has yet to be determined, but could help explain the variation in CRPS symptomology.

A transient breakdown in both the blood-spinal cord barrier and blood-brain barrier (BBB) has been shown to occur following damage or injury to peripheral nerves. [58] This may explain the leukocyte infiltration into the CNS that contributes to the remote neuroinflammation following nerve injuries. [59] This emigration of leukocytes from the periphery into the CNS communicates that there is peripheral nerve and tissue damage, which may be transmitted between leukocytes and neurons by neurotransmitters and cytokines, diffusible molecules produced by both cell types. [60] This exposure of neuronal axons and soma to inflammatory cells and mediators contributes to neuronal sensitization that enhances pain signal transmission. [61] Therefore, neuroimmune signaling is able to influence nociceptive processing at sites distant from the initial injury.

Patients with different chronic pain disease states experience reduction in the volume of specific brain regions. The volume of the hippocampus is reduced in patients with chronic back pain, osteoarthritis, or CRPS. Similarly, mice with sciatic neuropathic pain demonstrate decreased neurogenesis in the hippocampus. [62] Neuroinflammatory-induced microglial activation and prolonged production of TNFα may contribute to this reduction in gray matter volume, especially since increased TNFα has been associated with decreased neurogenesis during a neuropathic pain model. [63] Since microglia and neurons express both TNF receptor-1 (p55) and -2 (p75) (TNFR1 and TNFR2), and neuropathic pain development and maintenance is linked to signaling through TNFR1, it is likely that microglial activation by TNFα through TNFR1 mediates persistent TNFα production that contributes to the ongoing neuroinflammation and neuropathological consequences including synaptic transmission deficits and decreased neurogenesis. [15, 64-68]

CENTRAL SENSITIZATION

CRPS is both a PNS and a CNS disorder. [69, 70] Central sensitization refers to the neuroplastic changes in the CNS that are associated with the progression of acute CRPS-associated peripheral signs and symptoms to a chronic central pain state both mediated and perpetuated by neuroinflammatory dysregulation. In CRPS, development of central sensitization involves a complex set of neuroinflammatory responses, most likely including the release of pro-inflammatory cytokines from neurons, glial cells, and immune-effector cells such as macrophages. [52, 71] Whereas the role of pro-inflammatory cytokines in peripheral nociceptor sensitization is well-documented, their role in central sensitization is becoming recognized. [72, 73] Using an *ex vivo* system, spinal cord slices exposed to TNFα, IL-1β, or IL-6 demonstrated a positive influence on central sensitization through enhancement of excitatory neurotransmission and suppression of inhibitory neurotransmission as measured via patch-clamp recording. [74] Specifically, application of TNFα and IL-1β to spinal cord slices increased the frequency of spontaneous excitatory post-synaptic currents (sEPSC), suggesting presynaptic enhancement of glutamate release by these cytokines. IL-6 and IL-1β when added to spinal cord slices inhibited the frequency of inhibitory post-synaptic currents, suggesting suppression of inhibitory neurotransmission. [74] In the CCI sciatic nerve neuropathic pain model, enhanced expression of TNFα in hippocampal neurons is associated with greater inhibition of central norepinephrine release that is proposed to contribute to central sensitization through lack of engagement of spinal-mediated inhibitory synaptic transmission. [15, 21, 22] In chronic pain conditions, microglia and astrocytes in the spinal cord and brain have enhanced pro-inflammatory cytokine production that facilitates pain via glia-neuron interactions. [75, 76] Through the release of pro-inflammatory cytokines such as TNFα, long-term synaptic plasticity is induced by cAMP-response element binding (CREB)-mediated gene transcription, which favors excitatory over inhibitory synaptic transmission, as shown in the spinal cord. [74] Neuroplasticity following peripheral or central neuropathic injury also manifests itself in the form of aberrant neuron ion channel expression. Such abnormal expression occurs in the thalamus where voltage-gated sodium channels Nav1.3, which are normally absent in adult neurons in this region, permits neuronal firing at abnormally high frequencies. [77] Down-regulation of thalamic Nav1.3 expression in a neuropathic rodent model reversed the neuronal sensitization and alleviated pain behavior. [78] Introduction of antisense oligodeoxynucleotides to Nav1.3 via a catheter inserted into the lumbar intrathecal space was initiated 28 days following a contusive spinal cord injury, and animals were assessed four days later. Treatment with Nav1.3 antisense oligodeoxynucleotides knocked-down SCI-induced Nav1.3 expression in dorsal horn neurons, decreased the evoked hyper-responsiveness of dorsal horn neurons, reduced the number of thalamic neurons expressing Nav1.3, and reversed the increased spontaneous activity, hyper-responsiveness to peripheral stimulation, and after-discharge firing of thalamic neurons that was induced by the spinal cord injury. [79, 80] Sensitization in the thalamus due to increased spontaneous and enhanced firing of neurons as well as decreased firing thresholds can lead to synaptic potentiation in higher brain regions. This would be expected to impact integration of the nociceptive input and influence memory formation related to painful events. [81] The resultant induction of long-term plasticity in higher cortical regions allows for aberrant processing of nociceptive information along the descending pain pathways that would favor excitatory over inhibitory transmission. [56, 74]

CRPS AND THE NEURO-INFLAMMATORY REFLEX

The inciting injury leading to CRPS initiates neuroplastic changes that pathologically generate and amplify pain signals along the neuroaxis. Neuroimmune mediators that are produced by both neurons and immune cells have been shown to facilitate this miscommunication at multiple sites within the pain network, that is, at the injured primary afferent first order synapse, at the spinal cord second order synapse, and at the supra-spinal third order synapse level. In the CCI sciatic nerve neuropathic pain model, enhanced expression of TNFα in hippocampal neurons is associated with greater inhibition of central norepinephrine release that is proposed to contribute to central sensitization through subsequent lack of engagement of spinal-mediated inhibitory synaptic transmission. [15, 21, 22] CSF levels of TNFα, IL-1β, and IL-6 were found to be increased in chronic cases of CRPS, and a correlation was demonstrated between plasma pro-inflammatory cytokines, disease duration, and pain in a subgroup of CRPS patients. [71] Figure 2 illustrates the afferent and efferent arms of the neuro-inflammatory pain reflex and primary cytokine mediators implicated in the development of CRPS.

INFLAMMATORY-TO-NEURAL COMMUNICATION

An imbalance in cytokine activity that affects functioning of both the afferent and efferent arms of the neuroaxis is postulated to be involved in the pathogenesis of CRPS. For example, levels of IL-8 and soluble TNF receptors 1 and 2 were significantly elevated in venous blood taken from the affected arm of CRPS patients during the acute phase of the disorder, whereas all soluble forms of selectins were significantly suppressed. [29] Rodent peripheral nerve injury models show that TNFα is a product of the inciting injury that amplifies the inflammatory response by inducing an influx of macrophages to the site of injury. Consequently, these macrophages release cytokines, including TNFα [19], thereby amplifying the inflammatory response.

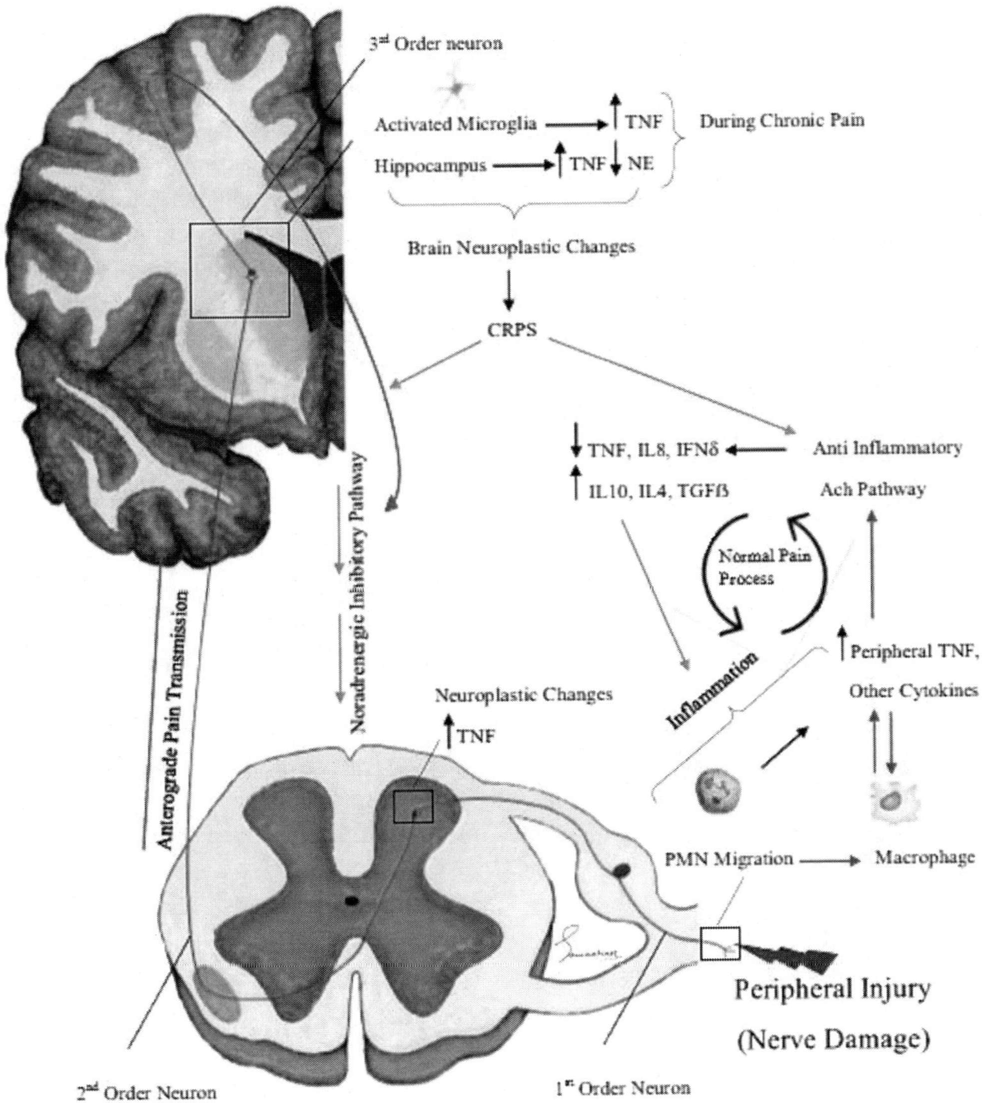

Figure 2. Proposed model for integration of multiple levels of the neuro-inflammatory reflex (inflammatory cells, primary afferent sensory nerve, and efferent (sympathetic and parasympathetic) systems), with emphasis on the role of TNFα, in the development of CRPS pain. Peripheral injury with nerve damage induces a local increase in TNFα and an influx of inflammatory cells (polymorphonuclear leukocytes, or PMNs, and macrophages) that further contribute to the local increase in TNFα concentration. [19] Neuroinflammation is precipitated by TNFα activation of inflammatory cells that produce TNFα and other pro-inflammatory cytokines, which sensitize primary afferent sensory nerve fibers. [18, 87, 89] Microglial cells at 1st, 2nd, and 3rd order synapses become activated and produce TNFα, indicating spread of the neuroinflammation along the neuroaxis. [53, 56] Altogether, the increased levels of TNFα, TNFα-induced neuroplastic changes, and loss of sensory gating along the neuroaxis leads to altered sympathetic outflow and potentially altered parasympathetic output, which fails to dampen inflammation at all levels of the reflex arc. Specifically, an increase in systemic norepinephrine (except in the affected limb, where sympathetic innervation is compromised and norepinephrine levels are decreased, but α-adrenergic receptors are increased either in number or function) and a predicted decrease in acetylcholine output would perpetuate an increase of TNFα levels and continual pain transmission. [92, 96]

Spread of inflammation along the neuroaxis may occur by retrograde transport of TNFα from the damaged nerve to the spinal cord, thereby initiating an inflammatory response within the CNS. [82-84] Subsequent activation of microglia and astrocytes at the level of the spinal cord results in the release of TNFα, which modulates synaptic transmission and neuroplasticity. In fact, TNFα controls glutamate release from astrocytes and regulates norepinephrine release from neurons. Thus, any alteration in the production of TNFα would be expected to negatively affect synaptic functioning in CRPS, as occurs during neuropathic pain conditions. [15, 85] Another mode by which neuroinflammation spreads from the periphery to the CNS is through direct stimulation of sensory afferent nerve fibers by TNFα, which results in signal transmission to the CNS. Many studies suggest that TNFα-induced ectopic activity, or abnormal neural activity, sensitizes primary afferent neurons after injury. [86-88] TNFα that was applied to rat dorsal root ganglions (DRG) *in vivo* mediated peripheral sensitization, or a reduction in the mechanical thresholds of fibers with an associated increase in their receptive field size. [88] Application of TNFα to rat DRG neuron cultures increased transient voltage-activated sodium channel currents through TNF receptor-1 (TNFR-1). [86] Direct application of TNFα to cultured DRG neurons from rats with chronic compression of lumbar ganglia evoked greater action potentials and enhanced neuronal excitability when compared to control neurons. [87] Both TNFα and its receptor (TNFR-1) are upregulated in glia and neurons following peripheral nerve injury. [89] Peripheral sensitization along with continued TNFα-induced anterograde transmission of information along the afferent pathway may, thus, contribute to the development of central sensitization at both the levels of the spinal cord and supra-spinal sites. Facilitation of nociceptive information along the pain pathway may result from consequent disinhibition of the descending analgesic pain pathway. In support of this pathologic plasticity, it was shown that proprioceptive spinal motor reflex circuits are disinhibited at the spinal level in CRPS dystonia. [90]

SYMPATHETIC NERVOUS SYSTEM

The sympathetic nervous system has long been implicated in playing a key role in maintaining pain and autonomic dysfunction in the afflicted extremity of CRPS patients. [91] Findings showing decreased serum norepinephrine levels in the affected versus non-affected limbs have, however, led to the contradictory proposal that adrenergic receptors are upregulated and hyper-responsive to circulating levels of catecholamines. [92] In particular, increased expression of α_2-adrenergic receptors on primary afferent sensory neurons has been postulated as a consequence of injury-induced cytokine production. [93] As a result, nociceptors are hypothesized to become hyperexcitable, due to stimulation of the upregulated α_2-adrenergic receptors, even though the local environment has less norepinephrine from the compromised sympathetic supply innervating the affected limb, and to circulating norepinephrine and epinephrine. [93] This continued sensory neuron excitation or 'afferent barrage' would contribute to the development of central sensitization that is typical of CRPS.

An animal model of CRPS in which rats were subjected to hind paw ischemia-reperfusion injury, termed chronic post-ischemia pain (CPIP), was used to compare the nociceptive and vascular sensitivity to norepinephrine. CPIP rats displayed exaggerated nociceptive behaviors and enhanced vasoconstrictive responses (decreased blood blow) to norepinephrine. [94] These findings parallel those observed in CRPS patients, whereby administration of norepinephrine evoked intense pain and increased vasoconstriction. [95, 96] Interestingly, both norepinephrine-induced augmented responses were reduced by α-adrenergic receptor antagonists, leading to the proposition that vascular α-adrenergic receptors are upregulated in CRPS. [94]

Both neurogenic inflammation and the sympathetic nervous system influence cytokine levels. [97] Whereas SP stimulates the production and release of TNFα, IL-1β, and IL-6 from immune cells such as macrophages, activation of norepinephrine and epinephrine sensitive adrenergic receptors on macrophages regulates the production of TNFα. [35, 43] In fact, stimulation of α_2-adrenergic receptors on activated macrophages increases TNFα production, whereas stimulation of β_2-adrenergic receptors inhibits TNFα production. [44, 45, 98] Therefore, during development of CRPS, an up-regulation (i.e., super-sensitization to catecholamines) of α_2-adrenergic receptors on macrophages due to neuroinflammatory-mediated deficiency of sympathetic innervation in the affected extremity would be expected to contribute to the aberrant increase in TNFα production. Likewise, the observation of autoantibodies to the β_2-adrenergic receptor in CRPS patients would be predicted to disinhibit TNFα production by macrophages. Together, these proposed changes in adrenergic receptor expression on inflammatory cells that support increased production of TNFα would serve to drive the neurogenic inflammation, as well as the peripheral and central sensitization, that all together contribute to development of CRPS. Taken together, these findings provide support for the use of non-selective α-adrenergic antagonists, such as phentolamine and phenoxybenzamine, which display the possible role of the α_1-adrenergic receptor, in the treatment of CRPS pain. [99, 100]

PARASYMPATHETIC NERVOUS SYSTEM

While impairment in the functioning of the sympathetic arm of the autonomic nervous system is well accepted in CRPS, changes in the functioning of the parasympathetic arm would likewise contribute to the autonomic dysfunction in CRPS. In support of impaired parasympathetic activity during CRPS, the efferent cholinergic anti-inflammatory pathway is implicated in playing a role in neuropathic pain syndromes. Following nerve injury, both pro-inflammatory and anti-inflammatory processes are initiated. [101] It is hypothesized, however, that during CRPS there is an imbalance between these processes such that inflammation is favored. [102] The afferent arc of the anti-inflammatory pathway serves as a sensory detector in that afferent vagal fibers are sensitive to stimulation by cytokines, such as TNFα, initially produced by the inciting injury. [103-105] Activation of afferent vagal fibers transmits the noxious signal via connections in the spinal cord and medulla oblongata to higher brain centers where central processing occurs. This processed ascending information is then relayed back through the brainstem and is communicated to the periphery via action potential transmission by the efferent vagus nerve. [103-105] The subsequent release of acetylcholine from efferent vagal fibers stimulates nicotinic acetylcholine receptors on immune cells to suppress the production of TNFα and other pro-inflammatory cytokines, but does not affect anti-inflammatory cytokine production. [103, 105] Impairment or disruption of this anti-inflammatory pathway could contribute to development and maintenance of

CRPS. For instance, the finding of autoantibodies to the m_2Ach receptor in CRPS patients may lead to disruption in efferent vagal outflow in CRPS. [106] Muscarinic-2-acetylcholine receptor agonists have been shown to reduce neurogenic inflammation and desensitize nociceptors. [42] Thus, autoantibody-mediated impediment in receptor signaling would account for the clinical finding of vasodilatation during CRPS. Failure in the efficacy of acetylcholine may counteract any anti-inflammatory mediated nicotinic receptor effect, leaving TNFα production unchecked with heightened levels contributing to the ongoing pathophysiologic mechanisms driving CRPS.

TREATMENT FOR CRPS

Unrelieved pain is maladaptive, and analgesics, such as morphine, non-steroidal anti-inflammatory drugs, and anticonvulsants that provide pain relief, if given early after injury, are rarely effective when treatment is initiated well-after CRPS development. Thus, advanced cases of CRPS that are more easily recognizable are not only severe in presentation, but are also difficult to treat. An important goal in CRPS pain management is to reduce the functional disability of the patient. This requires that the treatment prevents development of central sensitization and thereby minimizes the physical as well as the cognitive and emotional distress caused by pain. [4]

ANTIDEPRESSANTS, ANTICONVULSANTS, AND ADRENERGIC AGENTS

It is interesting that over time, patients experiencing CRPS may develop mood changes, disrupted sleep patterns, or enhanced level of disability. [107] Tricyclic antidepressants that are designed to treat depression have analgesic properties that are effective for neuropathic pain conditions; they can also improve sleep. [108] Whereas amitriptyline and nortriptyline are commonly used to treat CRPS, antidepressants that block the reuptake of both norepinephrine and serotonin may be more effective for CRPS management. [109] These same drugs have been shown to decrease levels of TNFα, both centrally and peripherally, at the time when nociceptive behavior is relieved. [21, 110] Since these classes of drugs do not effectively treat all patients, and side effects often limit their use, it may be more beneficial to target TNFα directly as a CRPS therapy. Exclusive inhibition of only TNFα production would not only prevent the inflammatory cascade, but would also enhance monoamine release, a mechanism that has been attributed to antidepressant and analgesic drug action. [21, 111] Pro-inflammatory cytokines, such as TNFα, influence monoamine turnover in the hippocampus. [11, 12] Therefore, pro-inflammatory dysfunction leads to deregulation of monoamines in the hippocampus, which suggests a possible mechanism underlying the pathophysiology of chronic pain conditions including CRPS. [112] Elevated levels of TNFα, as occurs in CSF during CRPS, would be predicted to suppress norepinephrine release in the hippocampus. [15, 22, 31, 111] TNFα production leads to remodeling of $α_2$-adrenergic regulation of norepinephrine release in the CNS, which contributes to the development of neuropathic pain central sensitization. [15] During peak hyperalgesia associated with CCI-induced neuropathic pain, TNFα and α$_2$-adrenergic inhibition of norepinephrine release is at its maximum in the hippocampus. [113] A decrease in norepinephrine release results in decreased activation of α$_2$-adrenergic receptors, which further increases TNFα levels in the brain; thus, low central levels of norepinephrine are maintained with subsequent enhanced production of TNFα. [15, 21] Furthermore, the identification of CRPS patient autoantibodies against β$_2$-adrenergic receptors suggests additional consequences to central regulation of norepinephrine release. The presynaptic β$_2$-adrenergic receptor functions to facilitate norepinephrine release; absence of this receptor-mediated response would contribute to the maintenance of neuropathic pain-induced low central norepinephrine levels.

Anti-seizure medications are useful in the treatment of neuropathic pain. Gabapentin and pregabalin are two commonly prescribed anticonvulsants for neuropathic pain conditions and are widely used "off-label" for the clinical management of CRPS. [114] Unfortunately, similar to the tricyclic antidepressants, anticonvulsant agents are not always effective, do not work for all patients, and may produce unwanted side-effects. In fact, the anti-convulsive drug gabapentin was shown to accentuate pro-inflammatory effects. [115] Anti-epileptic drugs, such as gabapentin (30 µg, intrathecal administration) and valproic acid (0.5-50 mg/kg, p.o.), decrease TNFα levels in rodent spinal cord (centrally) and hind paws (peripherally), respectively. Therefore, investigation into a more direct approach for decreasing TNFα, as a CRPS therapy, is warranted. [116, 117]

In practice, many physicians treat CRPS with sympatholytic agents (i.e., phentolamine, phenoxybenzamine, clonidine) with the intent to relieve dysfunctional autonomic symptoms. As reviewed by Rowbotham (2006), clinical investigation has shown that local injection of an α-adrenergic agonist in CRPS patients actually increases pain, which is not surprising given that TNFα levels are chronically increased. Stimulation of α$_2$-adrenergic receptors on neurons and on immune-effector cells (i.e., macrophages) also increases TNFα production. [45, 98, 118] However, the antinociceptive effect of clonidine was shown to be associated with increased production of TNFα during CCI-induced neuropathic pain. [113] In this pre-clinical study, treatment with clonidine for nociception switched the central presynaptic neuron response to TNFα and α$_2$-adrenergic agonists (i.e., from facilitation to inhibition of norepinephrine release). Paradoxically, this mechanism that expresses as antinociceptive requires the elevated production of TNFα, which is associated with development of thermal hyperalgesia. [14, 15, 22] Since there appears to be two forms of the α$_2$-adrenergic receptor, one that regulates TNFα synthesis, which is the form or configuration of the receptor that switches before the other α$_2$-adrenergic receptor (α$_2$-adrenergic autoreceptor) that regulates norepinephrine release, the overproduction of TNFα regulates the α$_2$-adrenergic autoreceptor culminating in the primed regulation of norepinephrine release. Therefore, normal physiological functioning is restored; this occurs during both clonidine- and amitriptyline-induced antinociception. [111] These neuroplastic changes in the noradrenergic system may reflect similar changes in other regions of the nervous system associated with pain. Thus, agents that act as α$_2$-adrenergic receptor agonists would be contraindicated as a sole treatment for patients with longstanding CRPS, while α$_1$-adrenergic antagonists, such as phentolamine and phenoxybenzamine, may be more effective in the management of CRPS pain. [99, 100] Consequently, the dynamics of the functioning of the α$_2$-adrenergic receptor is complex. It is intriguing to imagine how the different forms of these receptors interplay, offering fertile avenues for future research. Whether receptor populations change or their second messenger coupling in response to 'stress' changes is intriguing and may explain apparent contradictions.

NMDA ANTAGONISTS

Ketamine has been used for the management of pain in CRPS. [119] In addition to its anesthetic properties, ketamine has been reported to have anti-inflammatory properties, specifically inhibiting TNFα production from macrophages. [120] As an anti-inflammatory agent, ketamine also inhibits inflammatory cell recruitment. [121] These immunomodulatory properties of ketamine may contribute to its mechanism of analgesic action.

Memantine is another NMDA antagonist that is FDA approved for treatment of Alzheimer's disease, and it has shown promising initial results for the treatment of CRPS, such that pain was relieved in six treated patients. [122] Interestingly, memantine has been shown to decrease TNFα expression in the brain following administration to rats. [123] Whether the analgesic mechanism of action for memantine treatment of CRPS is due to inhibition of TNFα production has yet to be confirmed, and studies are warranted to determine whether this TNFα inhibition occurs locally and/or centrally.

ELECTRICAL STIMULATION

Non-pharmacological interventions are used for hard-to-treat chronic pain. Electroconvulsive therapy and vagal nerve stimulation are FDA-approved procedures for the treatment of refractory depression that reduce pain in patients suffering from chronic pain induced by migraines and cluster headaches and from chronic pelvic pain. [124-126] Interestingly, both electroconvulsive therapy and vagal nerve stimulation mediate anti-inflammation processes that decrease levels of TNFα in blood serum and plasma. [127, 128]. Whether vagal nerve stimulation will be useful for CRPS has yet to be determined. Based on the autonomic disturbances in CRPS and the concomitant elevated concentrations of TNFα, a favorable treatment outcome may ensue.

SPECIFIC ANTI-TNF MOLECULES

The discoveries of increased TNFα in CRPS patients, and its important role in CRPS pathogenesis, has led to a focus on targeting cytokines and their receptors to treat CRPS. [129] For example, infliximab, a chimeric monoclonal anti-TNFα antibody, when administered systemically or locally has been successful for treatment of CRPS, as reported in two separate case studies. [130, 131] Similarly, preliminary findings from a discontinued trial of infliximab for treatment of CRPS showed a promising trend toward decreasing the high TNFα concentrations in CRPS patients. [132] Interestingly, patients that received perispinal administration of etanercept, a human TNF receptor-2 antagonist, for stroke or traumatic brain injury (conditions that are often accompanied by development of CRPS) reported immediate alleviation of pain with improved mood and affect. [133] Perispinal administration involves injection (subcutaneous) at the cervical spine (C6–7) level; Trendelenburg positioning facilitates delivery into the brain. [134] Drugs injected posterior to the spine are absorbed by the external vertebral venous plexus, which drains into and is a component of the cerebrospinal venous system. [135, 136] This unique, bidirectional system provides a direct vascular pathway to the brain. [137] In all of these studies, no adverse effects were reported, warranting further clinical investigation of CRPS treatment with selective anti-TNFα antibody agents.

The immunomodulatory agent thalidomide and its potent analogue lenalidomide both inhibit TNFα production and provide some relief to CRPS patients. [138, 139] However, due to their teratogenic effects, the use of these drugs is restricted to patients beyond childbearing years. Pentoxifylline, a xanthine derivative and phosphodiesterase inhibitor that decreases the production of TNFα, was used to attenuate nociception and ameliorate TNFα expression in an animal model of CRPS. [140] Together, the finding that agents that reduce the availability of TNFα are effective in alleviating CRPS pain indicates that this cytokine may be the key mediator to target for effective treatment. Whether decreasing TNFα levels locally in the affected limb or in combination with central levels would result in better treatment outcomes is yet to be determined and warrants future investigation.

CONCLUSION

Based on the clinical and experimental evidence to date, CRPS is undoubtedly a complex, multisystem syndrome that is triggered by a peripheral insult involving neuroinflammatory injury and rapidly involves central changes that continue to drive the condition in its chronic form. Increased production of TNFα appears to be vital for the development and maintenance of CRPS both peripherally and centrally. Further clinical intervention studies and experimental investigations using anti-TNFα strategies hold much promise for illuminating the complexities underlying CRPS pathophysiology and pathogenesis, with subsequent promise of potential therapeutic options.

REFERENCES

[1]   Allen, G., B.S. Galer, and L. Schwartz, Epidemiology of complex regional pain syndrome: a retrospective chart review of 134 patients. *Pain*, 1999. 80(3): p. 539-44.

[2]   Watts, D. and M.J. Kremer, Complex regional pain syndrome: a review of diagnostics, pathophysiologic mechanisms, and treatment implications for certified registered nurse anesthetists. *AANA J.*, 2011. 79(6): p. 505-10.

[3]   Harden, R.N., et al., Validation of proposed diagnostic criteria (the "Budapest Criteria") for Complex Regional Pain Syndrome. *Pain*, 2010. 150(2): p. 268-74.

[4]   Harden, R.N., et al., Treatment of complex regional pain syndrome: functional restoration. *Clin. J. Pain*, 2006. 22(5): p. 420-4.

[5]   Birklein, F. and M. Schmelz, Neuropeptides, neurogenic inflammation and complex regional pain syndrome (CRPS). *Neurosci. Lett.*, 2008. 437(3): p. 199-202.

[6]   Uceyler, N., et al., Differential expression patterns of cytokines in complex regional pain syndrome. *Pain*, 2007. 132(1-2): p. 195-205.

[7]   Sommer, C. and F. Birklein, Resolvins and inflammatory pain. F1000 Med. Rep., 2011. 3: p. 19.

[8]   Bailey, J., et al., Imaging and clinical evidence of sensorimotor problems in CRPS: utilizing novel treatment approaches. *J. Neuroimmune Pharmacol.*, 2013. 8(3): p. 564-75.

[9]   Kohr, D., et al., Autoimmunity against the beta2 adrenergic receptor and muscarinic-2 receptor in complex regional pain syndrome. *Pain*, 2011. 152(12): p. 2690-700.

[10]   NINDS. NINDS Complex Regional Pain Syndrome Fact Sheet NINDS National Institute of Neurological Disorders and Stroke 2013 February 23, 2015 3.11.15; NIH Publication No. 13-4173. Available from: http://www.ninds.nih.gov/ disorders/reflex_sympathetic_dystrophy/detail_reflex_sympathetic_dystrophy.htm.

[11]   Maier, S.F. and L.R. Watkins, Cytokines for psychologists: implications of bidirectional immune-to-brain communication for understanding behavior, mood, and cognition. *Psychol. Rev.*, 1998. 105(1): p. 83-107.

[12]   Raison, C.L. and A.H. Miller, When not enough is too much: the role of insufficient glucocorticoid signaling in the pathophysiology of stress-related disorders. *Am. J. Psychiatry*, 2003. 160(9): p. 1554-65.

[13]   O'Connor, K.A., et al., Peripheral and central proinflammatory cytokine response to a severe acute stressor. *Brain Res.*, 2003. 991(1-2): p. 123-32.

[14]   Covey, W.C., et al., Expression of neuron-associated tumor necrosis factor alpha in the brain is increased during persistent pain. *Reg. Anesth. Pain Med.*, 2002. 27(4): p. 357-66.

[15]   Covey, W.C., et al., Brain-derived TNFalpha: involvement in neuroplastic changes implicated in the conscious perception of persistent pain. *Brain Res.*, 2000. 859(1): p. 113-22.

[16]   George, A., et al., Serial determination of tumor necrosis factor-alpha content in rat sciatic nerve after chronic constriction injury. *Exp. Neurol.*, 1999. 160(1): p. 124-32.

[17]   Myers, R.R., W.M. Campana, and V.I. Shubayev, The role of neuroinflammation in neuropathic pain: mechanisms and therapeutic targets. *Drug Discov. Today*, 2006. 11(1-2): p. 8-20.

[18]   Schafers, M., et al., Tumor necrosis factor-alpha induces mechanical allodynia after spinal nerve ligation by activation of p38 MAPK in primary sensory neurons. *J. Neurosci.*, 2003b. 23(7): p. 2517-21.

[19]   Shubayev, V.I., et al., TNFalpha-induced MMP-9 promotes macrophage recruitment into injured peripheral nerve. *Mol. Cell Neurosci.*, 2006. 31(3): p. 407-15.

[20]   Mueller, M., et al., Macrophage response to peripheral nerve injury: the quantitative contribution of resident and hematogenous macrophages. *Lab. Invest.*, 2003. 83(2): p. 175-85.

[21]   Sud, R., et al., Antinociception occurs with a reversal in alpha 2-adrenoceptor regulation of TNF production by peripheral monocytes /macrophages from pro- to anti-inflammatory. *Eur. J. Pharmacol.*, 2008. 588(2-3): p. 217-31.

[22]   Ignatowski, T.A., et al., Brain-derived TNFalpha mediates neuropathic pain. *Brain Res.*, 1999. 841(1-2): p. 70-7.

[23] Martuscello, R.T., et al., Increasing TNF levels solely in the rat hippocampus produces persistent pain-like symptoms. *Pain*, 2012. 153(9): p. 1871-82.

[24] Sabsovich, I., et al., TNF signaling contributes to the development of nociceptive sensitization in a tibia fracture model of complex regional pain syndrome type I. *Pain*, 2008. 137(3): p. 507-19.

[25] Ignatowski, T.A., B.A. Gerard, A. Bonoiu, S. Mahajan, P.R. Knight, B. Davidson, E.J. Bergey, P.N. Prasad, R.N. Spengler, Reduction of tumor necrosis factor (TNF) in the hippocampus alleviates neuropathic pain perception. Proceedings of the 4th International Congress on Neuropathic Pain 2013: p. 29-35.

[26] Huygen, F.J., et al., Evidence for local inflammation in complex regional pain syndrome type 1. *Mediators Inflamm.*, 2002. 11(1): p. 47-51.

[27] Lenz, M., et al., Local cytokine changes in complex regional pain syndrome type I (CRPS I) resolve after 6 months. *Pain*, 2013. 154(10): p. 2142-9.

[28] Maihofner, C., et al., Mechanical hyperalgesia in complex regional pain syndrome: a role for TNF-alpha? *Neurology*, 2005. 65(2): p. 311-3.

[29] Schinkel, C., et al., Inflammatory mediators are altered in the acute phase of posttraumatic complex regional pain syndrome. *Clin. J. Pain*, 2006. 22(3): p. 235-9.

[30] Kramer, H.H., et al., TNF-alpha in CRPS and 'normal' trauma--significant differences between tissue and serum. *Pain*, 2011. 152(2): p. 285-90.

[31] Parkitny, L., et al., Inflammation in complex regional pain syndrome: a systematic review and meta-analysis. *Neurology*, 2013. 80(1): p. 106-17.

[32] Coderre, T.J., et al., Chronic post-ischemia pain (CPIP): a novel animal model of complex regional pain syndrome-type I (CRPS-I; reflex sympathetic dystrophy) produced by prolonged hindpaw ischemia and reperfusion in the rat. *Pain*, 2004. 112(1-2): p. 94-105.

[33] Zubrzycka, M. and A. Janecka, Substance P: transmitter of nociception (Minireview). *Endocr. Regul.*, 2000. 34(4): p. 195-201.

[34] Guo, T.Z., et al., Substance P signaling contributes to the vascular and nociceptive abnormalities observed in a tibial fracture rat model of complex regional pain syndrome type I. *Pain*, 2004. 108(1-2): p. 95-107.

[35] O'Connor, T.M., et al., The role of substance P in inflammatory disease. *J. Cell Physiol.*, 2004. 201(2): p. 167-80.

[36] Holzer, P., Neurogenic vasodilatation and plasma leakage in the skin. *Gen. Pharmacol.*, 1998. 30(1): p. 5-11.

[37] Opree, A. and M. Kress, Involvement of the proinflammatory cytokines tumor necrosis factor-alpha, IL-1 beta, and IL-6 but not IL-8 in the development of heat hyperalgesia: effects on heat-evoked calcitonin gene-related peptide release from rat skin. *J. Neurosci.*, 2000. 20(16): p. 6289-93.

[38] Blaes, F., et al., Autoimmune etiology of complex regional pain syndrome (M. Sudeck). *Neurology*, 2004. 63(9): p. 1734-6.

[39] Kohr, D., et al., Autoantibodies in complex regional pain syndrome bind to a differentiation-dependent neuronal surface autoantigen. *Pain*, 2009. 143(3): p. 246-51.

[40] Hideshima, T., et al., The role of tumor necrosis factor alpha in the pathophysiology of human multiple myeloma: therapeutic applications. *Oncogene*, 2001. 20(33): p. 4519-27.

[41] van Rijn, M.A., et al., Spreading of complex regional pain syndrome: not a random process. *J. Neural Transm.*, 2011. 118(9): p. 1301-9.

[42] Bernardini, N., et al., Muscarinic M2 receptors on peripheral nerve endings: a molecular target of antinociception. *J. Neurosci.*, 2002. 22(12): p. RC229.

[43] Ignatowski, T.A. and R.N. Spengler, Regulation of macrophage-derived tumor necrosis factor production by modification of adrenergic receptor sensitivity. *J. Neuroimmunol.*, 1995. 61(1): p. 61-70.

[44] Ignatowski, T.A., S. Gallant, and R.N. Spengler, Temporal regulation by adrenergic receptor stimulation of macrophage (M phi)-derived tumor necrosis factor (TNF) production post-LPS challenge. *J. Neuroimmunol.*, 1996. 65(2): p. 107-17.

[45] Spengler, R.N., et al., Stimulation of alpha-adrenergic receptor augments the production of macrophage-derived tumor necrosis factor. *J. Immunol.*, 1990. 145(5): p. 1430-4.

[46] Spengler, R.N., et al., Endogenous norepinephrine regulates tumor necrosis factor-alpha production from macrophages in vitro. *J. Immunol.*, 1994. 152(6): p. 3024-31.

[47] Damon, D.H., Vascular-dependent effects of elevated glucose on postganglionic sympathetic neurons. *Am. J. Physiol. Heart Circ. Physiol.*, 2011. 300(4): p. H1386-92.

[48] Hodgkinson, C.P., et al., Advanced glycation end-product of low density lipoprotein activates the toll-like 4 receptor pathway implications for diabetic atherosclerosis. *Arterioscler. Thromb Vasc. Biol.*, 2008. 28(12): p. 2275-81.

[49] Straznicky, N.E., et al., Neuroadrenergic dysfunction along the diabetes continuum: a comparative study in obese metabolic syndrome subjects. *Diabetes*, 2012. 61(10): p. 2506-16.

[50] Takahashi, H.K., et al., Advanced glycation end products subspecies-selectively induce adhesion molecule expression and cytokine production in human peripheral blood mononuclear cells. *J. Pharmacol.* Exp Ther, 2009. 330(1): p. 89-98.

[51] Veloso, C.A., et al., TLR4 and RAGE: similar routes leading to inflammation in type 2 diabetic patients. *Diabetes Metab.*, 2011. 37(4): p. 336-42.

[52] Cooper, M.S. and V.P. Clark, Neuroinflammation, neuroautoimmunity, and the co-morbidities of complex regional pain syndrome. *J. Neuroimmune Pharmacol.*, 2013. 8(3): p. 452-69.

[53] Banati, R.B., et al., Long-term trans-synaptic glial responses in the human thalamus after peripheral nerve injury. *Neuroreport*, 2001. 12(16): p. 3439-42.

[54] Kreutzberg, G.W., Microglia: a sensor for pathological events in the CNS. *Trends Neurosci.*, 1996. 19(8): p. 312-8.

[55] Cooper, M.S. and A.S. Przebinda, Synaptic conversion of chloride-dependent synapses in spinal nociceptive circuits: roles in neuropathic pain. *Pain Res. Treat.*, 2011. 2011: p. 738645.

[56] Saab, C.Y. and B.C. Hains, Remote neuroimmune signaling: a long-range mechanism of nociceptive network plasticity. *Trends Neurosci.*, 2009. 32(2): p. 110-7.

[57] Zhao, P., S.G. Waxman, and B.C. Hains, Modulation of thalamic nociceptive processing after spinal cord injury through remote activation of thalamic microglia by cysteine cysteine chemokine ligand 21. *J. Neurosci.*, 2007. 27(33): p. 8893-902.

[58] Beggs, S., et al., Peripheral nerve injury and TRPV1-expressing primary afferent C-fibers cause opening of the blood-brain barrier. *Mol. Pain*, 2010. 6: p. 74.

[59] Stoll, G. and M. Bendszus, New approaches to neuroimaging of central nervous system inflammation. *Curr. Opin. Neurol.*, 2010. 23(3): p. 282-6.

[60] Franco, R., et al., The emergence of neurotransmitters as immune modulators. *Trends Immunol.*, 2007. 28(9): p. 400-7.

[61] Saab, C.Y., S.G. Waxman, and B.C. Hains, Alarm or curse? The pain of neuroinflammation. *Brain Res. Rev.*, 2008. 58(1): p. 226-35.

[62] Mutso, A.A., et al., Abnormalities in hippocampal functioning with persistent pain. *J. Neurosci.*, 2012. 32(17): p. 5747-56.

[63] Dellarole, A., et al., Neuropathic pain-induced depressive-like behavior and hippocampal neurogenesis and plasticity are dependent on TNFR1 signaling. *Brain Behav. Immun.*, 2014. 41: p. 65-81.

[64] Sakuma, Y., et al., Up-regulation of p55 TNF alpha-receptor in dorsal root ganglia neurons following lumbar facet joint injury in rats. *Eur. Spine J.*, 2007. 16(8): p. 1273-8.

[65] Harry, G.J., et al., Tumor necrosis factor p55 and p75 receptors are involved in chemical-induced apoptosis of dentate granule neurons. *J. Neurochem.*, 2008. 106(1): p. 281-98.

[66] Kuno, R., et al., Autocrine activation of microglia by tumor necrosis factor-alpha. *J. Neuroimmunol.*, 2005. 162(1-2): p. 89-96.

[67] Veroni, C., et al., Activation of TNF receptor 2 in microglia promotes induction of anti-inflammatory pathways. *Mol. Cell Neurosci.*, 2010. 45(3): p. 234-44.

[68] Zhang, H., H. Zhang, and P.M. Dougherty, Dynamic effects of TNF-alpha on synaptic transmission in mice over time following sciatic nerve chronic constriction injury. *J. Neurophysiol.*, 2013. 110(7): p. 1663-71.

[69] Janig, W., The fascination of complex regional pain syndrome. *Exp. Neurol.*, 2010. 221(1): p. 1-4.

[70] Janig, W. and R. Baron, Complex regional pain syndrome is a disease of the central nervous system. *Clin. Auton. Res.*, 2002. 12(3): p. 150-64.

[71] Alexander, G.M., et al., Changes in plasma cytokines and their soluble receptors in complex regional pain syndrome. *J. Pain*, 2012. 13(1): p. 10-20.

[72] Schafers, M., et al., Increased sensitivity of injured and adjacent uninjured rat primary sensory neurons to exogenous tumor necrosis factor-alpha after spinal nerve ligation. *J. Neurosci.*, 2003a. 23(7): p. 3028-38.

[73] Sommer, C. and M. Kress, Recent findings on how proinflammatory cytokines cause pain: peripheral mechanisms in inflammatory and neuropathic hyperalgesia. *Neurosci. Lett.*, 2004. 361(1-3): p. 184-7.

[74] Kawasaki, Y., et al., Cytokine mechanisms of central sensitization: distinct and overlapping role of interleukin-1beta, interleukin-6, and tumor necrosis factor-alpha in regulating synaptic and neuronal activity in the superficial spinal cord. *J. Neurosci.*, 2008. 28(20): p. 5189-94.

[75] DeLeo, J.A. and R.P. Yezierski, The role of neuroinflammation and neuroimmune activation in persistent pain. *Pain*, 2001. 90(1-2): p. 1-6.

[76] Watkins, L.R., E.D. Milligan, and S.F. Maier, Glial activation: a driving force for pathological pain. *Trends Neurosci.*, 2001. 24(8): p. 450-5.

[77] Cummins, T.R., et al., Nav1.3 sodium channels: rapid repriming and slow closed-state inactivation display quantitative differences after expression in a mammalian cell line and in spinal sensory neurons. *J. Neurosci.*, 2001. 21(16): p. 5952-61.

[78] Waxman, S.G. and B.C. Hains, Fire and phantoms after spinal cord injury: Na+ channels and central pain. Trends Neurosci, 2006. 29(4): p. 207-15.

[79] Hains, B.C., et al., Upregulation of sodium channel Nav1.3 and functional involvement in neuronal hyperexcitability associated with central neuropathic pain after spinal cord injury. *J. Neurosci.*, 2003. 23(26): p. 8881-92.

[80] Hains, B.C., C.Y. Saab, and S.G. Waxman, Changes in electrophysiological properties and sodium channel Nav1.3 expression in thalamic neurons after spinal cord injury. *Brain*, 2005. 128(Pt 10): p. 2359-71.

[81] Shyu, B.C. and B.A. Vogt, Short-term synaptic plasticity in the nociceptive thalamic-anterior cingulate pathway. Mol Pain, 2009. 5: p. 51.

[82] Myers, R.R. and V.I. Shubayev, The ology of neuropathy: an integrative review of the role of neuroinflammation and TNF-alpha axonal transport in neuropathic pain. *J. Peripher. Nerv. Syst.*, 2011. 16(4): p. 277-86.

[83] Shubayev, V.I. and R.R. Myers, Axonal transport of TNF-alpha in painful neuropathy: distribution of ligand tracer and TNF receptors. *J. Neuroimmunol.*, 2001. 114(1-2): p. 48-56.

[84] Shubayev, V.I. and R.R. Myers, Anterograde TNF alpha transport from rat dorsal root ganglion to spinal cord and injured sciatic nerve. *Neurosci. Lett.*, 2002. 320(1-2): p. 99-101.

[85] Santello, M. and A. Volterra, TNFalpha in synaptic function: switching gears. *Trends Neurosci.*, 2012. 35(10): p. 638-47.

[86] Czeschik, J.C., et al., TNF-alpha differentially modulates ion channels of nociceptive neurons. *Neurosci. Lett.*, 2008. 434(3): p. 293-8.

[87] Liu, B., et al., Increased sensitivity of sensory neurons to tumor necrosis factor alpha in rats with chronic compression of the lumbar ganglia. *J. Neurophysiol.*, 2002. 88(3): p. 1393-9.

[88] Ozaktay, A.C., et al., Effects of interleukin-1 beta, interleukin-6, and tumor necrosis factor on sensitivity of dorsal root ganglion and peripheral receptive fields in rats. *Eur. Spine J.*, 2006. 15(10): p. 1529-37.

[89] Ohtori, S., et al., TNF-alpha and TNF-alpha receptor type 1 upregulation in glia and neurons after peripheral nerve injury: studies in murine DRG and spinal cord. *Spine* (Phila Pa 1976), 2004. 29(10): p. 1082-8.

[90] Schouten, A.C., et al., Proprioceptive reflexes in patients with reflex sympathetic dystrophy. *Exp. Brain Res.*, 2003. 151(1): p. 1-8.

[91] Chelimsky, T.C., et al., Value of autonomic testing in reflex sympathetic dystrophy. Mayo Clin Proc, 1995. 70(11): p. 1029-40.

[92] Harden, R.N., et al., Norepinephrine and epinephrine levels in affected versus unaffected limbs in sympathetically maintained pain. *Clin. J. Pain.*, 1994. 10(4): p. 324-30.

[93] Perl, E.R., Causalgia, pathological pain, and adrenergic receptors. *Proc. Natl. Acad. Sci. U S A*, 1999. 96(14): p. 7664-7.

[94] Xanthos, D.N., G.J. Bennett, and T.J. Coderre, Norepinephrine-induced nociception and vasoconstrictor hypersensitivity in rats with chronic post-ischemia pain. *Pain*, 2008. 137(3): p. 640-51.

[95] Ali, Z., et al., Intradermal injection of norepinephrine evokes pain in patients with sympathetically maintained pain. *Pain*, 2000. 88(2): p. 161-8.

[96] Teasell, R.W. and J.M. Arnold, Alpha-1 adrenoceptor hyperresponsiveness in three neuropathic pain states: complex regional pain syndrome 1, diabetic peripheral neuropathic pain and central pain states following spinal cord injury. *Pain Res. Manag.*, 2004. 9(2): p. 89-97.

[97] Weber, M., et al., Facilitated neurogenic inflammation in complex regional pain syndrome. *Pain*, 2001. 91(3): p. 251-7.

[98] Ignatowski, T.A., S.L. Kunkel, and R.N. Spengler, Interactions between the alpha(2)-adrenergic and the prostaglandin response in the regulation of macrophage-derived tumor necrosis factor. *Clin. Immunol.*, 2000. 96(1): p. 44-51.

[99] Muizelaar, J.P., et al., Complex regional pain syndrome (reflex sympathetic dystrophy and causalgia): management with the calcium channel blocker nifedipine and/or the alpha-sympathetic blocker phenoxybenzamine in 59 patients. *Clin. Neurol. Neurosurg.*, 1997. 99(1): p. 26-30.

[100] Raja, S.N., et al., Systemic alpha-adrenergic blockade with phentolamine: a diagnostic test for sympathetically maintained pain. *Anesthesiology*, 1991. 74(4): p. 691-8.

[101] Austin, P.J. and G. Moalem-Taylor, The neuro-immune balance in neuropathic pain: involvement of inflammatory immune cells, immune-like glial cells and cytokines. *J. Neuroimmunol.*, 2010. 229(1-2): p. 26-50.

[102] Linnman, C., L. Becerra, and D. Borsook, Inflaming the brain: CRPS a model disease to understand neuroimmune interactions in chronic pain. *J. Neuroimmune Pharmacol.*, 2013. 8(3): p. 547-63.

[103] Rosas-Ballina, M. and K.J. Tracey, Cholinergic control of inflammation. *J. Intern. Med.*, 2009. 265(6): p. 663-79.

[104] Thayer, J.F. and E.M. Sternberg, Neural aspects of immunomodulation: focus on the vagus nerve. *Brain Behav. Immun.*, 2010. 24(8): p. 1223-8.

[105] Tracey, K.J., Understanding immunity requires more than immunology. *Nat. Immunol.*, 2010. 11(7): p. 561-4.

[106] Walker, S. and P.D. Drummond, Implications of a local overproduction of tumor necrosis factor-alpha in complex regional pain syndrome. *Pain Med.*, 2011. 12(12): p. 1784-807.

[107] Bruehl, S. and O.Y. Chung, Psychological and behavioral aspects of complex regional pain syndrome management. *Clin. J. Pain*, 2006. 22(5): p. 430-7.

[108] Saarto, T. and P.J. Wiffen, Antidepressants for neuropathic pain. *Cochrane Database Syst. Rev.*, 2007(4): p. CD005454.

[109] Sindrup, S.H., et al., Venlafaxine versus imipramine in painful polyneuropathy: a randomized, controlled trial. *Neurology*, 2003. 60(8): p. 1284-9.

[110] Ignatowski, T.A., et al., The dissipation of neuropathic pain paradoxically involves the presence of tumor necrosis factor-alpha (TNF). *Neuropharmacology*, 2005. 48(3): p. 448-60.

[111] Reynolds, J.L., et al., An antidepressant mechanism of desipramine is to decrease tumor necrosis factor-alpha production culminating in increases in noradrenergic neurotransmission. *Neuroscience*, 2005a. 133(2): p. 519-31.

[112] Blackburn-Munro, G. and R.E. Blackburn-Munro, Chronic pain, chronic stress and depression: coincidence or consequence? *J. Neuroendocrinol.*, 2001. 13(12): p. 1009-23.

[113] Spengler, R.N., et al., Antinociception mediated by alpha(2)-adrenergic activation involves increasing tumor necrosis factor alpha (TNFalpha) expression and restoring TNFalpha and alpha(2)-adrenergic inhibition of norepinephrine release. *Neuropharmacology*, 2007. 52(2): p. 576-89.

[114] Rowbotham, M.C., Pharmacologic management of complex regional pain syndrome. *Clin. J. Pain.*, 2006. 22(5): p. 425-9.

[115] Camara, C.C., et al., Oral gabapentin treatment accentuates nerve and peripheral inflammatory responses following experimental nerve constriction in Wistar rats. *Neurosci. Lett.*, 2013. 556: p. 93-8.

[116] Lee, B.S., et al., Intrathecal gabapentin increases interleukin-10 expression and inhibits pro-inflammatory cytokine in a rat model of neuropathic pain. *J. Korean Med. Sci.*, 2013. 28(2): p. 308-14.

[117] Ximenes, J.C., et al., Valproic acid: an anticonvulsant drug with potent antinociceptive and anti-inflammatory properties. *Naunyn Schmiedebergs Arch. Pharmacol.*, 2013. 386(7): p. 575-87.

[118] Renauld, A.E. and R.N. Spengler, Tumor necrosis factor expressed by primary hippocampal neurons and SH-SY5Y cells is regulated by alpha(2)-adrenergic receptor activation. *J. Neurosci. Res.*, 2002. 67(2): p. 264-74.

[119] Azari, P., et al., Efficacy and safety of ketamine in patients with complex regional pain syndrome: a systematic review. *CNS Drugs*, 2012. 26(3): p. 215-28.

[120] Chang, Y., et al., Suppressive effects of ketamine on macrophage functions. *Toxicol. Appl. Pharmacol.*, 2005. 204(1): p. 27-35.

[121] Loix, S., M. De Kock, and P. Henin, The anti-inflammatory effects of ketamine: state of the art. *Acta Anaesthesiol. Belg.*, 2011. 62(1): p. 47-58.

[122] Sinis, N., et al., Memantine treatment of complex regional pain syndrome: a preliminary report of six cases. *Clin. J. Pain*, 2007. 23(3): p. 237-43.

[123] Tsartsalis, S., et al., The effect of memantine on cerebral cortex tumor necrosis factor alpha exression in a rat model of acute hyperammonemia. *Annals of General Psychiatry*, 2010. 9(Suppl 1): p. S181-S181.

[124] Hord, E.D., et al., The effect of vagus nerve stimulation on migraines. *J. Pain*, 2003. 4(9): p. 530-4.

[125] Multon, S. and J. Schoenen, Pain control by vagus nerve stimulation: from animal to man...and back. *Acta Neurol. Belg.*, 2005. 105(2): p. 62-7.

[126] Napadow, V., et al., Evoked pain analgesia in chronic pelvic pain patients using respiratory-gated auricular vagal afferent nerve stimulation. *Pain Med.*, 2012. 13(6): p. 777-89.

[127] Bansal, V., et al., Vagal stimulation modulates inflammation through a ghrelin mediated mechanism in traumatic brain injury. *Inflammation*, 2012. 35(1): p. 214-20.

[128] Hestad, K.A., et al., Raised plasma levels of tumor necrosis factor alpha in patients with depression: normalization during electroconvulsive therapy. *J. ECT*, 2003. 19(4): p. 183-8.

[129] Kapoor, S., The evolution and progression of complex regional pain syndrome (CRPS): recent insights into the nociceptive role of cytokines and management of CRPS with anticytokine therapy. *Curr. Sports Med. Rep.*, 2010. 9(3): p. 183; author reply 183.

[130] Huygen, F.J., et al., Successful treatment of CRPS 1 with anti-TNF. *J. Pain Symptom Manage*, 2004. 27(2): p. 101-3.

[131] Bernateck, M., et al., Successful intravenous regional block with low-dose tumor necrosis factor-alpha antibody infliximab for treatment of complex regional pain syndrome 1. *Anesth. Analg.*, 2007. 105(4): p. 1148-51.

[132] Dirckx, M., et al., Report of a preliminary discontinued double-blind, randomized, placebo-controlled trial of the anti-TNF-alpha chimeric monoclonal antibody infliximab in complex regional pain syndrome. *Pain Pract.*, 2013. 13(8): p. 633-40.

[133] Tobinick, E., et al., Selective TNF inhibition for chronic stroke and traumatic brain injury: an observational study involving 629 consecutive patients treated with perispinal etanercept. *CNS Drugs*, 2012. 26(12): p. 1051-70.

[134] Ignatowski, T.A., et al., Perispinal etanercept for post-stroke neurological and cognitive dysfunction: scientific rationale and current evidence. *CNS Drugs*, 2014. 28(8): p. 679-97.

[135] Batson, O.V., The function of the vertebral veins and their role in the spread of metastases. *Ann. Surg.*, 1940. 112(1): p. 138-49.

[136] LaBan, M.M., et al., Paravertebral muscle metastases as imaged by magnetic resonance venography: a brief report. *Am. J. Phys. Med. Rehabil.*, 1998. 77(6): p. 553-6.

[137] Nathoo, N., et al., History of the vertebral venous plexus and the significant contributions of Breschet and Batson. *Neurosurgery*, 2011. 69(5): p. 1007-14; discussion 1014.

[138] Rajkumar, S.V., R. Fonseca, and T.E. Witzig, Complete resolution of reflex sympathetic dystrophy with thalidomide treatment. *Arch. Intern. Med.*, 2001. 161(20): p. 2502-3.

[139] Manning, D.C., 71 IMMUNOMODULATORY AGENTS FOR NEUROPATHIC PAIN SYNDROMES: FROM ANIMALS TO CRPS AND BEYOND. *European Journal of Pain*, 2006. 10(S1): p. S20b-S21.

[140] Wei, T., et al., Pentoxifylline attenuates nociceptive sensitization and cytokine expression in a tibia fracture rat model of complex regional pain syndrome. *Eur. J. Pain*, 2009. 13(3): p. 253-62.

[141] Blalock, J.E. and E.M. Smith, Conceptual development of the immune system as a sixth sense. *Brain Behav. Immun.*, 2007. 21(1): p. 23-33.

[142] Reynolds, J.L., T.A. Ignatowski, and R.N. Spengler, Effect of tumor necrosis factor-alpha on the reciprocal G-protein-induced regulation of norepinephrine release by the alpha2-adrenergic receptor. *J. Neurosci. Res.*, 2005b. 79(6): p. 779-87.

Chapter 4

DIAGNOSTICS AND EXPERIMENTAL DIAGNOSTIC STRATEGIES

James Hitt, MD, PhD [*]

Anesthesiology and Pain Management,
University at Buffalo, Buffalo, NY, US

CLINICAL DIAGNOSIS OF COMPLEX REGIONAL PAIN SYNDROME

Claude Bernard first mentioned a pain syndrome linked to the sympathetic nervous system in 1850, and later Weir-Mitchell and Evans coined the terms reflex sympathetic dystrophy (RSD) and causalgia. [1, 2] The terms RSD and causalgia have been the most commonly used historical terms for the condition now called complex regional pain syndrome (CRPS). Anecdotal clinical experience resulted in the initial attempts to formulate diagnostic criteria for the syndrome, but because of variability in clinical presentation, these efforts resulted in inconsistent and somewhat idiosyncratic definitions of the syndrome. The initial assumptions of RSD have also been called into question; namely, there does not appear to be a simple neural reflex circuit that underlies the disease, and not all patients present with dystrophic signs.

In 1993, a consensus panel convened, reviewed the taxonomy of reflex sympathetic dystrophy and causalgia, and coined the term CRPS. [3, 4] The previous conceptualization of RSD and causalgia did not fully capture patients, and some autonomic signs often seen in CRPS can also be seen in other chronic pain states, such as post-herpetic neuralgia, phantom limb pain, and metabolic neuropathies. The consensus paper divided CPRS into two types, whereby type I encompasses many of the features of RSD and type II is most similar to causalgia. The original consensus-derived diagnostic criteria for CRPS suggested that the signs and symptoms of CRPS cluster into two subgroups: pain or sensory findings and vasomotor, sudomotor, or edema changes. Table 1 summarizes the diagnostic criteria for CRPS that resulted from this 1993 Orlando conference. The sensory symptoms include

---

[*] Clinical Assistant Professor, jhitt@buffalo.edu.

chronic pain, including hyperalgesia or allodynia, which is disproportionate to the inciting noxious event in a distribution that exceeds the region of a dermatome or peripheral nerve. The criteria also include the presence of physical signs, edema, changes in cutaneous blood flow, or abnormal sudomotor activity, at some point during the course of the syndrome.

Table 1. International Association for the Study of Pain (Orlando) diagnostic criteria for CRPS

Criterion 1	*The presence of an initiating noxious event, visceral disease, or immobility.*
Criterion 2	Continuing pain, hyperalgesia, or allodynia with which the pain is disproportionate to any inciting event.
Criterion 3	Evidence at some time of edema, changes in skin blood flow, or abnormal sudomotor activity in the region of pain.
Criterion 4	This diagnosis is excluded by the existence of conditions that would otherwise account for the degree of pain and dysfunction

Subsequent to the development of the consensus-derived diagnostic criteria, validation research of the diagnostic criteria illuminated some strengths and weaknesses of the original criteria. A series of 123 patients who met the original IASP criteria for CRPS (Table 1) were examined using principal component factor analysis (PCA). [5] PCA is a form of factor analysis that can be used to identify coherent subsets of variables within a data set that best captures the variability in the data, and the analysis of the 123 CRPS patients showed that subgroupings of signs and symptoms of CRPS clustered in ways expected from clinical experience. Four subgroupings were identified, including sensory (hyperalgesia and hyperesthesia), vasomotor (temperature assymetry and color changes), edema or sudomotor (edema signs, edema symptoms, and sweating assymetry), and motor (decreased range of motion, motor dysfunction, and trophic changes). [5] This assessment of the internal validity of the Orlando CRPS criteria confirmed that sensory symptoms of CRPS cluster together, but the results also indicated that vasomotor and sudomotor changes should be considered separately. The analysis also indicated motor and range of motion changes should be included in the diagnostic workup.

An external validation study examined 117 patients with CRPS and 43 patients with other neuropathic pain conditions, including painful diabetic neuropathy, post-herpetic neuralgia, and radiculopathy. [6] Application of the original Orlando diagnostic criteria (1 or more sign or symptom in category 2 and 3 from Table 1) resulted in high sensitivity but low specificity (0.98 and 0.36 respectively, see Table 3), indicating that the original diagnostic criteria could lead to over diagnosis. The original Orlando diagnostic criteria only required sensory findings (continued pain, hyperalgesia or allodynia) and a single additional sign or symptom at any point in time, including edema, vasomotor, or sudomotor changes. This less stringent diagnostic algorithm results in many other neuropathic pain conditions qualifying for a diagnosis of CRPS.

Given the internal validation studies reported clustering of CRPS symptoms into 4 categories of physiological changes, modified diagnostic criteria were also proposed that included those 4 categories, sensory, vasomotor, sudomotor, and motor changes (Table 2). [6] The authors found that requiring clinical signs in 2 or more of the categories and symptoms in all 4 categories reduced the sensitivity to 0.70 but increased the specificity to 0.94. While that trade off of sensitivity for specificity is preferable for research applications, the lower sensitivity may be less useful in clinical practice. A requirement of symptoms in 3 of 4 categories and signs in 2 or more categories increased sensitivity to 0.85 and specificity to 0.69 (Table 3).

A second consensus panel convened in Budapest to reconsider the diagnostic criteria for CRPS and review the abovementioned results. The original Orlando classification of CRPS groups vasomotor, edema, and sudomotor changes in one criterion, but subsequent research implicated that those categories likely do not represent redundant information. In addition, the original diagnostic criteria do not consider any motor or trophic changes. These weaknesses in the original diagnostic construct likely result in high sensitivity but poor specificity. The Budapest consensus-panel recommended clinical diagnosis criteria that include at least 2 signs and at least 3 symptoms from categories shown in Table 2. [7]

Table 2. Modified Diagnostic Criteria for CRPS [6]

	Symptoms	*Signs*
Sensory	Reports of Hyperesthesia	Evidence of hyperalgesia or allodynia
Vasomotor	Reports of temperature asymmetry, skin color change or asymmetry	Evidence of temperature asymmetry or skin color changes
Sudomotor/edema	Reports of edema, sweating changes, or sweating asymmetry	Evidence of edema, sweating changes or asymmetry
Motor/trophic	Reports of decreased range of motion, motor dysfunction, or trophic changes	Evidence of reduced range of motion, motor dysfunction (weakness, tremor or dystonia), or trophic changes of the hair, nails, or skin

Table 3. Sensitivity and specificity of modified diagnostic criteria for CRPS diagnosis [6]

	Sensitivity	*Specificity*
Orlando criteria	0.98	0.36
2+ signs and 2+ symptoms	0.94	0.36
2+ signs and 3+ symptoms	0.85	0.69
2+ signs and 4+ symptoms	0.70	0.94

They did continue the distinction between CRPS type I and type II, reflecting the absence or presence of a peripheral nerve injury, but acknowledged that it is not known whether there is a clinical implication of that distinction. Given the reduced sensitivity of the Budapest criteria, a third classification of CRPS was proposed (CRPS-NOS) for patients who were not diagnosed by the new criteria who had pain not explained by another diagnosis.

STAGES OF CRPS

CRPS has been classically thought of as a progressive disease and is thought to progress through three stages. [8, 9] Stage I has been reported to be associated with persistent pain following a noxious insult that can include burning, throbbing, and aching qualities, typically in a distribution that is greater than a dermatomal or peripheral nerve distribution. The noxious insult need not involve significant tissue or neural injury (e.g., joint sprain, non-complicated surgery, or minor soft tissue injury), and CRPS has been observed following myocardial infarction or cerebrovascular accidents. [10, 11] Patients with stage I CRPS may have vasomotor changes (altered temperature and skin color) and radiographic findings are typically normal for patients with this presentation. Stage I disease can also include signs of vasomotor dysfunction, edema, or sudomotor disturbance.

Stage II (dystrophic) reportedly shows worsening of thepain and sensory symptoms along with progression of the vasomotor changes with increased soft tissue edema, skin temperature and color changes. Patients grouped in stage 2 also can show dystrophic signs, including thickening of the skin, thickening of the articular soft tissues, muscle wasting, and brawny edema (dermal atrophy, necrosis, and stasis ulceration surrounded by a rim of dry, scaling, and pruritic skin). Radiographs can show patchy demineralization in patients with this constellation of symptoms. Stage 2 has been reported to occur 3 to 6 months after initial onset.

Stage III (atrophic) has been associated with the most severe signs and symptoms, including limitations in range of motion, muscle atrophy or contracture, and more significant dystrophic changes of the skin and nails. Bone radiography can show significant demineralization. The advanced dystrophic changes associated with stage 3 CRPS appears to have a negative prognostic implications for response to treatment, but these patients should still undergo aggressive pharmacologic and rehabilitative treatment with the hopes of preserving or restoring some function.

The classical stages of CRPS are thought to represent a temporal progression of disease that initially presents with sensory and vasomotor symptoms and can progress to a severe syndrome that includes significant pain and trophic signs. Anecdotal clinical experience also indicates that CRPS can progress through stages of disease; however, the progression of the syndrome through the abovementioned stages has been called into question by some researchers. The classical concept of progression of CRPS through the various stages of disease has been challenged by the validation studies of the CRPS diagnostic schema. The original principal components analysis of CRPS diagnostic criteria published by Harden and colleagues failed to show a correlation between the duration of disease and likelihood of signs of edema, sudomotor signs, or trophic changes. [5] This observation questions the classic conception of CRPS as a progressive disease with vasomotor, motor, and trophic changes predominating in the late stages of disease.

The concept of the progressive stages of CRPS was examined by Bruehl and colleagues. [12] The authors examined the cases of 113 patients who qualified for the original (Orlando) criteria for CRPS proposed by Merskey and Bogduk. [3] The signs and symptoms of CRPS within each of the 4 categories (pain/sensory, vasomotor, sudomotor/edema, and trophic) were analyzed using K-means cluster analysis. The purpose of the analysis was to identify homogenous subgroups within the clinical categories outlined above. The authors did not find a temporal correlation in the patient subgroups with increasing levels of clinical symptoms, arguing against a typical progression of the disease. They did find 3 subgroups of patients with CRPS, but the constellation of symptoms was different from the classic definitions of the stages. They proposed 3 subtypes of CRPS that included subgroups with predominantly vasomotor signs, a subgroup with marked pain and sensory changes, and a florid presentation with advanced signs of trophic changes and motor dysfunction. The main limitation of this study is that it analyzed the frequency of CRPS signs or symptoms but did not quantify the severity of presentation.

QUANTIFYING CRPS SEVERITY

The Impairment Level SumScore (ISS) has been used to measure psychophysical impairment in patients suffering from CRPS, and it has been used to measure outcomes in some CRPS research. [13] The ISS quantifies pain intensity, McGill Pain ratings, goniometric measures of range of motion, temperature asymmetry, and edema, but the measure does not incorporate some aspects of CRPS diagnosis such as painandsensory changes (hyperalgesia or allodynia), vasomotor dysfunction, and sudomotor changes. As such, the measure does not truly reflect CRPS severity.

Harden and colleagues developed a CRPS severity score that includes all aspects of current CRPS diagnostic criteria. [14] The authors presented a score quantified based on 17 clinical signs and symptoms of CRPS (see table 4). The 17 components of the severity score are based on the updated Budapest clinical criteria for CRPS, and each sign or symptom is scored on the presence or absence of the finding. The analysis of the CRPS severity score showed high internal consistency and provides a measure of the spectrum of signs and symptoms associated with the disease and may help describe the magnitude of CRPS pathology. But the severity scale does not include a grading system for the severity of any individual factor and does not replace the need for evaluating the functional impact of the disease.

Table 4. CRPS Severity Score Components [14]

Self-reported symptoms
Allodynia or hyperpathia
Temperature asymmetry
Skin color asymmetry
Sweating asymmetry
Edema of affected side
Trophic changes
Motor changes
Decreased active range of motion
Observed clinical signs
Hyperpathia to pinprick
Allodynia
Temperature asymmetry by palpation
Skin color asymmetry
Sweating asymmetry
Edema of affected side
Trophic changes
Motor changes
Decreased active range of motion

ANCILLARY TESTING FOR CRPS

While CRPS remains a clinical diagnosis based on the signs and symptoms described above, investigators have examined other objective tests to aid in diagnosis of this syndrome. Ancillary tests such as sympathetic blocks, autonomic testing, and radiographic testing have been examined as adjuncts to traditional clinical diagnosis.

It has long been proposed that a significant but transient benefit from a sympatholytic intervention (intravenous regional anesthesia or stellate ganglion/lumbar sympathetic blocks) can confirm the diagnosis of CRPS and some have felt that a positive response is required to establish the diagnosis, but the exact role of sympathetic dysregulation is not well established in CRPS, calling into question the necessity of a positive response to a sympathetic block. A recent Cochrane review examined the results from 12 randomized controlled studies of local anesthetic sympathetic blockade for CRPS, including a total of 386 pooled patients. Many of the included studies had high or unclear risk of bias, but 3 studies included a placebo or sham treatment arm (N = 23). The analysis showed limited benefit associated with local anesthetic sympathetic blockade and reaffirmed an earlier position that questions the utility of sympathetic nerve blocks in the treatment of CRPS and questions the necessity of performing such blocks to establish the diagnosis. [15]

AUTONOMIC TESTING

Autonomic dysfunction has long been thought to be a central pathological mechanism in CRPS, although the true extent of that belief has been questioned. Objective autonomic testing has been proposed as a means to assist in making the clinical diagnosis of CRPS. Chelimsky and colleagues examined the utility of performing 3 autonomic tests in the diagnosis of CRPS (then called RSD), including resting sweat output (RSO), resting skin temperature (RST), and quantitative sudomotor axon reflex test (QSART). [16] The authors reported the results from a retrospective review of 396 patients diagnosed with RSD (prior to the adoption of CRPS diagnostic criteria), examining the relationship between abnormal autonomic test results and either a clinical diagnosis of RSD or a response to sympathetic block. They found the increased RSO predicted a diagnosis of RSD with high sensitivity and specificity, 0.94 and 0.98 respectively, but it is not clear if the sensitivity and specificity would remain high if the newer and more restrictive clinical criteria of CRPS were applied. They also reported that increased RST and QSART correlated very strongly with a positive response to sympathetic blockade, likely due to helping select for patients with a significant sympathetic pain generator.

Schurmann and colleagues developed a bedside test of sympathetic nervous system function that uses laser Doppler flowmetry to measure fingertip blood flow in response to sympathetic arousal stimuli (inspiratory gasp and contralateral cooling. [17] Peripheral sympathetic function was measured using laser Doppler flowmetry in a series of 50 patients who developed CRPS type I of the upper extremity after trauma or operation (utilizing the Orlando diagnostic criteria), and those patients were compared to 50 patients with a distal radius facture without signs of CRPS and 50 healthy age-matched control subjects. [18] The authors reported a significant reduction in the sympathetic vasoconstrictive response to provocative maneuvers in patients with CRPS at 8 weeks post trauma as compared to the non-CRPS control subjects. They did not find that sympathetic dysfunction correlated with any one functional category of CRPS (sensory, vasomotor, sudomotor, or motor changes) and felt that it was an independent marker of CRPS. Unfortunately, we do not know if incorporating a test of sympathetic nervous system function would aid in early recognition of patients with CRPS, and we do not know if utilizing autonomic testing earlier in the course of the disease would improve long-term outcomes.

PLAIN FILM RADIOGRAPHY

Diffuse osteoporosis and patchy demineralization of the periarticular areas, and subperiosteal bone resorption have been observed on plain film imaging, particularly in severe or late stage cases of CRPS. [19] Although these findings are common in patients with CRPS, the radiographic findings are not specific to the disease, as they can be seen in patients due to inactivity osteoporosis or age-related osteoporosis. A prospective study of patients with distal radius fractures found that radiographic findings in patients with CRPS were difficult to distinguish from control patients with trauma who did not develop the disease, with reported sensitivity of 36% and positive predictive value of 58%. The reported specificity and negative predictive values were higher (94% and 86% respectively), indicating that a lack of findings on plain film imaging could be used to question a diagnosis of CRPS. [20]

A study compared plain film radiography to scintigraphy in 37 adult patients with post traumatic CRPS (reported as RSD by the authors), reporting that delayed bone scintigraphy had improved sensitivity and positive predictive value as compared to plain film radiography (97% versus 73% and 95% versus 90% respectively). [21] When the authors performed a subgroup analysis, they found that the advantage of scintigraphy was only significant in patients with stage I disease, and improved accuracy of scintigraphy was lost in patients with stage II disease.

BONE SCINTIGRAPHY

Triple phase bone scintigraphy (TPBS) is performed by injecting a radiotracer (technetium-99m) and measuring its uptake at 3 time points. The first phase is immediately after injection and results in angiographic flow images. The second phase is 1 to 5 minutes after injection and reflects regional blood pool distributions, and the third phase is 1.5 to 4 hours after injection and shows bone turnover and periarticular uptake. It has been reported that CPRS is associated with increased blood flow to the affected extremity and increased periarticular uptake, but similar uptake can be seen in other conditions such as immobilization, denervation, stroke, cellulitis, and vascular or lymphatic obstruction. [22] Initial retrospective analysis of triple phase bone scintigraphy showed high variability in sensitivity and specificity (0.50 to 1.0 and 0.85 to 0.98 respectively) and positive and negative predictive values (67% to 95% and 61% to 100% respectively). [23] The early investigations of CRPS predated the consensus diagnostic criteria, so those data cannot be interpreted in light of current definitions of the disease.

A prospective study of 175 patients who suffered distal radial fractures examined the diagnostic utility of TPBS to aid in early diagnosis of CRPS. [20] This study utilized the more stringent Budapest research criteria (2 or more signs and symptoms in all 4 diagnostic categories) and followed the patient for 4 months following the trauma. The authors reported a low false positive rate in non-affected fracture patients (4% at 8 weeks and 0 at 16 weeks), but they found poor sensitivity in detecting the disease in patients with a clinical diagnosis of CRPS (19% and 14% at 8 and 16 weeks respectively). They also found a significant false-negative rate in patients diagnosed with CRPS, with TPBS only identifying 1 of 17 patients at 8 weeks (7%) and no patients at 16 weeks, possibly due to the fact that the typical scintigraphic pattern does not manifest in the early stages of CRPS type I.

A recent meta-analysis of 21 studies examining the effectiveness of TPBS in diagnosing CRPS found wide ranges in reported sensitivity and specificity (14% to 100% and 60% to 100% respectively), and the authors used analysis of variance to compare TPBS to magnetic resonance imaging (MRI) and plain film radiography. They found that TPBS had improved specificity and negative predicative value over MRI and plain film radiography, but sensitivity and positive predictive values did not show any statistical improvement over the other imaging techniques. [24] This meta-analysis performed by Cappello and colleagues must be interpreted with caution because it included studies published over a time span from 1975 to 2010, over which time period the clinical definition of CRPS underwent major changes. Much of the data included in the analysis was generated before the more restrictive clinical diagnosis of CRPS was agreed upon, so the analysis may overestimate the specificity if one assumes that some of the patients diagnosed with CRPS in the earlier studies would not qualify for diagnoses under the more restrictive research criteria of the Budapest conference.

MAGNETIC RESONANCE IMAGING

MRI has been used to identify pathologic disturbances in affected limbs, including spotted bone-marrow edema of carpal bones, skin edema, gadolinium uptake of the skin, joint effusion, and intra-articular gadolinium uptake. [25, 26] In the prospective study of patients with distal radial fractures, MRI findings suggestive of CRPS were found in 20 of 89 normal fracture patients (22% false positive results at 8 weeks, and only 3 of 10 patients with CRPS had positive MRI findings (70% false negative results). [20] While the sensitivity decreased from week 8 to week 16, the specificity increased from 78% to 98%, indicating that the early findings after trauma or surgery can mimic the MRI findings associated with CRPS. Data pooled from 3 studies examining MRI findings and CRPS diagnosis showed relatively high specificity ($91.00 \pm 13.89\%$) but poor sensitivity ($35.33 \pm 44.88\%$) with poor positive and negative predictive value (64.33 ± 33.71 and $51.76 \pm 28.59\%$ respectively). [24]

SUMMARY

Complex regional pain syndrome remains a clinical diagnosis based on 4 main categories of presenting signs and symptoms. The categories include sensory (pain, hyperpathia, and allodynia), vasomotor (temperature asymmetry and color changes), edema or sudomotor (edema signs, edema symptoms, and sweating asymmetry), and motor (decreased range of motion, motor dysfunction, and trophic changes). These symptom categories have been incorporated into the latest consensus-derived diagnostic criteria, with patients needing to exhibit signs in at least 2 of 4 categories and symptoms in at least 3 of 4 categories (with the exception of research criteria, which requires symptoms in 4 of 4 categories).

Early recognition and treatment of CRPS remains a focus of clinical efforts. While many of the signs and symptoms of CRPS can be difficult to distinguish from acute changes following trauma or surgery, utilizing the clinical diagnostic criteria remains the gold standard. Many patients who develop CRPS do not present to a pain specialist in the early phases of disease, so the challenge appears to be educating primary care providers on the clinical signs and symptoms of the disease.

Because the initial presentation of CRPS can resemble normal recovery after traumatic injury, various ancillary tests have been examined to aid in the diagnosis. Much of the data that exists on ancillary testing used old diagnostic criteria, and it is unknown to what extent those techniques could augment current clinical diagnosis. Of the various imaging techniques, delayed or triple phase bone scintigraphy appears to have the best specificity and negative predictive value over other techniques such as MRI or plain film radiography. No technique appears to have the ideal combination of sensitivity and specificity. Negative results on these tests may help exclude the diagnosis for patients who present with CRPS-NOS, but the tests do not have the ability to improve on the sensitivity of a careful clinical evaluation.

REFERENCES

[1]   Evans JA. Reflex sympathetic dystrophy. Surg Clin North Am. 1946;26:780-90.

[2]   Harden RN, Oaklander AL, Burton AW, Perez RS, Richardson K, Swan M, et al. Complex regional pain syndrome: practical diagnostic and treatment guidelines, 4th edition. *Pain medicine.* 2013;14(2):180-229.

[3]   Merskey H, Bogduk N. Classification of chronic pain: descriptions of chronic pain syndromes and definitions of pain terms,. 2nd ed. Seattle, WA: IASP Press; 1994.

[4]   Stanton-Hicks M, Janig W, Hassenbusch S, Haddox JD, Boas R, Wilson P. Reflex sympathetic dystrophy: changing concepts and taxonomy. *Pain.* 1995;63(1):127-33.

[5]   Harden RN, Bruehl S, Galer BS, Saltz S, Bertram M, Backonja M, et al. Complex regional pain syndrome: are the IASP diagnostic criteria valid and sufficiently comprehensive? *Pain.* 1999;83(2):211-9.

[6]   Bruehl S, Harden RN, Galer BS, Saltz S, Bertram M, Backonja M, et al. External validation of IASP diagnostic criteria for Complex Regional Pain Syndrome and proposed research diagnostic criteria. International Association for the Study of Pain. *Pain.* 1999;81(1-2):147-54.

[7]   Harden RN, Bruehl S, Stanton-Hicks M, Wilson PR. Proposed new diagnostic criteria for complex regional pain syndrome. *Pain medicine* (Malden, Mass). 2007;8(4):326-31.

[8]   Bonica JJ. Causalgia and other reflex sympathetic dystrophies. *Postgrad. Med.* 1973;53(6):143-8.

[9]   Veldman PH, Reynen HM, Arntz IE, Goris RJ. Signs and symptoms of reflex sympathetic dystrophy: prospective study of 829 patients. *Lancet.* 1993;342(8878):1012-6.

[10]   Pak TJ, Martin GM, Magness JL, Kavanaugh GJ. Reflex sympathetic dystrophy. Review of 140 cases. *Minn. Med.* 1970;53(5):507-12.

[11]   van Laere M, Claessens M. The treatment of reflex sympathetic dystrophy syndrome: current concepts. *Acta orthopaedica Belgica.* 1992;58 Suppl 1:259-61.

[12]   Bruehl S, Harden RN, Galer BS, Saltz S, Backonja M, Stanton-Hicks M. Complex regional pain syndrome: are there distinct subtypes and sequential stages of the syndrome? *Pain.* 2002;95(1-2):119-24.

[13]   Perez RS, Oerlemans HM, Zuurmond WW, De Lange JJ. Impairment level SumScore for lower extremity Complex Regional Pain Syndrome type I. *Disability and rehabilitation.* 2003;25(17):984-91.

[14]   Harden RN, Bruehl S, Perez RS, Birklein F, Marinus J, Maihofner C, et al. Development of a severity score for CRPS. *Pain.* 2010;151(3):870-6.

[15]   Stanton TR, Wand BM, Carr DB, Birklein F, Wasner GL, O'Connell NE. Local anaesthetic sympathetic blockade for complex regional pain syndrome. The Cochrane database of systematic reviews. 2013;8: CD004598.

[16]   Chelimsky TC, Low PA, Naessens JM, Wilson PR, Amadio PC, O'Brien PC. Value of autonomic testing in reflex sympathetic dystrophy. *Mayo Clin. Proc.* 1995;70(11):1029-40.

[17]   Schurmann M, Gradl G, Furst H. A standardized bedside test for assessment of peripheral sympathetic nervous function using laser Doppler flowmetry. *Microvasc. Res.* 1996;52(2):157-70.

[18]   Schurmann M, Gradl G, Andress HJ, Furst H, Schildberg FW. Assessment of peripheral sympathetic nervous function for diagnosing early post-traumatic complex regional pain syndrome type I. *Pain.* 1999;80(1-2):149-59.

[19]   Walker SM, Cousins MJ. Complex regional pain syndromes: including "reflex sympathetic dystrophy" and "causalgia." *Anaesth. Intensive Care.* 1997;25(2):113-25.

[20]   Schurmann M, Zaspel J, Lohr P, Wizgall I, Tutic M, Manthey N, et al. Imaging in early posttraumatic complex regional pain syndrome: a comparison of diagnostic methods. *The Clinical journal of pain.* 2007;23(5):449-57.

[21]   Todorovic-Tirnanic M, Obradovic V, Han R, Goldner B, Stankovic D, Sekulic D, et al. Diagnostic approach to reflex sympathetic dystrophy after fracture: radiography or bone scintigraphy? *Eur. J. Nucl. Med.* 1995;22(10):1187-93.

[22]   Intenzo C, Kim S, Millin J, Park C. Scintigraphic patterns of the reflex sympathetic dystrophy syndrome of the lower extremities. *Clin. Nucl. Med.* 1989;14(9):657-61.

[23]   Lee GW, Weeks PM. The role of bone scintigraphy in diagnosing reflex sympathetic dystrophy. *The Journal of hand surgery.* 1995;20(3):458-63.

[24]   Cappello ZJ, Kasdan ML, Louis DS. Meta-analysis of imaging techniques for the diagnosis of complex regional pain syndrome type I. *The Journal of hand surgery.* 2012;37(2):288-96.

[25] Graif M, Schweitzer ME, Marks B, Matteucci T, Mandel S. Synovial effusion in reflex sympathetic dystrophy: an additional sign for diagnosis and staging. *Skeletal Radiol.* 1998;27(5):262-5.

[26] Schweitzer ME, Mandel S, Schwartzman RJ, Knobler RL, Tahmoush AJ. Reflex sympathetic dystrophy revisited: MR imaging findings before and after infusion of contrast material. *Radiology.* 1995;195(1):211-4.

In: Complex Regional Pain Syndrome
Editors: Nader D. Nader and Ognjen Visnjevac

ISBN: 978-1-63483-130-7
© 2015 Nova Science Publishers, Inc.

Chapter 5

MEDICAL AND PHARMACEUTICAL MANAGEMENT

Vandana Sharma, MD*
Anesthesiology and Pain Management,
Upstate University, Syracuse, NY, US

INTRODUCTION

CRPS is a neuropathic pain syndrome that usually starts with a peripheral injury. A subset of CRPS involves sympathetic nervous system activation that explains the resolution of pain and clinical signs with sympathetic blocks. There is recent data to suggest that CRPS is not merely a disease of the peripheral nervous system, but also involves central nervous system. This is supported by the findings of bilateral hypersensitivity to chemical, mechanical and thermal stimuli in patients with unilateral CRPS, suggestive of the role of central sensitization in the evolution of chronic CRPS. [1-3] The role of various inflammatory pathways as evidenced by an increase in inflammatory markers in addition to changes in microcirculation and skeletal systems in the pathogenesis of CRPS is already proven. This explains the requirement of a multimodal treatment approach to the disease, with goal towards functional restoration of the affected patients.

Due to the scarcity of research data, the mechanisms of CRPS pathogenesis and pathophysiology are often not adequately understood and, as a result, the treatment options that are based on the underlying known pathophysiological mechanisms are still evolving. As per a recent Cochrane review looking at the regimens effective for the treatment of CRPS, the authors concluded that due to limited number of published trials, it is difficult to draw conclusions as to which treatment modalities should be offered to the patients. [4]

The management of CRPS is different from other well-explained pain syndromes for multiple other reasons as well. Our current knowledge about CRPS and its evolution indicates that it is distinct from other peripheral neuropathic states as the pathogenesis of CRPS involves multiple neural and biochemical pathways, both central and peripheral. Therefore there is no one single treatment for CRPS that is scientifically proven to cure the pain, motor

---

* Assistant Professor, Anesthesiology and Pain Management, Upstate University, Syracuse, NY sharmavandana912@gmail.com.

disability and psychological issues involved in CRPS. Successful treatment of CRPS involves a cluster of modalities that are geared towards the overall functional restoration of the patient. Stanton-Hicks et al. described an algorithm for treatment of CRPS involving psychological and physical therapy assisted by pharmacologic and interventional management to achieve "return of function." [5]

As per the multimodal paradigm suggested by Stanton Hicks et al., and still widely followed, the treatment of CRPS has three pillars with the common goal geared towards return of function:

1. Physical Therapy
2. Psychological Therapy
3. Medical management that includes medications and interventional management

In the following text, we will describe each of these therapies starting with pharmacologic management.

ANTI-INFLAMMATORY AGENTS

There is ample convincing evidence that inflammatory pathways are contributory in the pathogenesis of both acute and chronic CRPS. Inflammatory markers such as interlukin-6 and TNF-α have been seen to be elevated in the blister fluid of the affected limb in patients with CRPS [6] as are locally elevated neuropeptides such as calcitonin gene related peptide (CGRP) and substance P, suggesting the role of neurogenic inflammation. The inflammatory markers are believed to be responsible for peripheral sensitization and, as a result, the hyperalgesia and allodynia seen in CRPS. The role of anti-inflammatory agents such as corticosteroids, anti-TNF agents, NSAIDS and free radical scavengers has shown promise for symptomatic improvement of CRPS.

NON-STEROIDAL ANTI-INFLAMMATORY DRUGS (NSAIDS)

NSAIDS inhibit cyclooxygenase and therefore reduce the production of prostaglandins. They are worth consideration in the early stages as adjunct to other therapy, more so if there is skeletal structure involvement. [5] NSAIDS are the first line therapy in the WHO ladder when treating any pain condition mostly studied in cancer pain [7]. There is limited data testing their efficacy in the treatment of neuropathic states and CRPS, in particular. In a trial performed by Rico et al., comparing the course of CRPS under two therapeutic regimens in 26 patients, one group was administered 100 international units of calcitonin followed by 500 mg elemental calcium for 10 days a month separated by intervals free of therapy and another group was treated with 500 mg naproxen twice a day without interruption. In all the patients, a bone: soft tissue uptake index was measured by scintigraphic scanning before treatment and after 3 months of therapy. The calcitonin-calcium group showed a highly significant difference before and after therapy compared to the naproxen group, which also showed a statistically significant difference but was negative. [8] The results confirmed the efficacy of calcitonin-calcium in the treatment of CRPS and, at the same time, elucidated their superiority as a treatment compared with naproxen. It is worth considering that this was a small study conducted prior to the inception of IASP criteria for the diagnosis of CRPS. Similarly, in a recently conducted randomized controlled trial, effects of short term two day treatment with intravenous COX-2 inhibitor parecoxib 80 mg per day in patients diagnosed with CRPS did not reveal any significant reduction in blunt pressure hyperalgesia used as a surrogate marker for peripheral sensitization, or other markers of inflammation such as edema or pain. [9]

In addition to systemic use, NSAIDS have also been tried as adjuncts in IV regional anesthetics (bier blocks) in the treatment of CRPS and have shown somewhat better results compared to their systemic administration. In one trial evaluating the antinociceptive effect of regional or systemic parecoxib combined with lidocaine and clonidine IV regional analgesia showed that 5 mg IV regional parecoxib added to clonidine and lidocaine regional block produced significantly better pain scores in patients with CRPS I compared to clonidine and lidocaine regional block alone or systemic 20mg parecoxib over a 3 week period, when the blocks were performed once a week for 3 weeks. [10] Similarly, another trial evaluating ketorolac as an adjunct to lidocaine in intravenous regional block showed short-term improvement in pain scores compared to the local anesthetic alone. [11]

When prescribing NSAIDS, including the coxibs, we should be mindful of the side-effects especially those pertaining to renal injury in patients with existing or at a high risk for renal insufficiency, cardiovascular and thrombotic events, or gastrointestinal complications. [12-14] These effects are even more prominent in the geriatric population and therefore should be prescribed with caution if at all in this age group. [15] If no therapeutic reduction in symptoms is seen after an initial short course of NSAIDS, they should be replaced with other agents for pain control to minimize risk of complications.

CORTICOSTEROIDS

Owing to their anti-inflammatory properties, short course of oral corticosteroids has been shown to induce a positive response in the early stages of CRPS, when inflammation is most prevalent. Corticosteroids likely exert a dual anti-inflammatory effect, not only on the arachidonic acid pathway, but also regulate the neuropeptides such as substance P and CGRP. [16] A meta-analysis of various controlled clinical trials for peripheral neuropathic pain and CRPS performed by Kingery et al. looked at the existing evidence for various pharmacologic agents used in the treatment of CRPS. [17] This meta-analysis evaluated a total of 72 trials, out of which 26 controlled trials were specifically performed in CRPS patients. The authors assessed at least 10 different treatment modalities used for CRPS. The trial data only gave consistent support for corticosteroids as a treatment to provide analgesia, with evidence of long-term effectiveness. Most of the placebo-controlled trials evaluated the efficacy of different IV regional block agents including guanethidine, reserpine, droperidol, atropine, bretylium and ketanserin. The trials showed a limited support in favor of IV regional blocks as well as other treatment modalities such as topical dimethylsulfoxyde (DMSO) and epidural clonidine. The data also showed that intranasal calcitonin and IV Phentolamine were ineffective treatment options for CRPS. Another large meta-analysis looking at various trials concluded that oral corticosteroids are the only anti-inflammatory drugs for which there is positive direct clinical-trial evidence (Level 1) in CRPS. [18].

A high quality randomized control trial compared the effects of short course of oral prednisolone with piroxicam in CRPS I patients after stroke. They noted a significant improvement in the prednisolone group in terms of pain scores as well as activities of daily living. [19]

In addition to a short-term analgesic benefit, treatment with short course of low dose oral prednisone in conjunction with physical therapy has also shown continued long-term improvement in clinical and functional variables such as range of motion and grip strength persisting even up to a year. [20] Most of the studies evaluating the effects of corticosteroids utilized low doses of prednisone starting at 30-60 mg followed by a gradual taper over 2-3 weeks.

Systemic corticosteroids have been associated with several potential harmful effects such as hypertension, diabetes, peripheral edema and cerebrovascular events, but these effects have only been demonstrated in patients on high dose of corticosteroids. So far, no such association has been demonstrated in patients on short course of low dose oral corticosteroids. Da Silva et al. reported safety data of several RCTs of low dose (< 10mg per day oral prednisone equivalents) used in the treatment of rheumatoid arthritis. [21] They reported no excess cardiovascular events, including no incidence of hypertension, sudden death, arrhythmias, which seem to be more frequent in patients on high doses of steroids.

Considering the evidence (Level 1) for analgesic benefit with a short course of corticosteroids and the potential for adverse events with a prolonged course, current evidence implies that there is no role of chronic, long-term glucocorticoid therapy in the treatment of CRPS.

Anti TNF-α Agents

Locally elevated levels of TNF-α have been demonstrated in early stages of CRPS (see Chapter 3: Molecular Pathophysiology and the Role of TNF in the Neuro-Inflammatory Reflex). The rationale behind the early use of anti-TNF-α medications such as anti TNF α antibodies or TNF α antagonists is to limit the activity of inflammatory mediators associated with CRPS and, thereby, act as important tools in improvement of overall disability and progression of this syndrome.

Evidence for anti-TNF-α therapies is still growing. In 2004, Huygen et al. described two case studies of early CRPS, which were successfully treated with a TNF-α antibody (Infliximab). [22] More recently, a double blinded randomized controlled trial evaluating the role of infliximab in early CRPS was performed on 13 patients. The patients were randomly assigned infliximab 5mg/kg or placebo. The data looked at a reduction in the overall clinical signs of inflammation based on total impairment level sum score (ISS score). [23] The authors did not find a reduction in the ISS score, or a difference in the serum cytokine levels between the two groups, despite noting a trend towards lower TNF levels in the interventional group. The study was terminated early due to deterioration in health of the study group and the number of patients recruited did not reach statistical power.

Apart from CRPS, the role of anti-TNF α therapy has been promising in the treatment and symptom management in various other inflammatory disease states such as inflammatory bowel disease, ankylosing spondylitis, rheumatoid arthritis and psoriasis. The possible mechanism of action is related to inhibition of the cytokine cascade, reduction in the growth factor expression and induction of T-cell apoptosis.

In a case series recruiting 10 patients with CRPS I, the effects of TNF α antagonist drug adalimumab were studied. The patients were administered 3 biweekly doses of subcutaneous adalimumab and the pain scores were evaluated after 1 week and at 1, 3 and 6 months. [24]. The authors found that patients responded differently to the treatment and three subgroups of patients were identified on the basis of their response to the treatment: non-responders, responders, and robust responders in whom an improvement in all the parameters of CRPS was seen. The study group was small, thereby limiting analyses and more profound conclusions. Based on the results, the authors concluded that the anti-TNF α drug adalimumab could be used in some patients with CRPS I.

Although treatment of CRPS with anti-TNF α agents seems promising, especially in the early stages of the syndrome when inflammation is thought to be most pronounced, a plethora of good quality studies are needed before these therapies gain widespread acceptance.

FREE RADICAL SCAVENGERS

The role of free radical scavengers in the pathogenesis of CRPS has been studied in a number of trials. [25] With emerging evidence confirming the role of various inflammatory pathways in the pathogenesis of CRPS, there is a new interest in studying the potential prophylactic effect that free radical scavenger like vitamin C could have in alleviating the development of CRPS. [26-28] Vitamin C is an antioxidant, water-soluble vitamin that is inexpensive and without significant side effects at doses studied in the prevention of CRPS (500mg per day).

American Academy of Orthopedic Surgeons (AAOS), in their clinical guidelines published in 2009 supported the daily use of 500 mg per day vitamin C for 50 days after distal radius fractures to prevent CRPS with a "moderate" strength of evidence. [29] Malay et al. tested the validity of this recommendation by performing an extensive database search after which they included 4 studies and one systematic review. They concluded that the associative criteria were adequate to support the use of vitamin C as prophylactic agent in the perioperative period after distal radius fracture surgery. [30] Zollinger et al. prospectively investigated the rate of complications in 40 patients undergoing basal thumb prosthesis placement for trapeziometacarpal arthritis, a surgery known to have a high incidence of complications, with an incidence of CRPS as high as 8-19% in the postoperative period. [28] All of these patients were started on prophylactic vitamin C 500mg daily 1-2 days prior to the surgery and continued for 50 days after surgery. Interestingly, despite undergoing a surgery associated with high incidence of CRPS, none of the patients developed CRPS in this study. These patients were followed routinely for a year and then once a year for several years.

A more recent meta-analysis performed by Shibuya et al. studied 4 controlled trials involving prophylactic ascorbic acid administration during and after extremity surgeries. The authors concluded that prophylactic daily vitamin C administration could be beneficial in extremity surgery or injury to avoid CRPS. [27]

In addition to vitamin C, other free radical scavengers such as topical creams containing Dimethylsulfoxide (DMSO 50%) and N-Acetylcysteine are being used for treatment of cutaneous signs of inflammation and allodynia. They are thought to work by decreasing the concentration of toxic oxygen free radicals involved in early inflammation.

ANTICONVULSANTS

$\alpha2\delta$ ligand calcium channel modulators such as gabapentin and pregabalin have established role in the management of neuropathic states such as diabetic neuropathy and post herpetic neuralgia. A recent Cochrane database review evaluating the role of gabapentin in various neuropathic states including CRPS showed Level 2 evidence that gabapentin in doses of 1200mg per day or more was effective for some patients with painful neuropathic pain conditions. [31] The authors found that most of the trials evaluated the effect of gabapentin in post-herpetic neuralgia, painful diabetic neuropathy and mixed neuropathy. As a result, the evidence for gabapentin use in conditions such as CRPS was limited.

Overall, the efficacy of gabapentinoids such as gabapentin and pregabalin in CRPS treatment has not been proven. There are few trials in the literature that have evaluated the role of gabapentin in CRPS treatment, and none for pregabalin. In an initial case series involving a total of 6 patients with CRPS, the efficacy and mechanism of action of gabapentin in CRPS was evaluated. All six patients showed a significant pain relief and one of the patients demonstrated complete resolution of symptoms after gabapentin therapy. [32] The authors used gabapentin doses starting with 300mg once a day and titrated to 300mg three times a day.

A prospective study by Tan et al. investigating the role of gabapentin in conjunction with an exercise plan in the treatment of early stages of CRPS was published in 2007. [33] A total of 22 patients with early CRPS were started on gabapentin at an initial dose of 600mg per day with a gradual increase to effect. The mean maintenance dose was found to be 1145.46mg per day (range 900-1800mg per day). Gabapentin use resulted in significant improvement in pain intensity, but no improvement in functional parameters was seen. To date, there is only one published randomized controlled crossover trial evaluating the effectiveness of gabapentin in CRPS. [34] 58 patients with CRPS were treated with gabapentin or placebo over two three-week periods and then the groups were crossed over separated by a 2 week drug-free period. Gabapentin was started at 600 mg once a day and titrated to 600 mg three times a day. Gabapentin was found to reduce sensory deficits and mild pain relief with no difference in edema, discoloration or range of motion. No serious side effects of gabapentin were noted in either study.

So far, there is a lack of sufficient evidence supporting the use of gabapentin in CRPS. This was partly due to the lack of specific criteria for the diagnosis of CRPS until the IASP and then Budapest criteria came into view. But lack of published evidence doesn't actually equate to lack of efficacy of these medications. Gabapentin is widely used clinically in the management of neuropathic pain, especially the pain of burning or lancinating quality, which is often a component of CRPS. With a favorable side-effect profile in various patient groups (including the elderly) in addition to the lack of drug interactions, it is an attractive agent in the treatment of CRPS.

Gabapentin binds to the $\alpha2\delta$ subunit of the voltage gated calcium channels and therefore decreases the neuronal peak inward calcium currents. As a result of the diminished calcium transport, the release of neurotransmitters such as glutamate and substance P from the sensory neurons is impaired, which are calcium dependent processes. Based on gabapentin usage in other painful neuropathic states, gabapentin is often used as first line therapy and started at a dose of 300mg daily, gradually titrated to 300mg three times a day over a week to avoid side effects. If the patient is able to tolerate this well, then the dose is further titrated to a maximum dose of 1200mg three times a day over a period of 4-6 weeks. In the elderly, however, the titration is slower in order to minimize the risks of falls associated with sedation and dizziness. Common side effects associated with gabapentin are sedation, dizziness, ataxia, fatigue, blurriness of vision and nystagmus. [35] Serious side effects are rare with gabapentin use.

Pregabalin has not been studied independently in the management of CRPS. To date, there are no controlled trials in the literature evaluating the independent effect of pregabalin in treatment of CRPS. A recent case series showed successful pain control with gabapentin or pregabalin in conjunction with physical therapy in 7 children with CRPS. [36] Pregabalin has been extensively studied in other neuropathic states and has shown promising results as primary agent in alleviating neuropathic pain as well as additive to other anti-neuropathic agents such as duloxetine and tricyclic antidepressants. [37-40] Specifically with resect to CRPS, pregabalin at a daily mean dose of 316 mg added to other agents resulted in 61% improvement in VAS pain scores, significant reduction in anxiety and depression as well as improved sleep.

Furthermore, with a favorable pharmacokinetic profile and twice daily dosing, pregabalin offers benefits over gabapentin. Pregabalin follows a linear absorption with approximately 90% bioavailability irrespective of the dose with more predictable pharmacokinetics. In contrast, gabapentin follows zero order pharmacokinetics and the oral bioavailability is dose dependent with lower bioavailability (60-33%) at the higher doses. [41]

Another anticonvulsant used in the treatment of neuropathic states is carbamazepine, which is indicated for trigeminal neuralgia, postherpetic neuralgia and painful diabetic neuropathy. Both carbamazepine and oxcarbazepine have not been studied in CRPS. Oxcarbazepine is preferred in these neuropathic states over carbamazepine due to similar efficacy and better side effect profile. The absorption of oxcarbamazepine is rapid and complete with linear and dose-proportional pharmacokinetics. [42] While prescribing these drugs, it should be kept in mind that they are both inducers of CYP 3A4 enzymes and therefore could have potential drug interactions, with the inductive effect of carbamazepine being 46% that of oxcarbazepine. [43]

ANTIDEPRESSANTS

The role of tricyclic antidepressants in the management of various neuropathic states at doses lesser than those used for antidepressant effects is well known. [44] TCAs have been traditionally used in the management of CRPS as a part of a multimodal therapy, but no randomized controlled trials have been performed to evaluate their efficacy in CRPS associated neuropathic pain. TCAs act by inhibiting the monoamine reuptake in the presynaptic terminals and inhibiting cholinergic receptors and ion channels, particularly sodium channels (alike to local anesthetics). [45]

TCAs also provide the dual benefit of improving mood, sleep and decreased anxiety in patients with chronic neuropathic pain states. However, they may be associated with anticholinergic side effects. The most common adverse effects of tricyclic antidepressants (constipation, dry mouth, blurred vision, cognitive changes, tachycardia, urinary hesitation) are associated with their anticholinergic activity. Other common adverse effects are cardiac conduction defects, orthostatic hypotension, falls, weight gain, and sedation. In general, the secondary amines (e.g., desipramine, nortriptyline) exhibit fewer anticholinergic and sedative effects than do the tertiary amines (e.g., amitriptyline, imipramine, doxepin). Therefore, it is for these reasons that the secondary amines may be more desirable in the elderly population, which may be of greater consequence from such complications.

A recent Cochrane database review published in January 2015 evaluating the role of nortriptyline in various neuropathic pain states including CRPS. [46] The authors found six studies enrolling a total of 310 participants, with most studies enrolling only a small number of participants. They only found Level 3 evidence that nortriptyline was comparable in efficacy to other medications such as gabapentin, morphine and amitriptyline, but again efficacy could not be proven in individual neuropathic conditions. Overall, they found little evidence in support of nortriptyline for treatment of chronic neuropathic pain.

Other antidepressants include the selective serotonin reuptake inhibitors (SSRI) and serotonin and norepinephrine reuptake inhibitors (SNRI). Per the available literature, SSRIs have not consistently shown a significant analgesic efficacy. On the other hand, SNRIs such as duloxetine and venlafaxine are used in neuropathic pain syndromes, but again they are not backed up by literature validating their use in CRPS. Duloxetine has been more extensively studied in painful diabetic neuropathy and remains a FDA approved agent in addition to pregabalin in the treatment of this debilitating condition. The efficacy of duloxetine in treatment of painful diabetic neuropathy is confirmed at doses between 60-120mg per day. [47] In an observational trial, duloxetine at doses close to 60mg per day was found to be more effective in treating painful diabetic neuropathy compared to pregabalin or gabapentin at doses 173mg per day and 727mg per day, respectively. [48] It should be noted, however, that the doses used for both pregabalin and gabapentin were lower than those used to treat other neuropathic pain states and this apparent underdosing could be contributing to the observed lesser efficacy seen with these gabapentinoids. Based on the promising pain relief provided by SNRIs such as duloxetine in the management of other neuropathic pain states, they are used in CRPS, but there are no available trials supporting such use.

BISPHOSPHONATES

The findings of osteoporosis and increased activity on three-phase radioactive bone scintigraphy in the subacute stages of CRPS led to the assumption that the pathogenesis of CRPS likely also involved an osteoclast-mediated mechanism with increased bone turnover and bone resorption. This has not been well proven yet. Three-phase radioactive bone scintigraphy has traditionally been used to assist the diagnosis of CRPS. Interestingly the pattern of increased activity is also seen in many other conditions and sometimes in a normal limb as well and therefore the utility of bone scans in CRPS diagnosis remains controversial. In one of the studies, the three-phase bone scintigraphic analysis has been found to have 40% sensitivity and 76.6% specificity. [49]

Osteoclast resorbing drugs such as bisphosphonates and calcitonin have been successfully used in the treatment of CRPS, however the mechanism of action still remains unclear. The anti-osteoclastic role of bisphosphonates is well established in diseases such as paget's disease, metastatic bone disease and multiple myeloma. It has been proposed that bisphosphonates not only antagonize bone resorption and resulting osteoporosis, but also exert an anti-inflammatory action thereby suggesting another possible mechanism of action in the treatment of CRPS. [50] They inhibit the local synthesis of inflammatory mediators such as IL-6, TNF- α, PGE2 and thereby exerting their analgesic role. It is postulated that the bisphosphonate effects on microcirculation and inhibition of lactic acid production in the local tissues and bone lead to an inhibition of nociceptors and mechanoreceptors such as Transient Receptor Potential Vanilloid receptors (TRPV-1) and Acid sensing ion channels (ASICs) with a consequent analgesic effect. [51] Another suggested mechanism of analgesic action of bisphosphonates is believed to be mediated by the inhibition of macrophages and subsequently expression of nerve growth factor (NGF) [52] in the bone vicinity. NGF in turn propagates the vicious cycle of inflammation and hyperalgesia by facilitating neuropeptides, nociceptor activation and further differentiation of macrophages and monocytes. [53]

Of all the pharmaco-therapeutic options available for the management of CRPS, bisphosphonates are probably the most thoroughly studied so far with multiple trials assessing the efficacy of various preparations in CRPS. Bisphosphonates are available as both oral and intravenous preparation and have been studied in both forms in CRPS. Oral bisphosphonates have poor oral absorption (< 1%), which is further reduced by food intake. On the other hand, IV preparations have been found to provide rapid relief of bone pain. [50] Bisphosphonates are divided into non-nitrogen containing older compounds such as clodronate and etidronate; and nitrogen containing newer compounds such as palmidronate, alendronate, ibandronate and zoledronate. The last two are highly potent in their antiresorptive capability compared to the older bisphosphonates. The non-nitrogen compounds are thought to exert their action by anti-osteoclastic activity, whereas the nitrogen containing compounds affect the signaling proteins. [50]

A recent meta-analysis looked at all the randomized controlled trials comparing the analgesic agents used in the management of CRPS. [54] Overall, the authors found 16 studies meeting the criteria. Of all the medications used in the pain management of CRPS, bisphosphonates and calcitonin were found to be most effective. Of other treatment options evaluated, vasodilators and NMDA analogues showed better long-term effects as compared to the placebo. There are multiple randomized controlled trials evaluating the role of different bisphosphonates (IV and oral) in the treatment of pain associated with CRPS. [55-60]

A double blind control trial evaluated the effectiveness of oral alendronate in CRPS I at a dose of 40 mg per day for 8 weeks, a dose much higher than used in osteoporosis and comparable to the dose used in the treatment of Paget's disease. [56] They found that all the patients receiving alendronate showed significant improvement in pain, mobility, and pressure tolerance over 12 weeks after therapy. An earlier open label trial evaluated the role of intravenous alendronate in CRPS. Twenty patients were randomized to receive IV alendronate 7.5 mg iv infusion daily for 3 days or IV saline as placebo. Two weeks after initial treatment, both groups were given IV alendronate at same dose for 3 days. [55] The authors noted a significant reduction in pain scores, tenderness and swelling in the treatment group initially and later in all patients receiving alendronate hereby suggesting a rapid and early remission of disease in early CRPS. The patients who received two infusion showed better results than the ones who received only one infusion. Multiple small trials and case reports evaluating the role of IV palmidronate in differing doses have shown consistent promising effects in reducing pain in CRPS. Most of the studies included patients at different stages of CRPS with known bone changes verified by radiographic analysis, except the study by Robinson et al. where radiographic changes were not considered.

Per a recent Cochrane review evaluating various treatment modalities for CRPS, they concluded that there was low quality evidence that bisphosphonates were effective in the management of pain associated with CRPS accompanied by osteopenia. [4] Osteonecrosis of the jaw is a potential complication of long-term high dose bisphosphonate use and has been reported in a case report after use of IV bisphosphonates. [61]

Currently, the literature supporting the use of bisphosphonates in CRPS seems promising, but most of the studies available are small sized heterogenous trials and, thus, evidence is not sufficient for the results to be extrapolated to all patients with CRPS.

Larger randomized controlled trials are needed to support the use of bisphosphonates in CRPS. Nonetheless, it can probably be inferred from the literature that a small subset of bisphosphonate responsive CRPS patients may benefit from an early rather than later institution of this therapy for rapid and effective results.

NMDA ANTAGONISTS

As discussed, CRPS pathogenesis involves several different mechanisms at various levels including inflammation, peripheral sensitization and central sensitization all contributing to the development of state of severe hyperalgesia and disability. Central sensitization explains the progression of CRPS to a generalized peripheral response as evidenced by the hypersensitivity of the contralateral extremity or ipsilateral distant sites to various mechanical, thermal and chemical stimuli. [3] Central sensitization is mediated by the release of neuro-inflammatory peptides such as substance P, CGRP and the excitatory amino acid glutamate acting at the NMDA receptors in the dorsal horn and various supraspinal nuclei. With repetitive nociceptive stimuli and activation of slow conducting C fibers, the NMDA receptors are activated in the dorsal horn by the exaggerated release of neurotransmitters such as glutamate and aspartate leading to prolonged depolarization. [62] The magnesium plug, which otherwise obstructs the NMDA receptor, is released, thereby causing an increase in the calcium influx thus facilitating an intracellular cascade of reactions including phosphorylation of enzymes. The intracellular calcium increase also causes an increase in nitrous oxide synthase (NOS) and proto-oncogene transcription. The NOS generates nitric oxide, which in turn acts as a second messenger via cGMP and further propagates the phosphorylation and activation of ion channels. Nitric oxide also helps with the presynaptic release of glutamate and therefore starts a vicious cycle of further activation of receptors. All these phenomena result in amplification and prolongation of responses thereby contributing to the development of central sensitization. [63]

In vitro studies have shown that NMDA antagonists block this prolonged depolarization in the dorsal horn. [64] As explained, activation of the NMDA receptors is essential to the maintenance of pain, central sensitization and immunomodulation in CRPS and this explains the important role of NMDA receptor inhibition in decreasing the neuropathic pain component of CRPS. [63]

Ketamine is one of the most potent clinically available NMDA inhibitors and has been successfully used in the management of CRPS related pain using various therapeutic regimens. Ketamine was a drug primarily used for induction and maintenance of anesthesia, but has also found safe use in sedation protocols in operating rooms as well as outside the operating room due to the lack of cardio-respiratory depressive effects and opioid sparing analgesic benefit. It has also been used in the treatment of refractory depression and is becoming increasingly popular in pain management. The antidepressant effect of ketamine enhances the efficacy and utility of this medication in the treatment of debilitating neuropathic conditions such as CRPS that are invariably associated with depression. [65] It is widely accepted that analgesia in CRPS should be synchronized with aggressive psychiatric management of associated depression in order to achieve success. [66] Ketamine has been shown to be useful in conjunction with other antidepressants in a study in the treatment of bipolar depression. [67] In this randomized controlled cross over trial, patients with major depression already maintained on lithium or valproate were administered IV Ketamine infusion (0.5 mg/kg) or saline placebo. 71% of patients in the ketamine group showed rapid resolution of depression symptoms within 40 minutes of initiation of therapy that lasted at second evaluation after 3 days compared to 6% in the placebo group. No significant side effects were seen in the treatment group except for dissociative symptoms (at 40 minutes) that resolved spontaneously. This rapid antidepressant effect of ketamine is likely mediated through mammalian target of rapamycin (m-TOR) signaling pathway. [68, 69]

In the realm of CRPS management, ketamine has been used as a prolonged infusion either at sub-anesthetic doses or for inducing ketamine coma in the critical care setting. [70] In a case series including nine patients with refractory CRPS, inpatient ketamine infusion at anesthetic doses was administered for a period of 5 days and was shown to improve pain both at conclusion and 6 weeks after the therapy. The patients developed blood ketamine levels of 250-300mcg/dl for at least 4.5 days and Ramsay sedation score of 4 or 5 (medical coma). In addition, ketamine at anesthetic doses was not shown to produce any neurocognitive deficits at the end of therapy.

Several randomized controlled trials have assessed the efficacy of different prolonged sub-anesthetic ketamine infusion protocols. In one of the studies, ketamine was administered at a dose of 0.35mg/kg/hr over a 4-hour period daily for 10 days on an outpatient basis. [71] The results showed effective pain relief in chronic CRPS patients for 12 weeks. In another similar trial, ketamine was administered to 60 patients with CRPS at different stages at doses ranging 1.2-7.2 mcg/kg/min continuously for 5 days in an inpatient setting. [72] The authors reported significant pain relief over 10 weeks period in patients with CRPS irrespective of the duration of disease before ketamine therapy. In a systematic review by Azari et al. published in 2012, where they assessed the available literature for the efficacy of ketamine in the treatment of CRPS, the authors found three randomized controlled trials, seven observational studies and nine case reports. [71-74] Based on the results of the analysis, the authors concluded that ketamine is effective in the treatment of CRPS but, due to the lack of high quality randomized controlled trials, the current level of evidence is 2B (weak recommendation, moderate-quality evidence). There are no available randomized controlled trials supporting ketamine coma in the management of CRPS.

One of the major side effects of ketamine infusion is the development of psychomimetic effects, which can be effectively treated with pretreatment with midazolam and/or clonidine. Nausea, headache, fatigue and dysphoria are other common side effects that were reported in the above studies.

Liver toxicity is a major concern with ketamine therapy, as evidenced by reports of liver failure in ketamine abusers. There are reports of elevated liver enzymes with therapeutic use of low doses of ketamine, but the effect has been shown to be reversible. [75] None of the above mentioned trials reported liver dysfunction as a complication.

In addition to IV use, topical ketamine has also been studied in CRPS population and has shown promising results. A double-blind randomized cross over trial evaluated the effect of topical compounded 10% ketamine gel in CRPS patients (both types I and II). [73] The duration of pain in their participants ranged from 2 months to 19.2 years. The authors did not find a significant effect on overall pain in either group, but ketamine gel alleviated the allodynia and hyperalgesia components in the affected limb. There are successful case reports supporting the use of topical ketamine in early stages of CRPS, but not in long standing progressive disease. [76, 77]

Considering the current evidence, sub-anesthetic ketamine infusion offers promising treatment modality that may alleviate pain over a period of several weeks to months, but more randomized placebo controlled trials are required before this treatment option can be safely advocated for routine use in CRPS.

Other NMDA antagonists such as memantine, amantadine and magnesium have not been studied extensively in the management of CRPS pain. The overall lack of evidence for their safety and/or efficacy precludes support for their routine use in CRPS patients. [78]

A small (twenty patients) randomized controlled trial testing the efficacy of combination oral therapy of morphine (10-30mg) and memantine (titrated from 5 to 40mg) in CRPS involving upper extremity for a total of 56 days. [79] Functional MRI was performed to evaluate the changes in the cortical regions involved in the pain processing in CRPS patients. The authors found that a combination of morphine with memantine is more effective for pain control compared to morphine alone.

OPIOIDS

Opioids have proven efficacy as second or third line agents in the management of chronic neuropathic pain states and have been associated with functional improvement in these patients. Neuropathic pain is less responsive to the effects of opioids compared to nociceptive pain. Higher opioid doses are found to be more effective at reducing pain intensity and improving functional capacity, but at the cost of increased side effects. [80] Like anti-neuropathic agents, use of opioids in CRPS is derived from the results from the studies evaluating the efficacy of opioids in other neuropathic states such as diabetic neuropathy, peripheral polyneuropathies, and post-herpetic neuralgia. [81, 82] Though it would be assumptive to extrapolate the results from peripheral neuropathic pain states to CRPS, which is not considered an isolated peripheral neuropathic state, opioids are routinely prescribed in clinical practice.

A prospective open label trial studied the effects of transdermal Fentanyl in patients with various neuropathic states including peripheral neuropathy, CRPS and post-amputation pain. They found that there was significant reduction in the intensity of pain in all the three disease conditions, with most functional improvement seen in peripheral neuropathy patients. [83]

Tramadol, with its dual mechanism of action involving serotonin and norepinephrine reuptake inhibition and weak Mu antagonist action, may provide better efficacy compared to other opioids in treating neuropathic pain states, including those in CRPS. Methadone has NMDA antagonist activity in addition to the Mu receptor affinity that explains its use in certain neuropathic states. A newer analgesic, tapentadol, with activity at inhibiting norepinephrine reuptake along with weak opioid agonist action in the absence of active metabolites and slower development of tolerance compared to morphine, makes it a suitable agent in treating neuropathic pain states. It has been found to have utility in the management of neuropathic pain states such as diabetic peripheral neuropathy, but has not been studied in the management of CRPS. [84] The manufacturer recommends a dose of 50mg, 75mg or 100mg every 4-6 hours as needed per the pain intensity with a maximum dose not to exceed 600mg per day. Due to its relatively weak mu-opioid opioid action, tapentadol is considered to have less risk for dependence or abuse than pure mu-agonists. [85]

There is no evidence that any particular opioid may be better than the others in treating CRPS, but the agents must be selected carefully weighing their risks and benefits suited to the patient characteristics. Issues of opioid dependence, tolerance, addiction and opioid induced hyperalgesia are concerning and should be attended to. Opioids can be used in combination with oral anti-neuropathic agents for titration of effect to relieve pain and at the same time, improve functional capacity in patients with CRPS.

CONCLUSION

The current evidence base for pharmacological treatment of CRPS is limited and, thus, therapy is mostly speculative. The expert consensus suggests the use of a multidisciplinary approach utilizing pharmacologic therapy, physical and/or behavioral therapy and interventional therapy towards a common goal of decreasing pain and restoring functionality in CRPS patients so that they can return to baseline function in a pain free manner. The available therapeutic options should be carefully tailored to each phenotypic component of individual CRPS patients to mitigate their disability and distress. A plethora of prospective studies are needed to establish a stronger evidence base for the polypharmacologic treatment options in CRPS.

REFERENCES

[1]   Reinersmann, A., et al., Complex regional pain syndrome: more than a peripheral disease. *Pain Management*, 2013. 3(6): p. 495-502.

[2]   Schlereth, T. and F. Birklein, Complex Generalized Instead of Complex Regional? *Anesthesiology*, 2014. 120(5): p. 1078-1079 10.1097/ALN.0000000000000221.

[3]   Terkelsen, A.J.M.D.P.D., et al., Bilateral Hypersensitivity to Capsaicin, Thermal, and Mechanical Stimuli in Unilateral Complex Regional Pain Syndrome. *Anesthesiology*, 2014. 120(5): p. 1225-1236.

[4]   O'Connell NE, W.B., McAuley J, Marston L, Moseley GL., Interventions for treating pain and disability in adults with complex regional pain syndrome- an overview of systematic reviews. *Cochrane Database of Systematic Reviews*, 2013(4).

[5]   Stanton-Hicks, M.M.B.B.S., et al., Complex Regional Pain Syndromes: Guidelines for Therapy. *Clinical Journal of Pain*, 1998. 14(2): p. 155-166.

[6]   Huygen FJPM, d.B.A., de Bruin MT, Groeneweg JG, Klein J, Zijlstra FJ., Evidence for local inflammation in complex regional pain syndrome type 1. *Mediators Inflamm.*, 2002. 11: p. 47-51.

[7]   Ventafridda, V., et al., WHO guidelines for the use of analgesics in cancer pain. Int J Tissue React, 1985. 7(1): p. 93-6.

[8]   Rico H, M.E., Gomez-Castresana F, etai., Scintigraphic evaluation of reflex sympathetic dystrophy: Comparative study of the course of the disease under two therapeutic regimens. *Clin Rheumatol* 1987. 6: p. 233-237.

[9]   Breuer, A.J., et al., Short-term treatment with parecoxib for complex regional pain syndrome: a randomized, placebo-controlled double-blind trial. *Pain Physician*, 2014. 17(2): p. 127-37.

[10]   Frade, L.C., et al., The antinociceptive effect of local or systemic parecoxib combined with lidocaine/clonidine intravenous regional analgesia for complex regional pain syndrome type I in the arm. *Anesth Analg*, 2005. 101(3): p. 807-11, table of contents.

[11]   Eckmann, M.S.M.D., S.M.D. Ramamurthy, and J.G.P.T. Griffin, Intravenous Regional Ketorolac and Lidocaine in the Treatment of Complex Regional Pain Syndrome of the Lower Extremity: A Randomized, Double-blinded, Crossover Study. *Clinical Journal of Pain* March/April, 2011. 27(3): p. 203-206.

[12]   Trelle, S., et al., *Cardiovascular safety of non-steroidal anti-inflammatory drugs: network meta-analysis*. Vol. 342. 2011.

[13]   Roubille, C., et al., Cardiovascular adverse effects of anti-inflammatory drugs. *Antiinflamm Antiallergy Agents Med Chem*, 2013. 12(1): p. 55-67.

[14]   Fabule, J. and A. Adebajo, Comparative evaluation of cardiovascular outcomes in patients with osteoarthritis and rheumatoid arthritis on recommended doses of nonsteroidal anti-inflammatory drugs. *Ther Adv Musculoskelet Dis*, 2014. 6(4): p. 111-30.

[15]   Page, J.a.H., D., Consumption of NSAIDs and the development of congestive heart failure in elderly patients: an underrecognized public health problem. *Arch Intern Med.*, 2000(160): p. 777–784.

[16]   Smith GD, S.J., Sheward WJ, et al., Effects of adrenalectomy and dexamethasone on neuropeptide content of dorsal root ganglia in the rate. 1991; 564:27–30. *Brain Res* 1991. 564: p. 27-30.

[17]   Kingery, W.S., A critical review of controlled clinical trials for peripheral neuropathic pain and complex regional pain syndromes. *Pain*, 1997. 73(2): p. 123-39.

[18]   Harden, N.R.M.D., et al., Complex Regional Pain Syndrome: Practical Diagnostic and Treatment Guidelines, 4th Edition. *Pain Medicine*, 2013. 14(2): p. 180-229.

[19] Kalita, J., A. Vajpayee, and U.K. Misra, Comparison of prednisolone with piroxicam in complex regional pain syndrome following stroke: a randomized controlled trial. *Qjm*, 2006. 99(2): p. 89-95.

[20] Bianchi, C., et al., Long-term functional outcome measures in corticosteroid-treated complex regional pain syndrome. *Eura Medicophys*, 2006. 42(2): p. 103-11.

[21] Da Silva, J.A.P., et al., Safety of low dose glucocorticoid treatment in rheumatoid arthritis: published evidence and prospective trial data. *Annals of the Rheumatic Diseases*, 2006. 65(3): p. 285-293.

[22] Huygen, F.J.P.M., et al., Successful treatment of CRPS 1 with anti-TNF. *Journal of pain and symptom management*, 2004. 27(2): p. 101-103.

[23] Dirckx, M., et al., Report of a preliminary discontinued double-blind, randomized, placebo-controlled trial of the anti-TNF-alpha chimeric monoclonal antibody infliximab in complex regional pain syndrome. *Pain Pract*, 2013. 13(8): p. 633-40.

[24] Eisenberg, E., et al., Anti tumor necrosis factor - alpha adalimumab for complex regional pain syndrome type 1 (CRPS-I): a case series. *Pain Pract*, 2013. 13(8): p. 649-56.

[25] van der Laan, L. and R.J. Goris, Reflex sympathetic dystrophy. An exaggerated regional inflammatory response? *Hand Clin*, 1997. 13(3): p. 373-85.

[26] Ekrol, I., et al., The influence of vitamin C on the outcome of distal radial fractures: a double-blind, randomized controlled trial. *J Bone Joint Surg Am*, 2014. 96(17): p. 1451-9.

[27] Shibuya, N., et al., Efficacy and safety of high-dose vitamin C on complex regional pain syndrome in extremity trauma and surgery--systematic review and meta-analysis. *J Foot Ankle Surg*, 2013. 52(1): p. 62-6.

[28] Zollinger, P.E., et al., Clinical Results of 40 Consecutive Basal Thumb Prostheses and No CRPS Type I After Vitamin C Prophylaxis. *Open Orthop J*, 2010. 4: p. 62-6.

[29] Lichtman, D.M., et al., Treatment of distal radius fractures. *J Am Acad Orthop Surg*, 2010. 18(3): p. 180-9.

[30] Malay, S. and K.C. Chung, Testing the validity of preventing complex regional pain syndrome with vitamin C after distal radius fracture. *J Hand Surg Am*, 2014. 39(11): p. 2251-7.

[31] Moore, R.A., et al., Gabapentin for chronic neuropathic pain and fibromyalgia in adults. *Cochrane Database Syst Rev*, 2014. 4: p. Cd007938.

[32] Mellick, G.A. and L.B. Mellick, Reflex sympathetic dystrophy treated with gabapentin. *Archives of Physical Medicine and Rehabilitation*, 1997. 78(1): p. 98-105.

[33] Tan, A., et al., The effect of gabapentin in earlier stage of reflex sympathetic dystrophy. *Clinical Rheumatology*, 2007. 26(4): p. 561-565.

[34] van de Vusse, A.C., et al., Randomised controlled trial of gabapentin in Complex Regional Pain Syndrome type 1 [ISRCTN84121379]. *BMC Neurol*, 2004. 4: p. 13.

[35] Rosenquist, R.W.M.D., Gabapentin. *Journal of the American Academy of Orthopaedic Surgeons* May/June, 2002. 10(3): p. 153-156.

[36] Pedemonte Stalla, V., et al., Complex regional pain syndrome type i. *An analysis of 7 cases in children*. Neurologia, 2014.

[37] Moulin, D., et al., Pharmacological management of chronic neuropathic pain: Revised consensus statement from the Canadian Pain Society. *Pain Res Manag*, 2014. 19(6): p. 328-35.

[38] Mishra, A., et al., Pregabalin in Chronic Post-thoracotomy Pain. *J Clin Diagn Res*, 2013. 7(8): p. 1659-61.

[39] Iyer, S. and R.J. Tanenberg, Pharmacologic management of diabetic peripheral neuropathic pain. *Expert Opin Pharmacother*, 2013. 14(13): p. 1765-75.

[40] de la Calle, J.-L., et al., Add-On Treatment with Pregabalin for Patients with Uncontrolled Neuropathic Pain Who Have Been Referred to Pain Clinics. *Clinical Drug Investigation*, 2014. 34(12): p. 833-844.

[41] Bockbrader, H.N., et al., A comparison of the pharmacokinetics and pharmacodynamics of pregabalin and gabapentin. *Clin Pharmacokinet*, 2010. 49(10): p. 661-9.

[42] Lloyd, P., G. Flesch, and W. Dieterle, Clinical pharmacology and pharmacokinetics of oxcarbazepine. *Epilepsia,* 1994. 35 Suppl 3: p. S10-3.

[43] Andreasen, A.H., K. Brosen, and P. Damkier, A comparative pharmacokinetic study in healthy volunteers of the effect of carbamazepine and oxcarbazepine on cyp3a4. *Epilepsia*, 2007. 48(3): p. 490-6.

[44] Billings, J.A., Neuropathic pain. *Journal of Palliative Care*, 1994. 10(4): p. 40-43.

[45] Troels S. Jensen, C.S.M.a.N.B.F., Pharmacology and treatment of neuropathic pains. *Current Opinion in Neurology* 2009. 22: p. 467-474.

[46] Derry, S., et al., Nortriptyline for neuropathic pain in adults. *Cochrane Database Syst Rev*, 2015. 1: p. Cd011209.

[47] Tesfaye, S., et al., Painful diabetic peripheral neuropathy: consensus recommendations on diagnosis, assessment and management. *Diabetes/Metabolism Research and Reviews*, 2011. 27(7): p. 629-638.

[48] Happich, M., et al., Effectiveness of duloxetine compared with pregabalin and gabapentin in diabetic peripheral neuropathic pain: results from a German observational study. *Clin J Pain*, 2014. 30(10): p. 875-85.

[49] Moon, J.Y., et al., Analysis of patterns of three-phase bone scintigraphy for patients with complex regional pain syndrome diagnosed using the proposed research criteria (the 'Budapest Criteria'). *British journal of anaesthesia*, 2012: p. aer500.

[50] Jennifer Yanow, M.P., Letha Pillai, Complex Regional Pain Syndrome (CRPS/RSD) and Neuropathic Pain: Role of Intravenous Bisphosphonates as Analgesics *The scientific world journal*, 2008. 8: p. 229-236.

[51] Iannitti, T.P., et al., Bisphosphonates: Focus on Inflammation and Bone Loss. *American Journal of Therapeutics*, 2012. 19(3): p. 228-246.

[52] Radak, Z., et al., Oxygen consumption and usage during physical exercise: the balance between oxidative stress and ROS-dependent adaptive signaling. Antioxid Redox Signal, 2013. 18(10): p. 1208-1246.

[53] M. Varenna, S.A., L Sinigaglia, Bisphosphonates in Complex Regional Pain syndrome type I: how do they work? *Clin Exp Rheumatol*, 2014. 32: p. 451-454.

[54] Wertli, M.M., et al., Rational pain management in complex regional pain syndrome 1 (CRPS 1)--a network meta-analysis. *Pain Med*, 2014. 15(9): p. 1575-89.

[55] Adami, S., et al., Bisphosphonate therapy of reflex sympathetic dystrophy syndrome. *Annals of the Rheumatic Diseases*, 1997. 56(3): p. 201-204.

[56] Manicourt, D.-H., et al., Role of alendronate in therapy for posttraumatic complex regional pain syndrome type I of the lower extremity. *Arthritis & Rheumatism*, 2004. 50(11): p. 3690-3697.

[57] Robinson, J.N., J. Sandom, and P.T. Chapman, Efficacy of Pamidronate in Complex Regional Pain Syndrome Type I. *Pain Medicine*, 2004. 5(3): p. 276-280.

[58] Varenna, M., et al., Treatment of complex regional pain syndrome type I with neridronate: a randomized, double-blind, placebo-controlled study. *Rheumatology*, 2013. 52(3): p. 534-542.

[59] Littlejohn, G., THERAPY: Bisphosphonates for early complex regional pain syndrome. *Nature Reviews Rheumatology*, 2013. 9(4): p. 199-200.

[60] Breuer, B.P.M.P.H., et al., An Open-label Pilot Trial of Ibandronate for Complex Regional Pain Syndrome. *Clinical Journal of Pain*, 2008. 24(8): p. 685-689.

[61] Thomas Bittner, M., DMD, Natascha Lorbeer, DMD, Tobias Reuther, MD, DMD, PhD, Hartmut Böhm, MD, DMD, Alexander C. Kübler, Prof MD, DMD, PhD, and and M. Urs D.A. Müller-Richter, DMD, PhD, FEBOMFS, Hemimandibulectomy after bisphosphonate treatment for complex regional pain syndrome: A case report and review on the prevention and treatment of bisphosphonate-related osteonecrosis of the jaw. *Oral And Maxillofacial Surgery*, 2012. 113(1): p. 41-47.

[62] Hewitt, D.J., The use of NMDA-receptor antagonists in the treatment of chronic pain. *Clin J Pain*, 2000. 16(2 Suppl): p. S73-9.

[63] Oliveira, C.M.B.d., et al., Cetamina e analgesia preemptiva. *Revista Brasileira de Anestesiologia*, 2004. 54: p. 739-752.

[64] Woolf CJ, T.S., The induction and maintenance of central sensitization is dependent on N-methyl-D-aspartic acid receptor activation; implications for the treatment of post-injury pain hypersensitivity states. *Pain*, 1991. 44: p. 293-299.

[65] Rommel, O., et al., [Psychological abnormalities in patients with complex regional pain syndrome (CRPS)]. *Schmerz*, 2005. 19(4): p. 272-84.

[66] Tajerian, M., et al., Brain neuroplastic changes accompany anxiety and memory deficits in a model of complex regional pain syndrome. *Anesthesiology*, 2014. 121(4): p. 852-65.

[67] Diazgranados, N., et al., A randomized add-on trial of an N-methyl-D-aspartate antagonist in treatment-resistant bipolar depression. *Arch Gen Psychiatry*, 2010. 67(8): p. 793-802.

[68] Li, N., et al., mTOR-dependent synapse formation underlies the rapid antidepressant effects of NMDA antagonists. *Science*, 2010. 329(5994): p. 959-64.

[69] Paul, R.K., et al., (R,S)-Ketamine metabolites (R,S)-norketamine and (2S,6S)-hydroxynorketamine increase the mammalian target of rapamycin function. *Anesthesiology*, 2014. 121(1): p. 149-59.

[70] Koffler, S.P., et al., The neurocognitive effects of 5 day anesthetic ketamine for the treatment of refractory complex regional pain syndrome. *Arch Clin Neuropsychol*, 2007. 22(6): p. 719-29.

[71] Schwartzman, R.J., et al., Outpatient intravenous ketamine for the treatment of complex regional pain syndrome: a double-blind placebo controlled study. *Pain*, 2009. 147(1-3): p. 107-15.

[72] Sigtermans, M.J., et al., Ketamine produces effective and long-term pain relief in patients with Complex Regional Pain Syndrome Type 1. *PAIN*, 2009. 145(3): p. 304-311.

[73] Finch, P.M., L. Knudsen, and P.D. Drummond, Reduction of allodynia in patients with complex regional pain syndrome: A double-blind placebo-controlled trial of topical ketamine. *PAIN*, 2009. 146(1–2): p. 18-25.

[74] Azari, P., et al., *Efficacy and Safety of Ketamine in Patients with Complex Regional Pain Syndrome: A Systematic Review*. CNS Drugs, 2012. 26(3): p. 215-228.

[75] Noppers, I.M., et al., Drug-induced liver injury following a repeated course of ketamine treatment for chronic pain in CRPS type 1 patients: a report of 3 cases. *Pain*, 2011. 152(9): p. 2173-8.

[76] Takahiro Ushida, M.D., Toshikazu Tani, M.D., Tetsuya Kanbara, M.D., Vadim S. Zinchuk, M.D., Motohiro Kawasaki, M.D., and Hiroshi Yamamoto, M.D., Analgesic Effects of Ketamine Ointment in Patients With Complex Regional Pain Syndrome Type 1. *Regional Anesthesia and Pain management*, 2002. 27(5): p. 524-528.

[77] Sawynok, J.P., *Topical and Peripheral Ketamine as an Analgesic. Anesthesia & Analgesia*, 2014. 119(1): p. 170-178.

[78] Fischer, S.G.L.M.D., et al., Intravenous Magnesium for Chronic Complex Regional Pain Syndrome Type 1 (CRPS-1). *Pain Medicine*, 2013. 14(9): p. 1388-1399.

[79] Gustin, S.M., et al., NMDA-receptor antagonist and morphine decrease CRPS-pain and cerebral pain representation. *PAIN*, 2010. 151(1): p. 69-76.

[80] Rowbotham, M.C., et al., Oral Opioid Therapy for Chronic Peripheral and Central Neuropathic Pain. *New England Journal of Medicine*, 2003. 348(13): p. 1223-1232.

[81] Watson, C.P.N.M.D.F. and N.P. Babul, Efficacy of oxycodone in neuropathic pain: A randomized trial in postherpetic neuralgia. *Neurology*, 1998. 50(6): p. 1837-1841.

[82] Gimbel, J.S.M.D., P.M.D.P. Richards, and R.K.M.D. Portenoy, Controlled-release oxycodone for pain in diabetic neuropathy: A randomized controlled trial. *Neurology*, 2003. 60(6): p. 927-934.

[83] Agarwal, S., et al., Transdermal Fentanyl Reduces Pain and Improves Functional Activity in Neuropathic Pain States. *Pain Medicine*, 2007. 8(7): p. 554-562.

[84] Vadivelu, N., et al., Tapentadol extended release in the management of peripheral diabetic neuropathic pain. *Ther Clin Risk Manag*, 2015. 11: p. 95-105.

[85] Cepeda, M.S., et al., Comparison of the risks of opioid abuse or dependence between tapentadol and oxycodone: results from a cohort study. *J Pain*, 2013. 14(10): p. 1227-41.

In: Complex Regional Pain Syndrome
Editors: Nader D. Nader and Ognjen Visnjevac

ISBN: 978-1-63483-130-7
© 2015 Nova Science Publishers, Inc.

Chapter 6

INTERVENTIONAL TECHNIQUES AND NEUROMODULATION

Poupak Rahimzadeh[*], MD, FIPP*
and Seyed Hamid Reza Faiz[†], MD
Iran University of Medical Sciences, Tehran, Iran

INTRODUCTION

To date, there are no ubiquitously accepted evidence-based curative treatments for CRPS. [1, 2] This syndrome is a pathophysiologically multifaceted disease and should be managed with a multimodal approach. Part of the difficulty in establishing curative or evidence-based therapies in CRPS is likely due to a lack of adherence to the IASP diagnostic criteria for CRPS among clinicians and researchers. [3, 4] Some studies document a greater than 95% spontaneous remission in CRPS I, while other researches document persistent, disabling and debilitating symptoms despite aggressive treatment. [5] Currently, there is no international standard algorithm for the care and treatment of CRPS. In part, this is due to a lack of robust evidence regarding efficacy, costs, and the long-term implications to patients from varying degrees of procedural invasiveness. [6, 7]

Multiple modalities have been proposed for CRPS management but, despite a multitude of treatment options, a subgroup of CRPS patients remains refractory to all psychological, pharmaceutical, and physical therapies. As the consequence of such treatment failures in these patients, the disease may spread extraterritorially, which results in severe incapacitation. Uncontrolled allodynia and hyperalgesia can induce extreme morbidity, negatively impacting quality of life, and the failure of non-interventional therapeutic modalities leads physicians to more invasive strategies.

Interventional techniques are defined as either ''invasive procedures involving delivery of drugs into targeted areas,'' or ''ablation or modulation of targeted nerves'' for the treatment

---

[*] Associate Professor of Anesthesiology and Pain Medicine, Iran University of Medical Sciences, Tehran, Iran poupak_rah@hotmail.com.
[†] Associate Professor of Anesthesiology and Pain Medicine, Iran University of Medical Sciences, Tehran, Iran.

of pain. [8] These are often considered for patients with refractory CRPS, even though their effectiveness is often still debatable.

The role of intervention in the management of CRPS continues to evolve. [9] This chapter will discuss the options, techniques, and evidence for the following interventional modalities: sympathetic blockade and sympathectomy, intravenous regional blockade, peripheral and neuraxial blockade, spinal cord and peripheral nerve stimulation, intrathecal pump implantation, deep brain and motor cortex stimualtion, transcutaneous direct current stimulation, and dorsal root entry zone lesioning.

CHRONOLOGY

Past Interventional Modalities

Although a more thorough description of historical therapies for CRPS is provided in Chapter 1 (History and Epidemiology), this section will highlight some interventional techniques. Stellate ganglion blocks, sympathectomies, and intravenous regional blocks were among the first interventional approaches to the treatment of CRPS. [10] Various drug regimens, including local anesthetics, non-steroidal anti-inflammatory medications, sympathetic blocking agents and corticosteroids have also been trialed in conjunction with these procedures. Unfortunately, outcomes evidence does not support the effectiveness of these techniques and their use has diminished over time in lieu of newer modalities. Neurolytic procedures involving chemical neurolytic agents have also been performed in past years, but multiple adverse effects have led them to fall out of favor. [11]

Present Interventional Modalities

This chapter will discuss current interventional modalities in detail. Despite the implications of the evidence described herein, pain practitioners must recognize that regional and international guidelines vary, both in algorithmic approach to treating CRPS and in respect to considerations for cost-efficacy, procedural invasiveness, and insurance coverage. With respect to regional, governmental, or private health insurance policies, specifically, it is important to note that many such policies do not cover the costs of more complex interventions, despite growing evidence of improved efficacy with these therapeutic modalities.

Future Interventional Modalities

Potential interventional modalities and modalities currently in active research will be discussed in greater detail in Chapter 9 (Future Research and Advances in Technology), but some concepts and highlights are presented herein. Improved technology and a better understanding of the goals of stimulation have led to a new ability to stimulate the brain, spinal cord, or peripheral nervous system and increase the effectiveness of these therapies for CRPS pain.

New pathophysiological understanding about the targets of neuromodulation is leading a new wave of treatment of patients with novel neurostimulation approaches. This has led to a new rise in enthusiasm for spinal cord and supraspinal modulation for CRPS pain. By construction of new percutaneous paddle leads and other new technologies in neuromodulation, a number of potential candidates for spinal cord and central stimulation have been introduced. [12, 13]

Transcranial stimulatory techniques and functional neuroimaging tools are being developed and optimized, while multimodal therapeutic algorithms involving interventional techniques are already under investigation. Radiofrequency ablation is gaining a foothold in the treatment of CRPS, with an improved risk-benefit profile over traditional chemical neurolysis.

PERCUTANEOUS SYMPATHETIC BLOCKADE

The Role of the Sympathetic Nervous System in CRPS

Although discussed in greater detail in Chapter 2 (Pathophysiology and Related Mechanisms), the role of the sympathetic nervous system in CRPS pathophysiology can be broadly implicated to contribute to vascular and circulatory pathology, trophic changes, and sympathetically maintained pain (SMP). [11, 14, 15] Consequently, attempts at sympathetic blockade (SB) were logically considered for management of CRPS. [16, 17] In fact, SMP may be defined as pain relieved by SB. In this regard, SB has been performed for both diagnostic and therapeutic purposes and, when performed in a timely manner following onset of CRPS, SB may result in both pain relief and functional rehabilitation – the primary goals of CRPS therapy. [18]

Furthermore, recognizing that CRPS symptomatology is diverse and variable, a broad range of target sites and interventional techniques have been identified for inducing SB. SB can be performed via blocking sympathetic ganglia or via intravenous regional blockade (IVRB), which is done by injecting intravenous sympathetic blocking agents regionally into a limb. [19]

Sympathetic Ganglion Block

A 2002 systematic review reported that SB with a local anesthetic in patients with CRPS resulted in pain relief in approximately one third of patients. [20] Recent guidelines for CRPS management limit the role of SB, however, and they do not recommend this modality as a first-line therapy, considering it to be appropriate for select cases only, if patients are refractory to conservative treatment with pharmacologic therapy and physical rehabilitation. [1, 21] Success in response to sympathetic blockade has led some clinicians to perform destructive procedures targeting the sympathetic nervous system in an effort to produce a permanent interruption in the transmission of SMP. Multiple techniques have been employed to accomplish this goal, including chemical neurolysis, which involves the destruction of sympathetic neural ganglia and pathways through the injection of lytic agents such as phenol or alcohol, radiofrequency ablation (RFA), or surgical resection (sympathectomy). The evidence supporting the effectiveness of sympathetic chemical neurolysis is weak, favoring the RFA technique when SB is to be performed. [9, 18, 22]

Prognostication of Sympathetic Blockade

When a single procedure of SB of ganglia with a local anesthetic (diagnostic block) proves successful, typically defined by at least 50% pain reduction for the duration of action of the local anesthetic, repeated or more definitive SB (RFA, sympathectomy) may be indicated. [9, 21] Expectantly, some studies observed that the existence of sympathetically mediated signs such as temperature and color asymmetry between affected and unaffected limbs have been found to be predictive of positive response to sympathetic blockade. [9, 23] Mechanical allodynia, on the other hand, appears to be a poor predictor of success with conflicting evidence between studies. [24, 25] It is worth noting that a pain relief response in the absence of an adequate skin temperature change has been documented, leading researchers to hypothesize that the possible explanations for this phenomenon may involve spillover of the local anesthetic to somatic nerves, systemic action of absorbed local anesthetics, or even placebo response. [25]

Sympathetic Block of the Upper Extremity: Stellate Ganglion Block (SGB)

For treatment of upper extremity CRPS, stellate ganglion block (SGB) is commonly performed. This cervicothoracic ganglion is formed by joining of the last cervical and first thoracic ganglia, sending sympathetic afferents to the cervical trunks of the brachial plexus, and is typically located anterolaterally to the head of the first rib, just lateral to the longus colli muscle, and posteromedial to the vertebral artery. [26] This ganglion receives all preganglionic nerves that are traveling to more superior ganglia, covers sympathetic innervation to the upper extremities and head and neck region extending as low as C7-T1 nerve roots. Some sympathetic fibers arise from T2 and T3 levels, which do not pass through stellate ganglion and are named, "Kuntz's nerves." If Kuntz's nerves act as mediators for a patient's persistent pain in an upper limb, SGB may fail to alleviate symptoms.

TECHNIQUE

In order to make the procedure technically more reliable, supportive technology such as fluoroscopy, computed tomography (CT) and ultrasound have been investigated and often shown to be and reliable for localization of the stellate ganglion. [27-29] SGB may be performed by injection of local anesthetics alone or by RFA for ganglion denervation.

The patient is placed in a supine position with the head slightly extended. Immediate access to resuscitative drugs, suction, oxygen, and a defibrillator is needed as a precautionary measure. These precautionary measures are advised for all interventional procedures. Temperature monitors are placed on both hands in addition to routine hemodynamic monitors. Temperature changes are considered a surrogate for evaluating efficacy of SB. The C6-C7 level is identified with fluoroscopy in the anteroposterior position. After local disinfection, the skin is anesthetized with local anesthetic, followed by insertion of a 5-6 cm length needle at the junction of the transverse process and vertebral body of C6 or C7. After contact with the bone, the needle should be withdrawn to rest anteriorly to the precervical fascia. For confirming needle position anterior to the intervertebral foramen, an oblique fluoroscopy view can be used. Once the needle is in the correct position a small amount of contrast dye is injected in order to confirm needle tip placement and avoid intravascular injection. The contrast dye must spread craniocaudally in anteroposterior fluoroscopic view. (Figure 6.1)

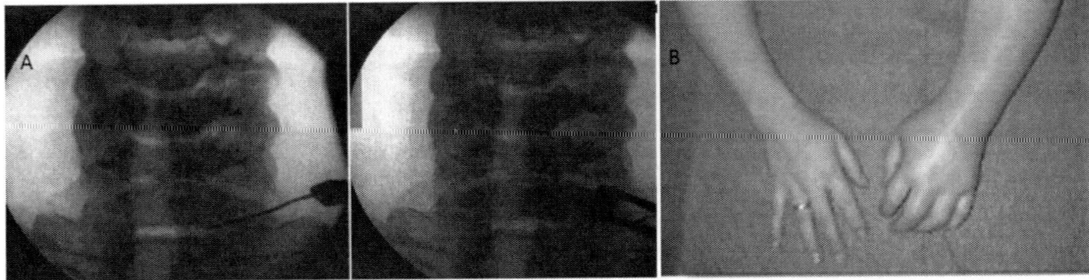

Figure 6.1. SGB in a CRPS patient. Anteroposterior fluoroscopic views of a needle while touching the left transverse process junction at the C7 vertebral body (A). Supine view of left (CRPS-afflicted) and right upper extremities (B).

For a diagnostic block, local anesthetic with or without corticosteroid is injected. For an ablative block using RFA, a 50-60 mm length, active tip RF needle may be used. After electrical stimulation typically at 50 Hz (sensory stimulation) and 2 Hz (motor stimulation) varying from 1 to 2 mA, local anesthetic is injected, after which a thermal lesion is carried out at a clinician-set temperature for a set period of time. Pulsed radiofrequency is can also be performed and RFA cycles can be repeated.

EVIDENCE

A Cochrane review by Cepeda et al. revealed the scarcity of published evidence to support the use of local anesthetic SB as the first-line therapy for CRPS. They attempted to assess the effectiveness of SB with local anesthetics in patients with CRPS to achieve greater than 50% pain relief immediately post-procedure and 48 hours later. This Cochrane review found only two small randomized double-blind studies that evaluated a total of 23 patients, with findings showing a relative risk (RR) of 1.17 [95% confidence interval (CI) 0.80–1.72] for attaining greater than 50% short term (30 min to 2 hour) reduction in pain immediately following SB. Despite intent for assessing effectiveness of SB pain relief at 48 hours, methodological differences between the two studies did not allow for such comparisons to be made. [16]

In one study by Yucel et al, they performed three SGB at weekly intervals in 22 patients with CRPS type I in one hand. The patients were divided into two groups depending on the time between symptom onset and treatment initiation. Pain intensity using a visual analog scale (VAS) and range of motion (ROM) for the wrist joint were assessed at baseline and at 2 weeks after treatment. They concluded that SGB successfully decreased VAS and increased ROM of wrist joints in patients with CRPS type I. Further, they found that duration between symptom onset and therapy initiation was a major factor predicting SB success. [30] Similarly, in a case series of 25 subjects who had 3 SGB at weekly intervals for upper-extremity CRPS reported that 40% of patients had complete pain relief, 36% had partial pain relief, and 24% had no pain relief over a 6-month observation period. Despite limitations in study design, these findings were promising regarding the effectiveness of SGB. [31]

In a pediatric case report, a boy who presented with severe resting pain over the right hand for last 6 months was scheduled for RFA of his SG. The research team performed SG RFA for him after a successful diagnostic block. Four lesions were made (each at 80°C for 60s) at the C7 level after confirming needle placement. Self-reported significant pain relief associated with both subjective and objective improvement in function was observed almost immediately after the procedure. The patient was followed-up for a period of 12 months and retained complete pain relief with normal function. [32]

When considering CT or ultrasound as alternatives to fluoroscopy, logistical considerations and evidence should be taken into account. Unfortunately, evidence is scarce. While CT induces a greater amount of radiation, this technique may improve SGB efficacy.

One study using CT guidance for SGB showed more than 50% pain relief for 2 years in 67% of the patients and concluded that this technique helps clinicians to obtain more precise placement of the needle for RFA. [33] On the other hand, a study by Yoo et al involving 42 patients also reported that US-guided SGB relieved pain in patients with CRPS following stroke. They reported a significant reduction in VAS values for all patients following the block. [34]

Sympathetic Block of the Upper Extremity: Thoracic Sympathetic Block (TSB)

Thoracic sympathetic block (TSB) is an alternative for SGB in management of upper extremity CRPS. Thoracic sympathetic ganglion cell bodies that supply the upper limbs are located parallel with the spinal cord from the T2 to T8 levels. Each ganglion has connection with the corresponding spinal nerve by white and gray rami communicans. The T2 and T3 sympathetic block is considered for patients who have CRPS with SMP in the upper extremity, thorax, or chest wall. It can be done either unilaterally or bilaterally. While considering anatomical variations in the sympathetic coverage of the upper limb, one must recognize the variable contribution of the Kuntz's nerves to SMP, which may limit the efficacy of thoracic sympathetic block in some cases. At the present time, TSB is generally utilized as an alternative choice to SGB in cases for which SGB fails to provide the desired clinical response.

TECHNIQUE

For performing this procedure, the patient must be positioned in prone position. Under C-arm guidance prior to the procedure, C7-to-T3 vertebra must be visualized using an anteroposterior view. Temperature monitors on both hands are needed in addition to other routine hemodynamic monitors to detect and measure the rise in temperature after the procedure. This rise in temperature indicates a successful block. [35] Appropriate pillows should be placed beneath the abdomen and chest.

The C-arm is directed to identify the T2-T3 vertebral body in an anteroposterior and ipsilateral oblique view. By rotating the C-arm in the cephalocaudal direction, the intervertebral space will open wider, which is better for visualization of the planned needle track. The needle is then introduced and advanced in close contact with the lateral edge of the T2-T3 vertebral body. A lateral view confirms needle placement, which should finally remain no deeper than the anterior aspect of the posterior half of T2 body while touching the lateral edge of the T2-T3 vertebral body. This close contact is important because it helps prevent perforation of the pleura. Radiocontrast dye is injected at this point to confirm needle placement and craniocaudal spread can be checked using the lateral view (Figure 6.2).

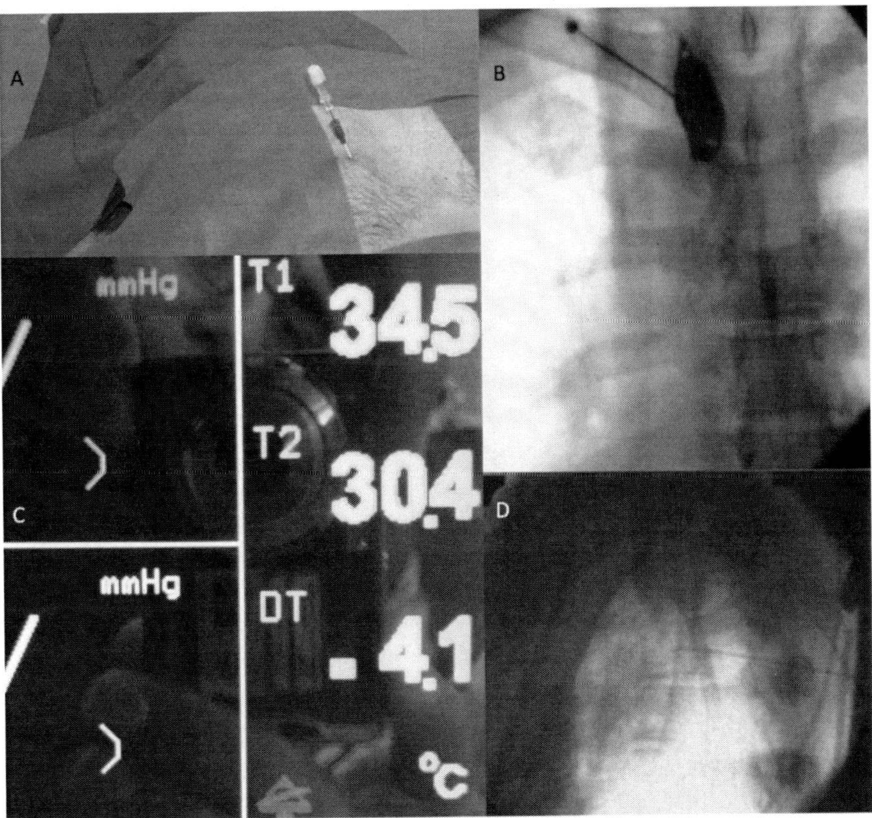

Figure 6.2. TSB in a CRPS patient with involvement of the left hand (A). Oblique (B) and lateral (C) view of the procedure after dye injection while shows the craniocaudal spreading of radiopaque dye in lateral aspect of body. Temperature difference of both hands after injecting local anesthetics (D).

For performing a diagnostic block, local anesthetic and/or steroid solutions are injected. Success is evaluated both by patients' subjective reports of changes in symptomatology and by objective measurements of temperature change in the affected extremity. If the block was beneficial, the patient may then be scheduled for RFA of the T2 and T3 sympathetic ganglia. [36, 37] In recent decades, there have been marked advancements in RFA applied via either conventional or pulsed modes, and long-lasting positive effects have been observed.

EVIDENCE

Several studies have evaluated the effect of TSB in CRPS management. In one study, 4 patients with CRPS due to brachial plexus injuries underwent T2 and T3 RF sympathectomy. The RF lesioning settings were set for 60 seconds at 80°C. The RF procedure was performed at both the T2 and T3 levels in this manner. The patients were assessed before the procedure and followed for 9 months after TSB. An acceptable 6-month pain relief was achieved in all 4 patients, defined in this study as a pain score less than 50% than that of initial score. All 4 patients were able to decrease their oral analgesic requirements. [38]

In another study, 36 patients with CRPS of upper limbs were randomized to undergo TSB procedures or a control procedure in addition to standardized physical therapy and pharmaceutical management for each group. At 1-month follow-up, the mean pain intensity was not significantly different after TSB. At 12 months, however, the mean pain scores were significantly lower in the TSB patients compared to controls. Quality of life was also improved in the TSB group. [39]

Sympathetic Block of the Lower Extremity: Lumbar Sympathetic Block (LSB)

Lumbar preganglionic sympathetic fibers arise from the dorsolateral aspect of the spinal cord and then synapse with the lumbar sympathetic ganglia located on the anterolateral aspect of the L2-4 vertebral bodies. The majority of sympathetic fibers pass through the L2 and L3 sympathetic ganglia. Lumbar sympathetic block (LSB) is frequently performed at the L2 to L4 lumbar levels for CRPS of the lower extremity. These ganglia are located at the anterolateral side of the lumbar vertebrae. Fluoroscopic, CT, and ultrasound-guided techniques have been described and their successful implementation has been documented. [40-42]

TECHNIQUE

The patient is placed in the prone position. Appropriate pillows should be placed beneath the abdomen and chest. Temperature monitors are needed on both legs, in addition to routine hemodynamic monitors, to measure the affected extremity's rise in temperature after procedure.

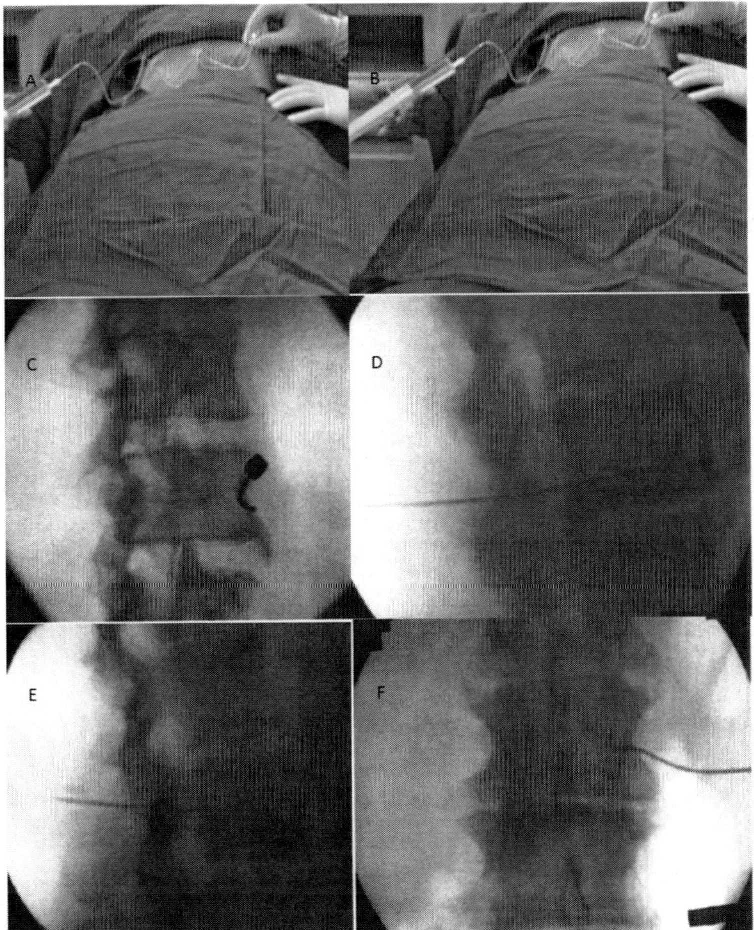

Figure 6.3. LSB in a patient with right lower extremity CRPS (A + B). oblique (C), lateral (D) and AP (E) view of the procedure after dye injection. F shows the craniocaudal spreading of radiopaque dye in anterolateral aspect of the vertebral body.

For identifying L2-L4 levels, the C-arm is usually used which is rotated in the craniocaudal direction until the vertebral end plates are squared off. Then the C-arm is positioned ipsilaterally until the distal end of the transverse process aligns with the lateral edge of the corresponding vertebral body. Often a 150mm length needle is inserted and guided using a tunnel view until the anterolateral border of the vertebral body in lateral view. After confirmation of the correct needle positioning by injecting the radiocontrast dye, local anesthetic with or without corticosteroid is injected (Figure 6.3). This may also be done under CT or ultrasound guidance.

In order to perform RFA, a 150 mm needle with 5-10 mm active tip is appropriate. After proper placement, electrical sensory and motor stimulation at allowable standard frequency (50 to 2 Hz) and current flow (1 to 2 mA) is induced. In order to confirm that there is no contact with a spinal segmental nerve root before the ablation can be started, the clinician must communicate with the patient in real time and the patient should only feel a vague sensation in the abdomen without any motor stimulation. For conventional ablative RF, local anesthetic is injected at each level after which a thermal lesion is carried out for a time and temperature selected by the clinician. The cycle can be repeated if necessary. Pulsed RF can also be used and cooled RF is emerging as a potential therapeutic option as well.

EVIDENCE

Evidence for LSB is sparse with a scarcity of large, high quality, randomized prospective trials. One study reported the effectiveness of different neurolytic regimens (RFA versus phenol). 20 participants with lower limb CRPS I were randomized to receive either percutaneous RF lumbar sympathectomy or lumbar sympathetic neurolysis with phenol 7%. After getting sensory and motor RF stimulation to identify proximity to target sympathetic ganglia, a subsequent RF lesioning has done for 90 seconds at a temperature of 80°C. Then they advanced the needle anteriorly by 5 mm, after repeating sensory-motor stimulation at new needle tip position a second lesion was made again. The above-mentioned procedure has been performed at L2-L4 levels. In patients randomized to receive phenol, the radiofrequency needle was guided just like the first group and the needle position has confirmed similar to the radiofrequency group, with the same sensory and motor stimulation at 50 and 2 Hz to maintain patient blinding between groups. Then, instead of performing RFA, an injection of 3 mL of 7% phenol at each level was made in the second group.

Their actual aim was pain score assessment and they found that within each group, there were statistically significant reductions in pain scores from baseline after performing each procedure. There were no statistically significant differences in mean pain scores between phenol and RF groups, however, leading to the conclusion that RF lesioning of lumbar sympathetics may be comparable to phenol lumbar sympathetic neurolysis. It is worth noting that the incidence of complication is thought to be lower with RFA than with phenol neurolysis, suggesting an improved risk-benefit profile with RFA. [43]

Scattered case reports describe the effects of RFA of the lumbar sympathetic chain in CRPS. For example, RF ablation of lumbar sympathetic ganglia was performed in a 55-year-old woman who had lower extremity neuropathic pain after T12-L1 disc herniation surgery. Diagnostic LSB was performed with bupivacaine, which resulted in marked decrease of pain and edema in the patient's affected extremity. Subsequently, percutaneous RF lumbar sympatholysis was performed with successful outcomes in pain, edema and color changes in the feet. [44] Similarly, there are case reports of CT-guided LSB being performed. One case presents a child who showed significant pain relief after 3 CT-guided LSB. The authors concluded that, in children and patients with low intra-abdominal fat, using CT could be safer than routine fluoroscopy. [45]

SUMMARY OF EVIDENCE REGARDING SYMPATHETIC BLOCKADE

There may be a correlation between shorter duration of symptoms and greater efficacy of sympathetic blockade, but further study to strengthen this observation is required. Existence of factors such as temperature asymmetry and color changes were also positive predictors to SB response, while as symptoms such as allodynia, hypoesthesia or hyperesthesia, and involvement of more than one limb were shown to be negative predictors to SB response. [25]

Despite the fact that the quality of evidence is low, advocating an inconclusive recommendation, the treatment alternatives for CRPS refractory to the other management strategies are limited. Given their simplicity of administration, relative safety, and long clinical history, sympathetic blocks have been proposed as a reasonable treatment choice to consider for patients who are refractory to pharmacologic modalities, psychiatric intervention, and physical therapy. Utilizing this modality early in the treatment course and considering it as a first line intervention before thought of other more invasive modalities (such as SCS) may be considered as it has a favorable risk-benefit profile, but one must consider the lack of evidence-based efficacy with this technique. [2] In a systematic review of 29 studies with 1144 CRPS-I patients, less than one third of the patients reported temporary relief of pain symptoms following a SB. [16] The authors also noted, however, that the placebo effect should also be considered in this setting, calling into question the apparent poor efficacy of SB. Others have emphasized this consideration for placebo effects in pain research as well. [46, 47] Thus, routine administration of percutaneous SB for patients with CRPS-I may not be as useful as previously predicted, but this modality still remains a viable interventional option for CRPS management and has been shown to effectively provide relief for some patients.

INTRAVENOUS REGIONAL BLOCK

Intravenous regional block (IVRB), also known as a "Bier block," is a classic technique that has fallen out of favor due to poor patient tolerance (dual tourniquet application and manual exsanguination of a painful CRPS-affected limb) and concurrent evidence suggesting poor outcomes following IVRB. [48, 49] Initially, IVRB for CRPS treatment was described with the utilization of guanethidine, a sympatholytic agent that acts by depleting norepinephrine stores from nerve terminals.

EVIDENCE

Unfortunately, a placebo-controlled randomized trial of 57 CRPS-I patients showed that patients receiving active IVRB with guanethidine had worsened pain and vasomotor symptoms after 6 months compared to controls. [48] Ramamurthy et al compared the effectiveness of guanethidine in another randomized double blind trial. These patients were enrolled to receive four intravenous regional blocks at 4-day intervals with various combinations of either guanethidine or 0.5% lidocaine. [50] Patients were randomized to receive one guanethidine and three lidocaine blocks, two guanethidine and two lidocaine blocks, or four guanethidine blocks without any lidocaine block. The outcomes did not exhibit any noteworthy differences between the intervention groups. With long term follow up, there were no distinctions in pain scores between groups receiving one, two, or four guanethidine injections. Generally, only 35% of patients experienced clinically significant long-term pain relief despite the fact that all were treated quite early following onset of their CRPS. This correlates to the outcomes data regarding ganglionic sympathetic blockade presented above, which showed approximately one third of patients found relief following SB. [16]

In a randomized cross-over study by Rocco et al, the effectiveness of adding guanethidine or reserpine to active control (lidocaine) was investigated in 12 patients suffering from CRPS. [51] At 2 to 14 months follow-up, pain relief was evident in two patients following reserpine administration, one following guanethidine, and none following lidocaine with no statistical significant difference between groups. In another crossover study, Hord et al. investigated the effectiveness of bretylium IVRB by administering either bretylium 1.5 mg/kg together with 0.5% lidocaine (active group) or 0.5% lidocaine without bretylium (control group). [52] Like guanethidine, bretylium obstructs the release of norepinephrine from nerve terminals, limiting peripheral sympathetic activity. In this study, the active treatment group exhibited statistically improved pain and temperature outcomes following IVRB compared to controls.

Another study compared SGB using 15 ml 0.5% bupivacaine every day up to a total of 8 blocks with IVRB using guanethidine 20mg every 4 days to a total of four blocks. [53] Outcomes were similar, with no statistical differences between groups. Data analyzed included pain scores and clinical signs (hyperesthesia, allodynia, vasomotor disturbances, trophic changes, edema and motor limitations).

Given the mixed results obtained with IVRB, several studies have sought to identify factors predictive for IVRB success or failure. Unfortunately, initially effective SB with local anesthetic does not predict long term pain relief. [54] Other factors that may result in apparent high rates of successful outcomes in active treatment are natural history, self-limited condition, personal and case to case variability and healthy psychological background. [55]

A 2010 review, however, found that IVRB had no added value for pain relief compared to placebo in CRPS-I patients. [1] The results suggest that about one third of CRPS patients obtain pain relief. This rate of success can be acceptable to many patients, yet its magnitude is consistent with a placebo response. [16] In fact, the placebo response, in addition to other factors such a rehabilitation programs and psychological variables, has been shown to have a great influence on pain outcomes and needs more attention. [56-59]

SGB for upper extremity CRPS is the first recommended intervention in more recent guidelines. Despite clinicians' preference for its application over IVRB, some studies continue to compare the effectiveness of SB with IVRB. In one study, 43 patients were selected and evaluated for the efficacy of IVRB produced by combining 70 mg lidocaine with 30 µg clonidine versus SGB produced by the injection of 70 mg lidocaine alone or combined with 30 µg clonidine into the stellate ganglion. Each method was repeated five times at 7-day interims.

The outcomes showed that after the first three blocks, a significant diminishment in pain scores and an improvement in sustained analgesic time occurred in all groups, but no further change was attained with the additional two blocks. Drowsiness and dry mouth were adverse effects seen only in patients receiving SGB with lidocaine plus clonidine. Thus, the authors concluded that IVRB may be desirable over SGB because of its easier administration and lower danger of undesirable events. [52] Thus, physicians and other clinicians must consider case characteristics and individual preferences as these may become some of the most important factors predicting and contributing to the treatment response.

SURGICAL SYMPATHECTOMY

While SB of ganglia or IVRB is now used prior to performing surgical sympathectomies, historically sympathectomy was a first line therapy for CRPS and ganglionic blockade only came into existence as a predictive tool for success of such procedures. In modern times, both new and old approaches to this technique are available. Open surgical sympathectomies take the classic approach, similar to any open surgical procedure. Thoracoscopic sympathectomies have gained some favor as a less invasive modality. Periarterial and perivenous sympathectomies, although old techniques, are also still applied in some situations.

Several observational studies have reported the effects of cervical, thoracic, or lumbar surgical sympathectomies for CPRS. In one study, 29 patients with CRPS-I had either transthoracic (lower third of stellate ganglia to T3) or lumbar (L2-L4) sympathectomy and were followed for 24 to 108 months postoperatively. Interestingly, the procedure gave lasting pain relief to all patients with CRPS of less than 12 months duration. [60] In another, larger case series with 73 CRPS patients who had documented SMP and underwent cervical or lumbar sympathectomy, only 25% of patients had significant pain relief one year postoperatively. [61] Moreover, the authors described their complication rates as follows: 33% of cervical sympathectomy and 20% of lumbar sympathectomy cases presented with transient postprocedural sympathalgia lasting less than 3 month; 10% of patients had no analgesia or disability reduction; 7% had new regional pain and sweating disturbance.

One study compared the outcomes of thoracoscopic versus open sympathectomies for CRPS. Although this study was not a randomized trial and patients were preferentially offered the thoracoscopic approach, all patients were reported to have improvements in symptoms. Furthermore, the authors reported that hospital stay was shorter and long-term positive outcomes were better with thoracoscopic sympathectomy. [62] Given the invasive nature of this procedure and the relatively common rates of unpleasant complications noted above, this procedure is rarely performed as a first line therapy.

In a report of local subcutaneous venous sympathectomy, 16 patients with CRPS-II of the upper or lower limb with no response to other modalities were included in this study. [63] After confining the most proximal region of pain, lidocaine was injected to provide local anesthesia to the subcutaneous tissues, followed by surgical removal of subcutaneous veins. 12 of 16 (75%) of these patients showed a significant analgesic effect and improvement in limb function.

SOMATIC AND CENTRAL NEURAXIAL BLOCKS

Brachial Plexus Block

Somatic nerve block of the brachial plexus can also lead to blockade the surrounding efferent sympathetic nerves. Somatic blockade, especially in case of shoulder involvement, improves the ability to tolerate physical therapy as well, but few studies exist regarding this interventional modality for CRPS management.

In one example, a retrospective case series reported the effects of serial interscalene blocks on CRPS patients. Bupivacaine 0.125% was used and injected every other day up to a total of 10 injections. In follow-up, the authors found improvement in pain and limb range of motion. Finally they recommended that this approach be considered if sympathetic blockade failed. [64] This recommendation was echoed by the findings of a randomized trial evaluating bupivacaine-based continuous SGB and continuous infraclavicular blocks, which showed similar positive outcomes (edema and range of motion) in each group. [65] 33 total patients were included and followed for 4 weeks.

Epidural Block

Continuous epidural infusion acts as an acceptable alternative to regional block or targeted SB. This technique also has the advantage of potential diversification of pharmaceutical options for multimodal targeted medical therapy, including opiates, ketamine, clonidine, or other adjuvants, in addition local anesthetics. Epidural blocks for patients with CRPS can be performed in outpatient settings and successful trials can be followed with placement of tunneled epidural catheters for providing prolonged somatic or sympathetic blockade. These interventions have been reported to be beneficial in controlling pain in patients with CRPS. [66-73]

In one study, 37 CRPS patients were enrolled to ascertain factors for success or failure of treatment. [72] After placement of an epidural catheter by the treatment team, patients were discharged home and closely monitored by home care nurses. All patients participated in a rehabilitation exercise program. Individually tailored psychological interventions were also provided as needed. Physician follow-up was performed every 2 to 3 weeks. While age and gender did not seem to have any influence on outcomes, the number of limbs with CRPS proved to be an inversely proportional predictor for success of treatment with epidural infusion. Although the authors concluded that this difference could be explained by a more intense wind-up phenomenon when more than one limb is involved, entrenchment of of central pain sensitization, patchy epidural spread of medications may also play a significant role in failure of epidural therapy. Furthermore, it was found that the longer length of treatment (8 versus 4 weeks) was associated with a higher success rate, suggesting a dose-time dependent process may play a role in success of therapy. Lastly, the authors found that early termination of the epidural catheter was either due to an uncontrolled side effect (intractable nausea, pruritis) or a complication (infection or dislodgment of the catheter), which resulted in their recommendation to aggressively treat adverse effects for the purpose of maximizing the potential period of active treatment in the hope of improving the rate of success with this treatment modality.

In another study, epidural clonidine was evaluated as a potential therapy and was infused for a mean of 43 days in 19 patients with CRPS refractory to other treatment modalities. While the authors concluded that epidural clonidine could cause significant analgesia, it was only demonstrated to give short-term pain relief in chronic CRPS, with signs of possible long-term efficacy based on small VAS reductions. Of note, the smaller clonidine dose (300 micrograms) was found to produce similar pain relief and hemodynamic changes as the larger 700 micrograms dose with fewer sedative sequelae. [69]

Scattered case reports also support the use of epidural catheters for CRPS patients, but it is important to recognize that such reports are often related to special situations (i.e., perioperative analgesia) or select populations (i.e., pediatrics). In one report, a 47-year-female with upper extremity CRPS presented for radical mastectomy of the right breast. [71] For postoperative analgesia and rehabilitation of affected limb, a cervical epidural catheter was placed and a continuous epidural infusion of 0.125% bupivacaine and 2.5 micrograms per ml clonidine solution was administered for 5 days. Physical therapy was started within 24 hour and the patient had good postoperative pain relief (>90% reduction) at hospital discharge. The patient did not have any complications in the postoperative period. Furthermore, during follow-up, the patient was very satisfied, and reported only slight discomfort in the affected limb and continued with regular physical therapy. In another report, a 15-year-old girl with severe CRPS pain in her right upper limb, without response to pharmacotherapy and stellate ganglion block, received continuous epidural analgesia for a period of 5 days, at which point all pain had dissipated. Finally the authors concluded that in the childhood setting, early initiation of such interventional treatment may be an appropriate choice for the management of CRPS. [73]

SPINAL CORD STIMULATION (SCS)

The Role of Neuromodulation

In conjunction with expert panel recommendations for CRPS management, which include pharmacologic, psychological, physical rehabilitation, and interventional pain management techniques, therapeutic interventions should be implemented as soon as possible, with delays likely resulting in compounded sequelae. [18] Among the many interventional techniques available to the pain practitioner, spinal cord stimulation (SCS) is generally thought of as a more invasive and costly treatment option that can be considered when other simpler treatments have failed, but some have advocated for its early implementation. [74-76]

The main mechanism of action of SCS is thought to be through the manipulation of the classic gate control theory of pain proposed by Melzack and Wall, which suggests that central processing of peripheral afferents is limited by peripheral competitive inhibition of small slower nociceptive fibers through a system of inhibitory interneurons activated by the larger myelinated high speed sensory nerve fibers. Following this theory, peripheral vibratory sensations would travel faster than concurrent painful stimuli, inhibit transmission of those smaller nociceptive fibers, and reduce the painful afferent input to supraspinal nuclei. [77, 78] Furthermore, dorsal horn stimulation of rats has been shown to induce an increase in the release of inhibitory transmitters like as gamma-amino butyric acid (GABA) and a decrease in the release of the excitatory neurotransmitters like glutamate. [79, 80] Other mechanistic theories have also been proposed to explain the antinociceptive effects of SCS, including direct blockade of the neuronal currents, inhibition of wide dynamic range (WDR) or "convergent" neuronal hyperactivity, activation of a spinal-brainstem-spinal loop, activation of supraspinal nuclei involved in both supraspinal and descending antinociceptive pathways, and supraspinal and segmental sympathetic outflow inhibition. [81-87] Considering that evidence has been presented for all of these potential mechanisms for SCS, it seems most likely that SCS functions through a complex set of interactions at several levels of both the peripheral and central nervous systems.

Neuropathic pain, along with other chronic pain conditions, is often thought to be mediated by the same neuronal circuits and pathways on which SCS is thought to act. For example, in the first hours after traumatic injury, nociception-induced central sensitization may be initiated, which, among other pathways, is mediated by glutamatergic activation of N-methyl-D-aspartate (NMDA) receptors, which may subsequently result in downstream CNS reconfiguration to coalesce into a state of chronic pain. [88] The pathogenesis of neuropathic pain is generally thought to be dependent of central sensitization, which can involve a diverse set of nuclei and neuronal pathways. Somatosensory neurons in the dorsal horn of the spinal cord, when sensitized, for example, exhibit a state of more frequent and spontaneous synaptic activity. [89] Initially (hours to days following injury), this process is thought to be mediated by more frequent glutamate discharge in the dorsal horn secondary to peripheral injury. [90] In neuropathic rat models, the inhibitory effects of SCS on pain perception have been investigated; with findings suggesting this process is largely mediated by a local decrease in glutamate concentrations in the dorsal horn. [91]

Considering the temporal component of post-traumatic neuropathic pain pathogenesis, early SCS intervention has been proposed to result in improved outcomes, including prevention or reversibility of the changes involved in the process of central sensitization. In an animal model with Seltzer injured rats, SCS placement within 24 hours after injury resulted in a lower incidence of neuropathic pain than when SCS was placed 16 days post-injury. [74] In clinical practice, however, it is quite difficult or even impossible to diagnose and treat CRPS patients with SCS within days after initiation of the disorder due to a delay in presentation and subsequent diagnosis, which may extend from months-to-years following CRPS onset. [92] Notwithstanding, a favorable outcome has been reported in some cases where SCS was implanted within the first year of CRPS onset. [92-94]

Technique

SCS implantation is performed in two stages. In the first stage, patients receive a trial of SCS with a temporary electrode for several days, sometimes exceeding one week's duration. If the trial is successful, the patient may become a candidate for permanent SCS implantation. While success is often defined as a reduction in pain score of at least 50% for research purposes and study designs, clinically patient satisfaction and individual preferences may play a greater role. Of course, patient selection is also of paramount importance and individual patient expectations also play a significant role in success of SCS therapy. [95, 96]

The procedure is performed with the patient in prone position. Prophylactic antibiotics may be given. The skin is prepped and draped, then generously anesthetized with a local anesthetic. Then, under direct fluoroscopy, a Tuohy needle is targeted to enter the epidural space. The SCS electrodes are then advanced through the needle until the electrode tip is at the level of C4 for cases of upper extremity CRPS, T3-T8 for thoracic or abdominal involvement, and T12 for lower extremity CRPS. After positioning the electrode at the desired level, stimulation is started and intensity manipulated under real-time patient feedback, with the typical goal of the patient reporting a sensation of paresthesia overlapping the area of pain. (Figure 6.4)

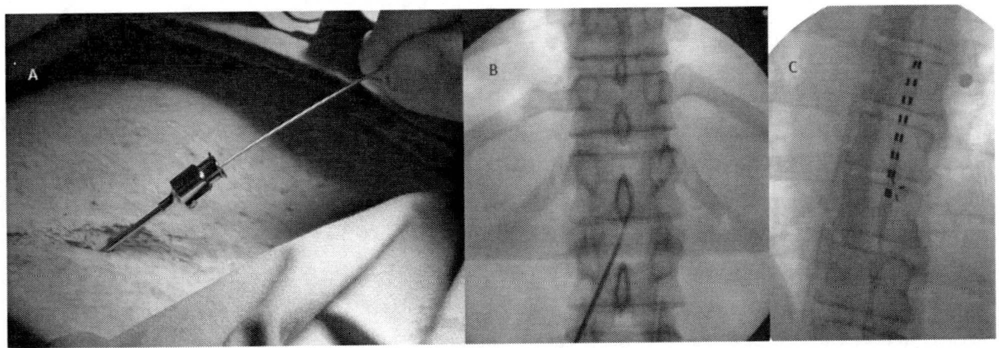

Figure 6.4. SCS implantation in a CRPS patient. Patient in prone position with electrode being introduced through a Tuohy needle (A). AP C-arm view of a Tuohy needle with the electrode tip protruding through (B). Electrode tip positions confirmed up to the T7 level following removal of Tuohy needles (C).

This procedure is often repeated on the contralateral side of the epidural space with a second Tuohy needle and second electrode. After successful positioning and satisfactory stimulation parameters, the needle is then withdrawn and the electrode connected to an external stimulator (trial stage) and the patient is encouraged to perform his or her normal daily activities.

Conversion of successful trials to permanent stimulators involves a very similar procedure, but requires the additional surgical creation of two pockets: one for securing and coiling electrode leads, and the other for placement of the implantable pulse generator. A midline incision is typically performed and a small pocket is created to coil the leads within it, providing slack and removing tension from the active stimulating portion of the electrode within the epidural space. The lead extension is tunneled to a pocket created to house the internal pulse generator, to which the electrode is connected and fixed. The internal pulse generator may be placed in the lower abdomen or upper buttocks – a choice that is often case-specific. The skin is then sutured and the patient is discharged home with appropriate follow-up.

EVIDENCE

In the majority of cases, SCS for CRPS has been considered late in the treatment course of this syndrome. This decision has traditionally been related to the invasiveness of these interventional procedures and their associated costs, but some have begun to advocate for early use of SCS in the treatment of CPRS. [97-101] A recent review on the clinical and cost-effectiveness of SCS in the management of chronic neuropathic or ischemic pain suggests that this treatment is effective in reducing the chronic neuropathic pain of CRPS I. [102] Another systematic review reported SCS to be both a clinically-effective and a cost-effective therapy in the management of patients with CRPS I (Level A evidence) and clinically effective for CPRS II (Level D evidence). [103]

To date, only one randomized controlled trial has been conducted with CRPS patients to evaluate SCS efficacy, with results originally extending to a period of 2-years follow-up. This study represents the highest level of evidence available specifically for SCS in CRPS. In this trial, the combined effect of SCS with physiotherapy (SCS-PT) was compared with physiotherapy alone in patients with refractory CRPS-1. [104] Of 36 patients randomly allocated to the SCS-PT group, 12 failed the SCS trial and a permanent SCS was placed in the remaining 24 patients. VAS-measured pain scores and health-related quality of life were significantly improved in the SCS-PT group compared to controls at 6-months, with similar findings at 2 years follow-up. Of note, 9 of the 24 patients with an implanted SCS (38%) experienced complications requiring further surgery within two years. [95, 101] Subsequent 5-year follow-up revealed that the previously significant differences were no longer present, but patients in the SCS-PT group were generally satisfied and reported that they would undergo the procedure again for similar results. [105] Following this trial, an investigation of factors predictive of SCS success identified brush-stroke allodynia as a negative predictor of SCS success at 1-year time. [106]

While other data for SCS use in CRPS exist, quality of evidence is limited by sample size or study design. Ranging from non-randomized prospective observational studies or open label designs to retrospective chart reviews and case reports, the evidence is generally supportive of SCS efficacy in CRPS, suggesting that there is significant potential for future research and clinical applicability in this arena. [25, 76, 92, 99, 100, 107, 108]

Of note, there are several unique findings from among these reports. One retrospective review of 10 military personnel with CRPS of 5 to 12 months duration who were treated with SCS resulted not only in a reduction of oral morphine equivalents, but also resulted in 6 of 10 returning to active military duty – a functional status requiring a greater-than-average level of physical activity. [100] In another study, Forouzanfar et al investigated the long-term effects of cervical and lumbar SCS in 36 patients with CRPS I, finding no significant analgesic differences between cervical and lumbar SCS groups and noting that both groups showed a significant reduction in pain intensity at 6 months, 1 year, and 2 years follow-up. [99] Kumar et al reported similar findings in follow-up comparisons of SCS in lower extremity and upper extremity CRPS. [76] In a study on CRPS patients with SMP with more than one-year duration, SCS induced vasodilation and increased limb blood flow in the affected limb. [109] In patients with CRPS associated sympathetically independent pain this vascular effect could not be demonstrated. [110]

While traditional SCS is rapidly advancing in scope, science, and versatility through research and diversification of clinical practice, dorsal root ganglion (DRG) stimulation has recently emerged as a potential therapeutic option in CRPS. Deer et al describe the results of their pilot study on DRG stimulation in CRPS patients with 8 of 9 patients reporting reduced pain and 7 of 9 decreasing their medication consumption. [111] Although subsequent case reports and observational studies support these positive findings, much additional research will be needed to elucidate DRG stimulation safety and efficacy in CRPS. [112, 113] Of note, Van Buyten et al report excellent lower extremity pain-paresthesia concordance with the use of their modified DRG neuromodulation system in locations which are typically difficult to target with traditional SCS. [113] Similarly, Liem et al reported good safety and efficacy with DRG stimulation, but this multicenter study was inclusive of a broader chronic pain population. [114]

The European Federation of Neurological Societies 2007 report concluded that there was moderate evidence of efficacy of SCS in patients with CRPS I, while the lack of evidence for patients with CRPS II warranted an "inconclusive" recommendation. [115] More recently, the Neuromodulation Appropriateness Consensus Committee guidelines of 2014 recommend the implementation of SCS for CRPS of 3 months duration or greater if a CRPS patient is not responsive to more conservative measures. [116] While some would argue the conservative approach, advocating that it remains prudent to reserve SCS for patients with CRPS who do not respond adequately to noninvasive treatments and sympathetic nerve blocks or for whom nerve blocks are determined to be ineffective, others would point to emerging evidence of success with SCS attributed to its early implementation. [75, 76, 116]

PERIPHERAL NERVE STIMULATION (PNS)

Invasive treatments such as peripheral nerve stimulation (pNS) with an implantable programmable generator and peripheral nerve electrode have been reported in the literature mainly as case reports or series. In one case series study, six patients with CRPS showed a good response to pNS and SCS. [97] In another series, 32 patients with symptoms entirely or mainly in the distribution of one major peripheral nerve underwent paddle-type electrodes trials and 30 patients received permanent pNS placement on the affected nerves. 63% reported "good" or "fair" relief and 20% had an improvement in functional outcome and could return to part-time or full-time work. [98] In a third series, 41 pNS devices were implanted in 38 patients with pain in a peripheral nerve distribution. Over 60% of patients had significant improvement of their pain of more than 50% following implantation of the pNS. [117]

It is important to recognize, however, that this interventional procedure can only be applied if the pain is in the distribution of a peripheral nerve, thus making pNS less suitable for most CRPS I patients. Per a task force launched by the European Federation of Neurological Societies to evaluate evidence for all neurostimulation techniques and to produce relevant recommendations, evidence for implanted peripheral stimulations is still inadequate to select a definitive approach. [115]

IMPLANTABLE INTRATHECAL PUMPS

Intrathecal (IT) therapy using implantable drug administration systems is an invasive pain management technique so it has been reserved for CRPS patients whose condition is refractory to other modalities or those who have become intolerant of the side effects of their systemic therapies. It can also be used in patients with spasticity, contractures, dystonia, or those with palliative care requirement.

Proper catheter placement is of utmost importance as this modality relies of targeted drug delivery directly into the cerebrospinal fluid. Needless to say, once properly placed, it is of almost equal importance to carefully secure the catheter in place to minimize migration and maximize long-term outcomes. The FDA has approved few drugs for IT pumps. These agents are morphine and ziconotide for the treatment of pain, and baclofen for the treatment of spasticity. Medications such as hydromorphone, clonidine, bupivacaine, fentanyl, sufentanil, ketamine, and midazolam have also been used clinically and studied on an off-label basis.

TECHNIQUE

In many ways, IT catheter-pump placement is similar to SCS implantation, but a greater depth of anesthesia is often required than with SCS implantation. The patient is often positioned prone or lateral, prepped and draped, and the intrathecal catheter is placed through a needle under fluoroscopy in a fashion similar to that of SCS electrode placement. Once placement is confirmed fluoroscopically, the catheter extension is tunneled to a surgically created pocket which will house the pump and medication reservoir, typically to the lower abdomen or upper buttocks, again similar to that which is done with SCS placement. (Figure 6.5)

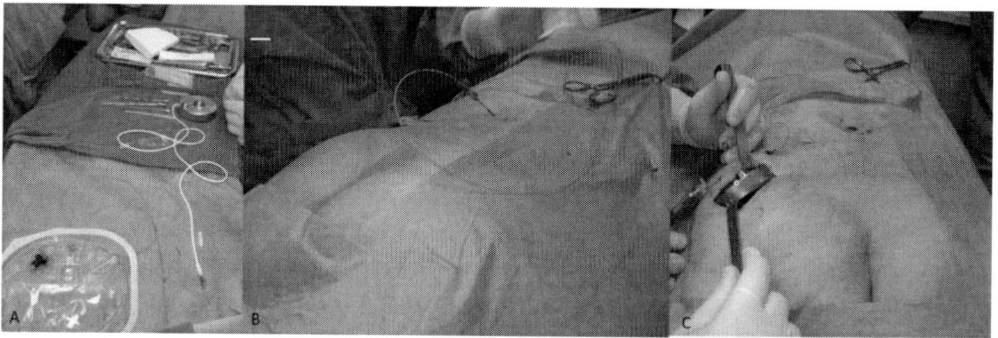

Figure 6.5. IT pump placement procedure. IT catheter-pump equipment kit (A). Catheter being placed through the needle (B). Surgical creation of a pocket for the IT pump and reservoir (C).

EVIDENCE

There is a paucity of high quality data regarding IT therapy for CRPS. The highest level of evidence comes from several case series published between 1994 and 2013, but varied in drug of choice, study design, and reported complications. [118-123] Kanoff described success in 11 of 15 chronic pain patients (5 with CRPS) using IT morphine therapy with 2-44 month follow-up, noting a general need for increasing morphine dosing over time. [118] CRPS-related dystonia has been treated with IT baclofen (dose range 25 to 450 micrograms per day) with mixed but generally positive results. [121-123] Goto et al described a case series of IT baclofen in combination with SCS therapy for refractory CRPS with dystonia, concluding that combined SCS and ITB can decrease unpleasant movement impairment and pain intensity, to some degree, in refractory CRPS cases. [116] One additional case series described successful IT baclofen therapy in two patients who previously failed IT morphine therapy. Of note, one patient required the additional of IT clonidine as IT baclofen alone was not well tolerated. [124] Similarly, in the study by van Rijn et al, baclofen-related complications were reported in 19 of 89 adverse events. 52 of 89 were secondary to catheter-pump system defects, while 18 could not be specified. [122]

Lundborg et al. described a case series of 3 CRPS patient who received IT bupivacaine with or without IT buprenorphine, noting that while there were some improvements in refractory pain, this treatment modality did not prevent the progression of CRPS, nor did it have a significant impact on the associated signs and symptoms of this syndrome. [123]

Hence, Lundborg et al emphasized that IT bupivacaine therapy should not replace any established therapeutic modalities for CPRS, especially if there is evidence of efficacy with such modalities.

Lastly, IT ziconotide has shown some promise in the treatment of CRPS. As a selective N-type voltage-gated calcium channel blocker, it reduces the release of excitatory neurotransmitters like substance P, calcitonin gene-related peptide, and glutamate, inducing an inhibitory effect to nociceptive pathways in the spinal cord and brain, thereby resulting in analgesia. Kapural et al described a series of 7 CPRS patients treated with IT ziconotide for a mean duration of 3.1 years, 5 of which showed substantial clinical signs of improvement, including 2 of those 5 who were able to discontinue IT ziconotide with remission of CRPS-related pain. [119] Supporting the findings of this series is a pediatric CRPS case report effectively treated with a slow up-titration of IT ziconotide to 24 micrograms per day. [125]

DORSAL ROOT ENTRY ZONE (DREZ)

Destructive procedures such as dorsal root entry zone (DREZ) lesioning should be considered as a treatment option in intractable severe cases and not as a first-line treatment option in the management of CRPS. [126] In this procedure, a destructive surgical lesion would be applied to the dorsal root entry region and is also known as a posterior selective rhizotomy. [127] This technique has also been described using RF and targeting the nucleus caudalis. [128] It is a therapeutic option in cases with severe refractory CRPS, despite the fact that this resultant lesion is potentially irreversible and also leads to severe complication such as limb ataxia and weakness. [129]

While no large randomized trials are available for establishing efficacy of DREZ procedures, multiple case reports outline successful outcomes following DREZ lesioning. One such report described two cases of refractory CRPS in the right hand following blunt trauma: one in a 12-year-old boy and the other in a 35-year-old woman. [129] Various types of interventions were tried prior to DREZ lesioning but were not successful, including SGB, transcutaneous electrical nerve stimulation, morphine IT pump combined with oral opioids, and pNS. During 60 months of follow-up, the 12-year-old boy was totally pain free and no episodes of recurrence. The 35-year-old woman was pain-free until the 6th month, when she required psychological support, followed by partial satisfactory pain control (VAS=4), which was controlled by oral pregabalin and risperidone. Transient ipsilateral lower extremity ataxia occurred in both cases, but improved within approximately 3 months.

DEEP BRAIN STIMULATION (DBS)

Deep brain stimulation (DBS) has been carried out using a variety of brain targets including brain stimulation of periaqueductal gray, periventricular gray, ventral posterolateral and ventral posteromedial nuclei and internal capsule, each of which has been shown to be effective for pain relief in select patient populations. One must remember, however, that this neurosurgical procedure requires target identification, often employing a stereotactic approach at the initiation of the procedure followed in the operating room by electrophysiological monitoring to identify optimal target sites. Once the implanter is satisfied with the correct target, a trial may be performed and permanent leads may be placed.

Overall, a review of the literature demonstrates that DBS could be considered for refractory conditions including nociceptive and/or neuropathic pain and shows that 30-40% of patients with intractable neuropathic pain have been adequately controlled. [130] There are not enough studies evaluating DBS for pain indications as of yet and, to date, there is no reported case of its use in CRPS. Furthermore, when considering this option (discussed in greater detail in Chapter 9: Future Research and Advances in Technology), one must consider that a number of major complications, including death, have occurred with this technique. [130, 131]

MOTOR CORTEX STIMULATION (MCS)

Motor cortex stimulation has provided early promising results for the treatment of CRPS pain. The epidural motor cortex, also being used for the treatment of central pain, is safer, less invasive and technically easier to access than DBS. [132] Although central pain syndromes are the classic MCS indications, CRPS patients have also been treated with this modality. The exact mechanism through which MCS is able to produce analgesia is not clear, but reciprocal connections between the primary motor and the primary sensory area are believed to play a role. It is believed that MCS produces its effect by restoring inhibitory fields that would normally surround primary sensory neurons but that have been lost as a result of deafferentation.

TECHNIQUE

In order to perform this procedure it is critical to have the patient keep a good pain diary prior to the implant and during the course of the trial. Since the patient cannot feel a sensory change during the trial, the ability to keep proper records is critical in determining the success of the trial.

The surgical approach to motor cortex stimulation differs from deep brain stimulation in several ways. For one, a craniotomy, rather than a burr hole, is performed for entry into the cranium and access to the motor cortex. [133, 134] This may be done under local or general anesthesia. [135-138] Neuronavigation is still employed and thin-cut MRI imaging is still typically required, but the approaches are different. Functional MRI is employed to identify the area of the motor strip area correlating with pain and intraoperative neuronavigation is often frameless with localization of the precentral gyrus, along with the central sulcus, being done physiologically. [136, 139, 140]

This involves the use of an epidural grid electrode to record cortical surface electrical activity. Once simulated, a waveform with negative inflection is seen, then reverses form negative to positive at the central sulcus, a phenomenon known as phase reversal. Once the target is identified, with or without a trial, the craniotomy site is closed and the lead cables are externalized for connection to the pulse generator. Electrodes have historically been positioned in a variety or arrangements and there is no absolute recommendation for electrode positioning at this time.

Unlike deep brain stimulation, for which trials are almost always performed, trialing for motor cortex stimulation is not always done. While the benefits reflect the predictive value for success of the implant, the ideal trial period is unclear and controversial because the onset and peak effect of analgesia with this therapeutic modality are often delayed longer than 2 weeks, a period exceeding the duration of most MCS trials. [130, 131] Raslan et al have suggested that trials could be extended upward of 6 months to optimize permanent implant results, but recognized that any prolongation of trial time would involve increased risk of infection. [141] Further still, one must consider that stimulation parameters have varied greatly across the literature, with pulse widths from 60 to 450 microseconds, rates from 5 to 130 Hertz, and voltage amplitudes form 0.5 to 10V. [142]

In its first reported uses for pain, motor cortex stimulation employed the use of paddle electrodes from spinal cord stimulators. [143, 144] More recently, an octopolar lead was trialed, but lead design and optimization remain a broad and expansive field of research and development. [145] Irrespective of lead type, most leads are sutured epidurally to the target area. [130, 131] Some have secured leads subdurally, however, within the interhemispheric fissure or central sulcus in an attempt to optimize cortical stimulation to specific desired homuncular target areas. [146-148]

EVIDENCE

Unfortunately, there is a paucity of strong evidence regarding this intervention in CRPS management. MCS for treatment of CRPS has been reported for 10 patients to date and has proven efficacious in all except one in which the stimulator trial failed. [149-152] Starting with the description of a successful case report of MCS for a CRPS II patient with hemibody allodynia in 2003, MCS was described in two randomized, blinded, crossover studies of mixed neuropathic and CRPS I and II patients in 2008 and 2009, with a total of 7 CRPS patients between the two studies. These to randomized trials together represent the highest level of evidence for MCS in CRPS to date. In one trial, 2 of 2 CRPS patients had successful lasting analgesia, while in the other trial, 4 of 5 patients had a successful MCS trial and received permanent implants with lasting relief. [149, 151] These were followed in 2011 with another report of 2 successfully treated CRPS Type I patients, with both patients again retaining lasting analgesia, improvements in motor function, allodynia, hyperesthesia, and sympathetic signs at 27 and 36 months post implant. [152]

Velasco et al noted several other important findings. [151] Primarily, the success of MCS appeared to be related to the degree of avulsion injury and motor deficit, if avulsion injury was the cause of CRPS (i.e., brachial plexus avulsion). Patients presented with motor function that was in part or fully preserved with no areas of anesthesia dolorosa or paralysis for all cases in which motor cortex induced effective analgesia, along with relief in sensory and sympathetic signs. For all cases in which paralysis and/or anesthesia were present, MCS was not effective at providing analgesia or improving sympathetic signs to the denervated area. This observation encompasses one case in this trial in which a patient had paralysis in thumb and index finger due to a brachial plexus avulsion injury, noting CRPS pathology present in other areas of the upper extremity as well. In this case, MCS was effective in areas that had retained motor function, but was ineffective for the denervated thumb and index finger within the same individual.

Considering the invasive nature of this procedure and temporal difficulty of trialing MCS, and that validated criteria for choosing appropriate candidates for this procedure are still to be developed, great emphasis has been placed on identifying predictive tools. One such potential tool is repetitive transcranial magnetic stimulation (rTMS).

In a prospective randomized trial of active versus sham rTMS (not exclusive to CRPS patients), 79% of 33 patients who responded to the active rTMS trial responded well to MCS. While a positive outcome to MCS may be predicted by a positive response to rTMS, rTMS unresponsiveness was not found to be highly predictive of failure and, thus, has little value in excluding patients from MCS therapy. [153]

REPETITIVE TRANSCRANIAL MAGNETIC STIMULATION (RTMS)

Repetitive transcranial magnetic stimulation (rTMS) involves a magnetic induction subthreshold to motor evoked potentials in site-specific neurons. This relatively new technology has been applied to the treatment of both pain and psychiatric components of CRPS pathology and will be discussed in greater detail in Chapter 9 (Future Research and Advances in Technology). Despite mounting evidence of its efficacy, including 2 randomized controlled trials totaling 33 CRPS patients, differences in logistical and stimulatory parameters between studies reflect an evolving understanding of this technology in the medical community at-large and allude to a yet-to-be optimized analgesic tool with much potential. [22, 154-159] It is also worth noting that rTMS has been studied as a non-invasive predictive tool for success of surgical MCS implantation, not only in CRPS but in other pain states as well. [153, 160]

DIRECT CURRENT STIMULATION (DCS)

This neuromodulatory technique acts by applying direct current stimulation through the skin in a non-invasive manner in one of two directions: transcranial or spinal. The transcranial manner is named tDCS and the spinal is named sDCS. This modality uses weak electrical currents for inducing inhibitory effects on ascending and descending spinal pain pathways. Despite promise for potential use, it is a new modality for CRPS and future studies will be needed to assess outcomes and subsets of CRPS patients for whom it will induce the greatest effects.

COMPLICATIONS OF INTERVENTIONS

No procedure is devoid of complications, whether it is being performed for CRPS or for other indications. While there is an expansive set of procedures available for CRPS management, perhaps the most common ones involve the SB. For sympathetic ganglia ablation, a review by Stanton-Hicks et al. emphasized that complications of SB vary depending on the location, the approach, and the agents used. [161]

In spite of the invasive nature of some SB procedures, no serious complication was reported in the reviewed studies, a fact that suggests the need for more thorough reporting of side effects. The literature on all forms of analgesic interventions tends to define and evaluate the amount of pain relief and related outcomes more carefully than side effects. The following sections describe potential complications specific to each procedure.

COMPLICATIONS AFTER SGB

Some serious problems have been reported following SGB, the most important of which are inadvertent subarachnoid injection or injection into the vertebral or carotid arteries, all of which are potentially life-threatening complications. This makes hemodynamic and ECG monitoring and placement of an intravenous line prior to performing the procedure mandatory. [162]

A more common side effect is the occurrence of Horner's syndrome caused by the local anesthetic spreading to the cervical sympathetic trunk. Hoarseness can also occur via spread to the recurrent laryngeal nerve. Lung collapse and puncture of adjacent structures such as esophagus is one of the other complications of SGB. [29]

COMPLICATIONS AFTER LSB

Orthostatic hypotension is a potential adverse effect of LSB due to lower extremity vasodilatation after blocking the lumbar sympathetic ganglia. Another possible complication is damage to the genitofemoral (most common), lateral femoral cutaneous, or ilioinguinal nerves - a complication that should be considered especially in cases of planned neurolysis or permanent ablation. [163, 164]

COMPLICATIONS AFTER ABLATIVE PROCEDURES

Although ablative procedures are thought to be generally safe, patients may develop post-ablation pain conditions that can sometimes be worse than the original pain. Ablative procedures of autonomic structures for CRPS management should be cautiously selected given the weak evidence and potential for serious sequelae associated with these interventions.

COMPLICATIONS AFTER EPIDURAL INFUSIONS

Post-dural puncture headache is one of the classic problems following epidural catheter placement, but this can be treat with oral analgesics, rest, hydration and caffeinated beverages, or epidural blood patch. Some of the other reported complications are as follows:

infection at the catheter insertion point, catheter or pump failure, and, rarely, epidural abscess. [98]

COMPLICATIONS AFTER IT INFUSIONS

Although infrequent, some of the most common reported complications of IT infusion are as follows: infections, catheter and pump system failures, post-dural puncture headache, drug overdose and the formation of intrathecal granulomas, which have the potential danger of producing spinal cord compression. [165]

COMPLICATION AFTER SCS

Electrode dislocation or pain from the implanted pulse generator pocket are complications of SCS which require reoperation. [101] Meningitis is a potential life-threatening complication, but occurs rarely. In 34% of the SCS patients, other adverse events have been reported, including infection, dural puncture, pain in the region of a stimulator component, equipment failure, revision procedures other than battery change and removal operations. [166] One multicenter retrospective review from the United States reported the collective experience with SCS, finding that 15% of the systems had to be removed due to lack of lasting pain relief. [96]

In a retrospective study performed on 160 patients after SCS implantation followed up to 10 years, a significantly lower rate of complications was described including a 4.4% incidence of infection and a 3.1% incidence of seroma, while no neural injury or death was reported. [104] In an extensive analysis of the literature, the safety and efficacy of SCS over a period of 20 years was reviewed. [167] In this study, which evaluated 2972 cases, the rate and incidence of biologic complications observed was as follows: (3.4%), skin erosion (0.03%), hematoma (0.3%), cerebrospinal fluid (CSF) leak (0.3%), allergic reaction (0.1%), and paralysis (0.03%). In another retrospective review of complications associated with placement of post laminotomy paddle leads, complication rates as follows: major motor deficit (0.25%), limited motor deficit (0.14%), sensory deficit (0.10%), CSF leak (0.047%), and autonomic changes (0.013%). [168] The authors concluded that this small incidence of complication could further be reduced by considering approaches that improve procedural safety (such as appropriate preoperative imaging to rule out spinal stenosis) and by careful patient follow-up and complication management.

COMPLICATIONS OF PNS

There are some possible complications related to the pNS equipment design requiring reoperation. These include migration of the electrode (33%) and the need for placement in an alternative location (11%). There are other complications related to the surgical technique such as infection with the incidence upward of 15%. [169]

COMPLICATIONS OF BRACHIAL PLEXUS BLOCK

Although rare, the most common complications after brachial plexus blockade are infection of the catheter skin insertion site, transient paralysis, and ipsilateral partial sensory or motor deficit. Interestingly, there is one case report of CRPS onset following interscalene block in the perioperative setting. [170]

COMPLICATIONS OF MCS

The majority of studies report few or no complications, but serious complications have occurred. Seizures (12%), intracranial bleeding (2.5%), infection (5.7%), and both transient and permanent neurological deficits have been reported. [132, 134, 140, 171-174] Seizures are the most common adverse effect (0-41%) and can occur at various times, including the intraoperative implantation, stimulator programming and reprogramming, or after chronic stimulation. [130]

A case of transient facial droop and speech deficits was reported to resolve with a decrease in pulse generator stimulation. [175] It is worth noting that like other implantable devices, the efficacy of motor cortex stimulators may recede with time or stop altogether with an inciting event such as traumatic lead displacement, a fact that may be considered a downstream complication of this therapy.

CONCLUSION

- There is a paucity of high quality evidence for outcomes of most interventional procedures in CRPS, both in regard to short and long term efficacy, and complications.
- Although interventional techniques have been previously reserved for CRPS patients with severe pain who do not respond to medication and physical therapy, some evidence suggests that early intervention may lead to improved patient outcomes.
- For symptoms predictive of SMP, a diagnostic block of the stellate ganglion or the lumbar sympathetic nervous system can be performed.
- In the case of at least 50% pain reduction during diagnostic block, radiofrequency ablative therapy of the stellate or the lumbar sympathetic ganglia may be a suitable option.
- SCS can be used after multidisciplinary evaluation of the patient.
- Somatic brachial plexus block, epidural analgesia and pNS can be considered for select patients but are generally not recommended as first line therapy.
- In cases refractory to all other therapy, IT therapy, deep brain or motor cortex stimulation can be considered, as can the DREZ lesioning procedure, but the potential for morbid complications should lead each practitioner to choose these therapeutic modalities with great caution.

REFERENCES

[1] Perez, R. S., et al., Evidence based guidelines for complex regional pain syndrome type 1. *BMC Neurol*, 2010. 10: p. 20.

[2] O'Connell, N.E., et al., Interventions for treating pain and disability in adults with complex regional pain syndrome. *Cochrane Database Syst Rev*, 2013. 4: p. CD009416.

[3] Merskey, H., N. Bogduk, and International Association for the Study of Pain. Task Force on Taxonomy. *Classification of chronic pain:* descriptions of chronic pain syndromes and definitions of pain terms. 2nd ed. 1994, Seattle: IASP Press. xvi, 222 p.

[4] Harden, R. N., et al., Complex regional pain syndrome: are the IASP diagnostic criteria valid and sufficiently comprehensive? *Pain*, 1999. 83(2): p. 211-9.

[5] Inhofe, P. D. and C.A. Garcia-Moral, Reflex sympathetic dystrophy. A review of the literature and a long-term outcome study. *Orthop Rev*, 1994. 23(8): p. 655-61.

[6] Krames, E., Spinal Cord Stimulation: Indications, Mechanism of Action, and Efficacy. *Curr Rev Pain*, 1999. 3(6): p. 419-426.

[7] Krames, E., et al., Rethinking algorithms of pain care: the use of the S.A.F.E. principles. *Pain Med*, 2009. 10(1): p. 1-5.

[8] Dworkin, R. H., et al., Interventional management of neuropathic pain: NeuPSIG recommendations. *Pain*, 2013. 154(11): p. 2249-61.

[9] Nelson, D. V. and B. R. Stacey, Interventional therapies in the management of complex regional pain syndrome. *Clin J Pain*, 2006. 22(5): p. 438-42.

[10] Dunningham, T. H., The treatment of Sudeck's atrophy in the upper limb by sympathetic blockade. *Injury*, 1980. 12(2): p. 139-44.

[11] Stanton-Hicks, M., et al., Reflex sympathetic dystrophy: changing concepts and taxonomy. *Pain*, 1995. 63(1): p. 127-33.

[12] Krames, E., et al., Implementing the SAFE Principles for the Development of Pain Medicine Therapeutic Algorithms That Include Neuromodulation Techniques. *Neuromodulation*, 2009. 12(2): p. 104-13.

[13] Poree, L., et al., Spinal cord stimulation as treatment for complex regional pain syndrome should be considered earlier than last resort therapy. *Neuromodulation*, 2013. 16(2): p. 125-41.

[14] Jorum, E., et al., Catecholamine-induced excitation of nociceptors in sympathetically maintained pain. *Pain*, 2007. 127(3): p. 296-301.

[15] Raja, S. N., et al., Systemic alpha-adrenergic blockade with phentolamine: a diagnostic test for sympathetically maintained pain. *Anesthesiology*, 1991. 74(4): p. 691-8.

[16] Cepeda, M.S., D. B. Carr, and J. Lau, Local anesthetic sympathetic blockade for complex regional pain syndrome. *Cochrane Database Syst Rev*, 2005(4): p. CD004598.

[17] Perez, R. S., et al., Treatment of reflex sympathetic dystrophy (CRPS type 1): a research synthesis of 21 randomized clinical trials. *J Pain Symptom Manage*, 2001. 21(6): p. 511-26.

[18] Stanton-Hicks, M.D., et al., An updated interdisciplinary clinical pathway for CRPS: report of an expert panel. *Pain Pract*, 2002. 2(1): p. 1-16.

[19] Forouzanfar, T., et al., Treatment of complex regional pain syndrome type I. *Eur J Pain*, 2002. 6(2): p. 105-22.

[20] Cepeda, M. S., J. Lau, and D.B. Carr, Defining the therapeutic role of local anesthetic sympathetic blockade in complex regional pain syndrome: a narrative and systematic review. *Clin J Pain*, 2002. 18(4): p. 216-33.

[21] van Eijs, F., et al., Evidence-based interventional pain medicine according to clinical diagnoses. 16. Complex regional pain syndrome. *Pain Pract,* 2011. 11(1): p. 70-87.

[22] Schwenkreis, P., et al., Bilateral motor cortex disinhibition in complex regional pain syndrome (CRPS) type I of the hand. *Neurology*, 2003. 61(4): p. 515-9.

[23] Hartrick, C. T., J.P. Kovan, and P. Naismith, Outcome prediction following sympathetic block for complex regional pain syndrome. *Pain* Pract, 2004. 4(3): p. 222-8.

[24] Dellemijn, P.L., et al., The interpretation of pain relief and sensory changes following sympathetic blockade. *Brain,* 1994. 117 (Pt 6): p. 1475-87.

[25] van Eijs, F., et al., Predictors of pain relieving response to sympathetic blockade in complex regional pain syndrome type 1. *Anesthesiology,* 2012. 116(1): p. 113-21.

[26] Hogan, Q. H., et al., Success rates in producing sympathetic blockade by paratracheal injection. *Clin J Pain*, 1994. 10(2): p. 139-45.

[27] Abdi, S., et al., A new and easy technique to block the stellate ganglion. *Pain Physician*, 2004. 7(3): p. 327-31.

[28] Erickson, S. J. and Q. H. Hogan, CT-guided injection of the stellate ganglion: description of technique and efficacy of sympathetic blockade. *Radiology,* 1993. 188(3): p. 707-9.

[29] Narouze, S., A. Vydyanathan, and N. Patel, Ultrasound-guided stellate ganglion block successfully prevented esophageal puncture. *Pain Physician,* 2007. 10(6): p. 747-52.

[30] Yucel, I., et al., Complex regional pain syndrome type I: efficacy of stellate ganglion blockade. *J Orthop Traumatol,* 2009. 10(4): p. 179-83.

[31] Ackerman, W. E. and J. M. Zhang, Efficacy of stellate ganglion blockade for the management of type 1 complex regional pain syndrome. *South Med J,* 2006. 99(10): p. 1084-8.

[32] Roy, C. and N. Chatterjee, Radiofrequency ablation of stellate ganglion in a patient with complex regional pain syndrome. *Saudi J Anaesth,* 2014. 8(3): p. 408-11.

[33] Kastler, A., et al., CT-guided stellate ganglion blockade vs. radiofrequency neurolysis in the management of refractory type I complex regional pain syndrome of the upper limb. *Eur Radiol,* 2013. 23(5): p. 1316-22.

[34] Yoo, S.D., et al., Efficacy of ultrasonography guided stellate ganglion blockade in the stroke patients with complex regional pain syndrome. *Ann Rehabil Med,* 2012. 36(5): p. 633-9.

[35] Skaebuland, C. and G. Racz, Indications and Technique of Thoracic(2) and Thoracic(3)Neurolysis. *Curr Rev Pain,* 1999. 3(5): p. 400-405.

[36] Wilkinson, H. A., Percutaneous radiofrequency upper thoracic sympathectomy. *Neurosurgery,* 1996. 38(4): p. 715-25.

[37] Wilkinson, H. A., Radiofrequency percutaneous upper-thoracic sympathectomy. Technique and review of indications. *N Engl J Med,* 1984. 311(1): p. 34-6.

[38] Chen, C. K., et al., Percutaneous t2 and t3 radiofrequency sympathectomy for complex regional pain syndrome secondary to brachial plexus injury: a case series. *Korean J Pain*, 2013. 26(4): p. 401-5.

[39] de Oliveira Rocha, R., et al., Thoracic sympathetic block for the treatment of complex regional pain syndrome type I: A double-blind randomized controlled study. *Pain*, 2014. 155(11): p. 2274-81.

[40] Redman, D. R., P.N. Robinson, and M.A. Al-Kutoubi, Computerised tomography guided lumbar sympathectomy. *Anaesthesia*, 1986. 41(1): p. 39-41.

[41] Konig, C. W., et al., MR-guided lumbar sympathicolysis. *Eur Radiol*, 2002. 12(6): p. 1388-93.

[42] Kirvela, O., E. Svedstrom, and N. Lundbom, Ultrasonic guidance of lumbar sympathetic and celiac plexus block: a new technique. *Reg Anesth*, 1992. 17(1): p. 43-6.

[43] Manjunath, P.S., et al., Management of lower limb complex regional pain syndrome type 1: an evaluation of percutaneous radiofrequency thermal lumbar sympathectomy versus phenol lumbar sympathetic neurolysis--a pilot study. *Anesth Analg*, 2008. 106(2): p. 647-9, table of contents.

[44] Akkoc, Y., et al., Complex regional pain syndrome in a patient with spinal cord injury: management with pulsed radiofrequency lumbar sympatholysis. *Spinal Cord*, 2008. 46(1): p. 82-4.

[45] Nordmann, G. R., G. R. Lauder, and D. J. Grier, Computed tomography guided lumbar sympathetic block for complex regional pain syndrome in a child: a case report and review. *Eur J Pain*, 2006. 10(5): p. 409-12.

[46] Turner, J. A., et al., The importance of placebo effects in pain treatment and research. *JAMA*, 1994. 271(20): p. 1609-14.

[47] Hrobjartsson, A. and P.C. Gotzsche, Placebo interventions for all clinical conditions. *Cochrane Database Syst Rev*, 2010(1): p. CD003974.

[48] Livingstone, J. A. and R. M. Atkins, Intravenous regional guanethidine blockade in the treatment of post-traumatic complex regional pain syndrome type 1 (algodystrophy) of the hand. *J Bone Joint Surg Br*, 2002. 84(3): p. 380-6.

[49] Lake, A. P., Intravenous regional sympathetic block: past, present and future? *Pain Res Manag*, 2004. 9(1): p. 35-7.

[50] Ramamurthy, S. and J. Hoffman, Intravenous regional guanethidine in the treatment of reflex sympathetic dystrophy/causalgia: a randomized, double-blind study. Guanethidine Study Group. *Anesth Analg*, 1995. 81(4): p. 718-23.

[51] Rocco, A.G., et al., A comparison of regional intravenous guanethidine and reserpine in reflex sympathetic dystrophy. A controlled, randomized, double-blind crossover study. *Clin J Pain*, 1989. 5(3): p. 205-9.

[52] Hord, A.H., et al., Intravenous regional bretylium and lidocaine for treatment of reflex sympathetic dystrophy: a randomized, double-blind study. *Anesth Analg*, 1992. 74(6): p. 818-21.

[53] Bonelli, S., et al., Regional intravenous guanethidine vs. stellate ganglion block in reflex sympathetic dystrophies: a randomized trial. *Pain*, 1983. 16(3): p. 297-307.

[54] Perez, R. S., et al., Evidence based guidelines for complex regional pain syndrome type 1. *BMC Neurol*, 2010. 10(1): p. 20.

[55] Margalit, D., et al., Complex regional pain syndrome, alexithymia, and psychological distress. *J Psychosom Res*, 2014. 77(4): p. 273-7.

[56] Marx, C., et al., Preventing recurrence of reflex sympathetic dystrophy in patients requiring an operative intervention at the site of dystrophy after surgery. *Clin Rheumatol*, 2001. 20(2): p. 114-8.

[57] Moseley, G. L., Is successful rehabilitation of complex regional pain syndrome due to sustained attention to the affected limb? A randomised clinical trial. *Pain*, 2005. 114(1-2): p. 54-61.

[58] Benson, H. and R. Friedman, Harnessing the power of the placebo effect and renaming it "remembered wellness." *Annu Rev Med*, 1996. 47: p. 193-9.

[59] Gotzsche, P.C., Is there logic in the placebo? *Lancet*, 1994. 344(8927): p. 925-6.

[60] Schwartzman, R.J., et al., Long-term outcome following sympathectomy for complex regional pain syndrome type 1 (RSD). *J Neurol Sci*, 1997. 150(2): p. 149-52.

[61] Bandyk, D.F., et al., Surgical sympathectomy for reflex sympathetic dystrophy syndromes. *J Vasc Surg*, 2002. 35(2): p. 269-77.

[62] Singh, B., et al., Sympathectomy for complex regional pain syndrome. *J Vasc Surg*, 2003. 37(3): p. 508-11.

[63] Happak, W., S. Sator-Katzenschlager, and L.K. Kriechbaumer, Surgical treatment of complex regional pain syndrome type II with regional subcutaneous venous sympathectomy. *J Trauma Acute Care Surg*, 2012. 72(6): p. 1647-53.

[64] Gibbons, J. J., et al., Interscalene blocks for chronic upper extremity pain. *Clin J Pain*, 1992. 8(3): p. 264-9.

[65] Toshniwal, G., et al., Management of complex regional pain syndrome type I in upper extremity-evaluation of continuous stellate ganglion block and continuous infraclavicular brachial plexus block: a pilot study. *Pain Med*, 2012. 13(1): p. 96-106.

[66] Borg, P.A. and H.J. Krijnen, Long-term intrathecal administration of midazolam and clonidine. *Clin J Pain*, 1996. 12(1): p. 63-8.

[67] Glynn, C. and K. O'Sullivan, A double-blind randomised comparison of the effects of epidural clonidine, lignocaine and the combination of clonidine and lignocaine in patients with chronic pain. *Pain*, 1996. 64(2): p. 337-43.

[68] Lin, T. C., et al., Long-term epidural ketamine, morphine and bupivacaine attenuate reflex sympathetic dystrophy neuralgia. *Can J Anaesth*, 1998. 45(2): p. 175-7.

[69] Rauck, R. L., et al., Epidural clonidine treatment for refractory reflex sympathetic dystrophy. *Anesthesiology*, 1993. 79(6): p. 1163-9; discussion 27A.

[70] Takahashi, H., et al., The NMDA-receptor antagonist ketamine abolishes neuropathic pain after epidural administration in a clinical case. *Pain*, 1998. 75(2-3): p. 391-4.

[71] Jadon, A. and P.S. Agarwal, Cervical Epidural Anaesthesia for Radical Mastectomy and Chronic Regional Pain Syndrome of upper limb-A Case Report. *Indian J Anaesth*, 2009. 53(6): p. 696-9.

[72] Moufawad, S., O. Malak, and N.A. Mekhail, Epidural infusion of opiates and local anesthetics for Complex Regional Pain Syndrome. *Pain Pract*, 2002. 2(2): p. 81-6.

[73] Saito, Y., et al., Complex regional pain syndrome in a 15-year-old girl successfully treated with continuous epidural anesthesia. *Brain Dev*, 2015. 37(1): p. 175-8.

[74] Truin, M., et al., Increased efficacy of early spinal cord stimulation in an animal model of neuropathic pain. *Eur J Pain*, 2011. 15(2): p. 111-7.

[75] Stanton-Hicks, M., Complex regional pain syndrome: manifestations and the role of neurostimulation in its management. *J Pain Symptom Manage*, 2006. 31(4 Suppl): p. S20-4.

[76] Kumar, K., S. Rizvi, and S.B. Bnurs, Spinal cord stimulation is effective in management of complex regional pain syndrome I: fact or fiction. *Neurosurgery*, 2011. 69(3): p. 566-78; discussion 5578-80.

[77] Melzack, R. and P.D. Wall, Pain mechanisms: a new theory. *Science,* 1965. 150(3699): p. 971-9.

[78] Kunnumpurath, S., R. Srinivasagopalan, and N. Vadivelu, Spinal cord stimulation: principles of past, present and future practice: a review. *J Clin Monit Comput,* 2009. 23(5): p. 333-9.

[79] Cui, J. G., et al., Effect of spinal cord stimulation on tactile hypersensitivity in mononeuropathic rats is potentiated by simultaneous GABA(B) and adenosine receptor activation. *Neurosci Lett,* 1998. 247(2-3): p. 183-6.

[80] Meyerson, B.A., et al., Modulation of spinal pain mechanisms by spinal cord stimulation and the potential role of adjuvant pharmacotherapy. *Stereotact Funct Neurosurg,* 1997. 68(1-4 Pt 1): p. 129-40.

[81] Larson, S. J., et al., Neurophysiological effects of dorsal column stimulation in man and monkey. *J Neurosurg,* 1974. 41(2): p. 217-23.

[82] Saade, N.E., et al., Supraspinal modulation of nociception in awake rats by stimulation of the dorsal column nuclei. *Brain Res,* 1986. 369(1-2): p. 307-10.

[83] Linderoth, B., I. Fedorcsak, and B.A. Meyerson, Is vasodilatation following dorsal column stimulation mediated by antidromic activation of small diameter afferents? *Acta Neurochir Suppl* (Wien), 1989. 46: p. 99-101.

[84] Oakley, J. C. and J.P. Prager, Spinal cord stimulation: mechanisms of action. *Spine* (Phila Pa 1976), 2002. 27(22): p. 2574-83.

[85] Barchini, J., et al., Spinal segmental and supraspinal mechanisms underlying the pain-relieving effects of spinal cord stimulation: an experimental study in a rat model of neuropathy. *Neuroscience,* 2012. 215: p. 196-208.

[86] Linderoth, B. and B. A. Meyerson, Spinal cord stimulation: exploration of the physiological basis of a widely used therapy. *Anesthesiology,* 2010. 113(6): p. 1265-7.

[87] Guan, Y., et al., Spinal cord stimulation-induced analgesia: electrical stimulation of dorsal column and dorsal roots attenuates dorsal horn neuronal excitability in neuropathic rats. *Anesthesiology,* 2010. 113(6): p. 1392-405.

[88] Wilder-Smith, O. H. and L. Arendt-Nielsen, Postoperative hyperalgesia: its clinical importance and relevance. Anesthesiology, 2006. 104(3): p. 601-7.

[89] Cook, A. J., et al., Dynamic receptive field plasticity in rat spinal cord dorsal horn following C-primary afferent input. Nature, 1987. 325(7000): p. 151-3.

[90] Ji, R.R., et al., Central sensitization and LTP: do pain and memory share similar mechanisms? *Trends Neurosci,* 2003. 26(12): p. 696-705.

[91] Cui, J. G., et al., Spinal cord stimulation attenuates augmented dorsal horn release of excitatory amino acids in mononeuropathy via a GABAergic mechanism. *Pain,* 1997. 73(1): p. 87-95.

[92] van Eijs, F., et al., Spinal cord stimulation in complex regional pain syndrome type I of less than 12-month duration. *Neuromodulation,* 2012. 15(2): p. 144-50; discussion 150.

[93] Harney, D., J.J. Magner, and D. O'Keeffe, Early intervention with spinal cord stimulation in the management of a chronic regional pain syndrome. *Ir Med J,* 2005. 98(3): p. 89-90.

[94] Saranita, J., D. Childs, and A.D. Saranita, Spinal cord stimulation in the treatment of complex regional pain syndrome (CRPS) of the lower extremity: a case report. *J Foot Ankle Surg,* 2009. 48(1): p. 52-5.

[95] Kemler, M.A., et al., Spinal cord stimulation in patients with chronic reflex sympathetic dystrophy. *N Engl J Med,* 2000. 343(9): p. 618-24.

[96] Oakley, J.C., Spinal cord stimulation: patient selection, technique, and outcomes. *Neurosurg Clin N Am,* 2003. 14(3): p. 365-80, vi.

[97] Ebel, H., et al., Augmentative treatment of chronic deafferentation pain syndromes after peripheral nerve lesions. *Minim Invasive Neurosurg,* 2000. 43(1): p. 44-50.

[98] Hassenbusch, S.J., et al., Long-term results of peripheral nerve stimulation for reflex sympathetic dystrophy. *J Neurosurg,* 1996. 84(3): p. 415-23.

[99] Forouzanfar, T., et al., Spinal cord stimulation in complex regional pain syndrome: cervical and lumbar devices are comparably effective. *Br J Anaesth,* 2004. 92(3): p. 348-53.

[100] Verdolin, M.H., E.T. Stedje-Larsen, and A.H. Hickey, Ten consecutive cases of complex regional pain syndrome of less than 12 months duration in active duty United States military personnel treated with spinal cord stimulation. *Anesth Analg,* 2007. 104(6): p. 1557-60, table of contents.

[101] Kemler, M. A., et al., The effect of spinal cord stimulation in patients with chronic reflex sympathetic dystrophy: Two years' follow-up of the randomized controlled trial. *Ann Neurol,* 2004. 55(1): p. 13-18.

[102] Simpson, E. L., et al., Spinal cord stimulation for chronic pain of neuropathic or ischaemic origin: systematic review and economic evaluation. *Health Technol Assess,* 2009. 13(17): p. iii, ix-x, 1-154.

[103] Taylor, R. S., J.P. Van Buyten, and E. Buchser, Spinal cord stimulation for complex regional pain syndrome: a systematic review of the clinical and cost-effectiveness literature and assessment of prognostic factors. *Eur J Pain,* 2006. 10(2): p. 91-101.

[104] Kumar, K., et al., Complications of spinal cord stimulation, suggestions to improve outcome, and financial impact. *J Neurosurg Spine,* 2006. 5(3): p. 191-203.

[105] Kemler, M. A., et al., Effect of spinal cord stimulation for chronic complex regional pain syndrome Type I: five-year final follow-up of patients in a randomized controlled trial. *J Neurosurg,* 2008. 108(2): p. 292-8.

[106] van Eijs, F., et al., Brush-evoked allodynia predicts outcome of spinal cord stimulation in complex regional pain syndrome type 1. *Eur J Pain,* 2010. 14(2): p. 164-9.

[107] Calvillo, O., et al., Neuroaugmentation in the treatment of complex regional pain syndrome of the upper extremity. *Acta Orthop Belg,* 1998. 64(1): p. 57-63.

[108] Kemler, M. A., et al., Electrical spinal cord stimulation in reflex sympathetic dystrophy: retrospective analysis of 23 patients. *J Neurosurg,* 1999. 90(1 Suppl): p. 79-83.

[109] Harke, H., et al., Spinal cord stimulation in sympathetically maintained complex regional pain syndrome type I with severe disability. A prospective clinical study. *Eur J Pain,* 2005. 9(4): p. 363-73.

[110] Kemler, M. A., et al., Pain relief in complex regional pain syndrome due to spinal cord stimulation does not depend on vasodilation. *Anesthesiology,* 2000. 92(6): p. 1653-60.

[111] Deer, T. R., et al., A prospective study of dorsal root ganglion stimulation for the relief of chronic pain. *Neuromodulation,* 2013. 16(1): p. 67-71; discussion 71-2.

[112] van Bussel, C. M., D. L. Stronks, and F.J. Huygen, Successful Treatment of Intractable Complex Regional Pain Syndrome Type I of the Knee With Dorsal Root Ganglion Stimulation: A Case Report. *Neuromodulation,* 2014.

[113] Van Buyten, J. P., et al., Stimulation of dorsal root Ganglia for the management of complex regional pain syndrome: a prospective case series. *Pain Pract*, 2015. 15(3): p. 208-16.

[114] Liem, L., et al., A multicenter, prospective trial to assess the safety and performance of the spinal modulation dorsal root ganglion neurostimulator system in the treatment of chronic pain. *Neuromodulation*, 2013. 16(5): p. 471-82; discussion 482.

[115] Cruccu, G., et al., EFNS guidelines on neurostimulation therapy for neuropathic pain. *Eur J Neurol*, 2007. 14(9): p. 952-70.

[116] Deer, T. R., et al., The appropriate use of neurostimulation of the spinal cord and peripheral nervous system for the treatment of chronic pain and ischemic diseases: the Neuromodulation Appropriateness Consensus Committee. *Neuromodulation*, 2014. 17(6): p. 515-50; discussion 550.

[117] Mobbs, R. J., S. Nair, and P. Blum, Peripheral nerve stimulation for the treatment of chronic pain. *J Clin Neurosci*, 2007. 14(3): p. 216-21; discussion 222-3.

[118] Kanoff, R. B., Intraspinal delivery of opiates by an implantable, programmable pump in patients with chronic, intractable pain of nonmalignant origin. *J Am Osteopath Assoc*, 1994. 94(6): p. 487-93.

[119] Kapural, L., et al., Intrathecal ziconotide for complex regional pain syndrome: seven case reports. *Pain Pract*, 2009. 9(4): p. 296-303.

[120] Goto, S., et al., Spinal cord stimulation and intrathecal baclofen therapy: combined neuromodulation for treatment of advanced complex regional pain syndrome. *Stereotact Funct Neurosurg*, 2013. 91(6): p. 386-91.

[121] van Hilten, B. J., et al., Intrathecal baclofen for the treatment of dystonia in patients with reflex sympathetic dystrophy. *N Engl J Med*, 2000. 343(9): p. 625-30.

[122] van Rijn, M. A., et al., Intrathecal baclofen for dystonia of complex regional pain syndrome. *Pain*, 2009. 143(1-2): p. 41-7.

[123] Lundborg, C., et al., Clinical experience using intrathecal (IT) bupivacaine infusion in three patients with complex regional pain syndrome type I (CRPS-I). *Acta Anaesthesiol Scand*, 1999. 43(6): p. 667-78.

[124] Zuniga, R. E., S. Perera, and S.E. Abram, Intrathecal baclofen: a useful agent in the treatment of well-established complex regional pain syndrome. *Reg Anesth Pain Med*, 2002. 27(1): p. 90-3.

[125] Stanton-Hicks, M. and L. Kapural, An effective treatment of severe complex regional pain syndrome type 1 in a child using high doses of intrathecal ziconotide. *J Pain Symptom Manage*, 2006. 32(6): p. 509-11.

[126] Kanpolat, Y., et al., Spinal and nucleus caudalis dorsal root entry zone operations for chronic pain. *Neurosurgery*, 2008. 62(3 Suppl 1): p. 235-42; discussion 242-4.

[127] Sindou, M., et al., Selective posterior rhizotomy in the dorsal root entry zone for treatment of hyperspasticity and pain in the hemiplegic upper limb. *Neurosurgery*, 1986. 18(5): p. 587-95.

[128] Nashold, B. S., Jr., et al., A new design of radiofrequency lesion electrodes for use in the caudalis nucleus DREZ operation. Technical note. *J Neurosurg*, 1994. 80(6): p. 1116-20.

[129] Kanpolat, Y., et al., A curative treatment option for Complex Regional Pain Syndrome (CRPS) Type I: dorsal root entry zone operation (report of two cases). *Turk Neurosurg*, 2014. 24(1): p. 127-30.

[130] Parmar, V. K., et al., Supraspinal stimulation for treatment of refractory pain. *Clin Neurol Neurosurg*, 2014. 123: p. 155-63.

[131] Levy, R., T. R. Deer, and J. Henderson, Intracranial neurostimulation for pain control: a review. *Pain Physician*, 2010. 13(2): p. 157-65.

[132] Nguyen, J. P., et al., Chronic motor cortex stimulation in the treatment of central and neuropathic pain. Correlations between clinical, electrophysiological and anatomical data. *Pain*, 1999. 82(3): p. 245-51.

[133] Meyerson, B. A., et al., Motor cortex stimulation as treatment of trigeminal neuropathic pain. *Acta Neurochir Suppl* (Wien), 1993. 58: p. 150-3.

[134] Nguyen, J. P., et al., Treatment of deafferentation pain by chronic stimulation of the motor cortex: report of a series of 20 cases. *Acta Neurochir Suppl*, 1997. 68: p. 54-60.

[135] Katayama, Y., C. Fukaya, and T. Yamamoto, Poststroke pain control by chronic motor cortex stimulation: neurological characteristics predicting a favorable response. *J Neurosurg*, 1998. 89(4): p. 585-91.

[136] Pirotte, B., et al., Combination of functional magnetic resonance imaging-guided neuronavigation and intraoperative cortical brain mapping improves targeting of motor cortex stimulation in neuropathic pain. *Neurosurgery*, 2005. 56(2 Suppl): p. 344-59; discussion 344-59.

[137] Rainov, N. G., et al., Epidural electrical stimulation of the motor cortex in patients with facial neuralgia. *Clin Neurol Neurosurg*, 1997. 99(3): p. 205-9.

[138] Roux, F. E., et al., Chronic motor cortex stimulation for phantom limb pain: a functional magnetic resonance imaging study: technical case report. *Neurosurgery*, 2001. 48(3): p. 681-7; discussion 687-8.

[139] Gharabaghi, A., et al., Volumetric image guidance for motor cortex stimulation: integration of three-dimensional cortical anatomy and functional imaging. *Neurosurgery*, 2005. 57(1 Suppl): p. 114-20; discussion 114-20.

[140] Nuti, C., et al., Motor cortex stimulation for refractory neuropathic pain: four year outcome and predictors of efficacy. *Pain*, 2005. 118(1-2): p. 43-52.

[141] Raslan, A. M., et al., Motor cortex stimulation for trigeminal neuropathic or deafferentation pain: an institutional case series experience. *Stereotact Funct Neurosurg*, 2011. 89(2): p. 83-8.

[142] Bonicalzi, V. and S. Canavero, Motor cortex stimulation for central and neuropathic pain (Letter regarding Topical Review by Brown and Barbaro). *Pain*, 2004. 108(1-2): p. 199-200; author reply 200.

[143] Tsubokawa, T., et al., Chronic motor cortex stimulation for the treatment of central pain. *Acta Neurochir Suppl* (Wien), 1991. 52: p. 137-9.

[144] Tsubokawa, T., et al., Treatment of thalamic pain by chronic motor cortex stimulation. *Pacing Clin Electrophysiol*, 1991. 14(1): p. 131-4.

[145] Lefaucheur, J. P., Y. Keravel, and J.P. Nguyen, Treatment of poststroke pain by epidural motor cortex stimulation with a new octopolar lead. *Neurosurgery*, 2011. 68(1 Suppl Operative): p. 180-7; discussion 187.

[146] Saitoh, Y., et al., Motor cortex stimulation for deafferentation pain. *Neurosurg Focus*, 2001. 11(3): p. E1.

[147] Saitoh, Y., et al., Primary motor cortex stimulation within the central sulcus for treating deafferentation pain. *Acta Neurochir Suppl*, 2003. 87: p. 149-52.

In: Complex Regional Pain Syndrome
Editors: Nader D. Nader and Ognjen Visnjevac

ISBN: 978-1-63483-130-7
© 2015 Nova Science Publishers, Inc.

Chapter 7

PHYSICAL THERAPY AND FUNCTIONAL REHABILITATION

Kellie Jaremko[1,], PhD and Bernard Hsu[2], MD*
[1]Jefferson Medical College, Philadelphia, PA, US
[2]Clinical Assistant Professor, Anesthesiology and Pain Management,
University at Buffalo, Buffalo, NY, US

INTRODUCTION

The goal of physiotherapy has always been and will always be to re-establish function with a prominent secondary objective of pain reduction. The challenge arises in modality selection to optimize functional outcomes without causing unnecessary discomfort to our patients. Over the years, as our understanding of complex regional pain syndrome (CRPS) pathophysiology has deepened, so has our repertoire of established treatment techniques in the realm of non-medicinal and non-surgical rehabilitation. Conversely, early physical interventions without substantiated scientific backing or published clinical benefit have fallen out of practice. This chapter will explore both the historical underpinnings of physical therapy and rehabilitation in CRPS, as well as delve into the clinical evidence to support or negate these treatments in addition to emerging and promising therapies of the future.

STANDARD PHYSICAL AND OCCUPATIONAL THERAPY: THE ROLE OF EXERCISE

It is unsurprising that laying hands on someone to heal them was one of many historical treatments for CRPS. Given the ease of application and apparent increased blood flow resultant from connective tissue massage (CTM), its use was one of the predecessors to physical therapy (PT) in chronic pain. CTM was found to induce local analgesia, in addition to nondescript autonomic effects when applied to the thorax. This was noted in a case report

---

[*] Medical student; E-mail: kmjaremko@gmail.com.

by Frazer and advocated by some clinical expert opinions. [1-3] The efficacy and feasibility of broad compression massage to lessen pain in spinal cord injuries was recently assessed. Chase et. al. demonstrated non-inferiority of massage to controlled light contact touch, despite excellent safety and tolerability. [4] Neither the efficacy nor harm of massage, however, was further documented for use in CRPS, nor were consistent long-term benefits observed in control subjects. [5]

Transcutaneous electrical nerve stimulation (TENS), in the 1980s, was developing a reputation for improving pain tolerance and case reports suggested that in CRPS TENS elicited pain relief. [6-8] The proposed mechanism of relief in CPRS was via decreased sympathetic tone. Presumably this led to vasomotor dilation and potential temperature normalization in the affected limb. Thacker and Gilford astutely put, however, this possible benefit assumes a purely peripheral sympathetic dysfunction that is correctable. [9, 10] Ultimately the intermittent exacerbation of allodynia associated with TENS use, in the absence of clear clinical support, has led to a trend of discontinued use. Similarly treatments, such as vasomotor challenge and splinting, while well-meaning at the time, are without definitive clinical evidence. [9, 10] In fact, these therapeutic interventions are now considered relatively contraindicated in light of studies showing the role of hypoxia and immobilization in the generation of the pathologic state of an affected limb (discussed further in physiology section of this chapter). [11-16]

In the late 1990s and early 2000s, primarily driven by review of evidence-based medicine (EBM), there was a shift away from splinting, CTM, and TENS in CRPS to a paradigm starting at desensitization. Progression through passive flexibility and isometric exercises follows to active range of motion (ROM), aerobic exercise, and finally specific vocational and occupational rehabilitation. [10, 17, 18] Desensitization can be described as the process of gradually applying tactile stimuli with an increasing intensity of textural, pressure, and sensory activation. For example, a desensitization tactic may employ the application of silk to an area of allodynia, transitioned to cotton cloth, followed by sandpaper. Immersion of the affected extremity sequentially into contrast baths of different temperatures with an expanding divergence of temperature over time is another form of desensitization. Incorporation of vibration and passive movement constitute additional applications of desensitization treatment. [9, 18] Overall the intent of desensitization is a gradual normalization of sensory input to "reset the central nervous system." [19] More recent utilization of this concept has been incorporated to reduce pain-related fear associated with movement (discussed further in section three of this chapter). [20] Concern of re-injury is not without merit in aggressive and abrupt range of motion challenges, whether passively (often facilitated by regional anesthesia) or actively, which necessitate gentle progression toward active movement. This anecdotal but logical concept has been relatively unstudied in a focused manner but the benefits of safely reaching the point of active movement in the affected limb are nearly unanimously accepted to be of long-term functional benefit. Persistent allodynia agitating ineffectively desensitized areas is a poor prognostic indicator of CRPS recovery and highlights the conceivable importance of correcting this abnormality. [21] The remainder of this section will focus on the physiological basis for the favorable outcomes of exercise and activity, as well as the efficacy, limitations, and implications of its use in clinical studies and our patients.

PHYSIOLOGY

Both the importance of extremity mobility in the maintenance of normal function and, conversely, role of immobilization in the pathophysiology of CRPS was shown by 28-day scaphoid cast immobilization in a cohort of healthy controls by Terkelson et. al. [14] While no subjects had spontaneous pain upon cast removal, 90% of participants had joint-related pain that persisted for an average of 6.3 days at sites proximal to the cast and up to 2.1 days as distally as the elbow joint with maximal duration of movement-induced pain out to two weeks. Further, pain threshold at skin folds were decreased, cold hyperalgesia increased, and there was a temperature discrepancy between the skin of the casted and control hand that persisted for 3 days after cast removal. Uncasted control patients exhibited none of these signs or symptoms. While this study does not recapitulate all of the Budapest CRPS diagnostic criteria (discussed in Chapter 4), it does implicate physiologic changes during immobilization that likely contribute to the development of CRPS. Pepper et. al. demonstrated similar pathologic findings after elective wrist surgery and although without a control group, this study probes within the most common site for CRPS development, according to the three existing population-based studies in the USA, Netherlands, and Taiwan; injury to the upper limb. [16, 22-24] In this study, vascular and trophic changes were observed with moderate to severe pain that persisted within the post-surgical hand for up to a month and exhibited neuropathic characteristics in 23% at onset and in 35% one-month later (assessed with the Leeds Assessment of Neuropathic Symptoms and Signs). Skin biopsies likewise showed increased concentrations of pro-inflammatory mediators, interleukin-6 (IL-6) and tissue necrosis factor alpha (TNF-α), compared to the contralateral hand to surgery. Animal studies of fracture and nerve injury with immediate immobilization likewise showed evidence of allodynia and hyperalgesia, in addition to pro-inflammatory up-regulation in the injured limb, including IL-6, TNF-α, and substance P. [15, 25]

The consequential pro-inflammatory findings from immobilization and nerve injury have been hypothesized to contribute to CRPS pathophysiology (discussed in detail in Chapters 2 and 3) and evidence in exercise trials, of both animals and patients, suggest possible reversibility of this state by exercise. A 12-week flexibility and muscle strengthening training program in individuals with knee osteoarthritis (OA) was conducted and compared to non-exercise controls with OA. This study displayed subjective improvement in pain on a visual analog scale (VAS) and the Western Ontario and McMaster Universities questionnaire subscale following an extended exercise regimen. [26] Aguiar et. al. additionally confirmed that serum levels of IL-6 were significantly reduced in the participants that underwent exercise. TNF-α levels were not appreciably changed in this model, which may be due to the short 2-hour half-life of TNF-α in blood, dilution throughout the body of the individual versus a sample isolated from the site of inflammation, or may be a consequence of the modality and load applied during exercise, as the authors note in their discussion. [26] Furthermore, exercise appeared to have a beneficial impact on pain perception and some markers of systemic inflammation. Assessment of localized changes in inflammatory markers was undertaken by Helmark et. al., again in knee OA, with acute resistance exercise and microdialysis catheters in the intraarticular and synovial spaces. [27] Over the three hours following exercise fluid was collected and normalized to relative recovery rate by a radioactively-labeled glucose perfusion of catheters. Anti-inflammatory interleukin-10 (IL-

10) was significantly elevated in the exercise group alone. IL-6, conversely was increased in both locations regardless of exercise participation, suggesting that exercise may be therapeutic but also noting that inactivity is not the sole causative source of inflammation (as assessed by IL-6 concentrations) in this OA model. [27]

Animal experiments have paralleled these clinical studies and suggest exercise, specifically aerobic treadmill running, is protective against post-operative pain and systemic inflammatory conditions. A chronic heart failure rat model ran for 50 minutes a day, five days a week for two months and resulted in significantly reduced pro-inflammatory IL-6, TNF-α and increased anti-inflammatory IL-10 than their sedentary counterparts. [28] Analogous work in a post-incisional rat model with a month of comparable exercise intensity showed a quicker recovery from mechanical hypersensitivity at the surgical site and attenuated upregulation of IL-6, substance P, and interleukin-1β within the dorsal root ganglion, where the cell body of afferent neurons reside, by day 28 compared to non-exercised controls. [29] Aggravation of local damage and ensuing inflammatory infiltration may be partially modified by reactive oxygen species (ROS). ROS while necessary for modulation and priming of muscle contraction, antioxidant protection, and oxidative injury repair, in excess may cause muscular damage. In biopsy samples from CRPS patients that underwent amputation, a disrupted system of mitochondrial function was identified and found to result in decreased ATP production, substrate oxidation rates, and increased ROS. [30, 31] This is consistent with prior reports of increased serum lipid peroxidation induced by ROS in CRPS. Regular exercise does generate ROS but is presumed to act as a preconditioning tool to enhance the adaptive zone between functional and biological limitations, such that there is a protective effect when ROS are reintroduced. Inactivity conversely may trigger a decreased adaptive zone and predispose to ROS mediated injury, which suggests that regular non-exhaustive exercise in CRPS may reverse or stave off the ROS injury prone state in muscles themselves. [32]

Exercise has been implicated to counteract additional putative CRPS pathophysiology mechanisms, such as vasomotor control, adrenergic tone, and cortical plasticity. Unsurprisingly 8-10 weeks of treadmill training in rats increased the functional vasodilation of limb arterioles (20%) and improved the capillary–to-muscle fiber ratio by 15%. [33] Even in aging arteries, exercise has been demonstrated to restore vasodilatory properties through maintenance of large-conductance calcium-activated potassium channel (MaxiK) protein levels in mesenteric arteries of a rat model that are normally down-regulated with advancing age. [34] Adrenergic tone within blood vessels is known to modulate arteriole dilation and initial decreases in catecholamine circulation within the CRPS site is postulated to up-regulate peripheral activating alpha-1-adrenergic receptors. This causes heightened sensitivity to subsequent epinephrine exposure through compensatory denervation-induced dysfunction of the peripheral sympathetic system. [35] Exercise may thwart this change by engaging opposing inhibitory alpha-2-adrenergic receptors (α2-AR) in the periphery. In support of this hypothesis, wild-type rats and mice who underwent aerobic and resistance exercise demonstrated higher nociceptive thresholds as opposed to α2-AR knockout mice or those exposed to peripheral and specific α2-AR receptor antagonists. [36] Exercise also causes a breakdown of ATP, resulting in increased serum and therefore extracellular adenosine, which can in turn regulate blood flow, epinephrine release, and pain transmission. [37] Peripherally this was validated in an animal model of CRPS that found high intensity swimming to decrease mechanical allodynia only in the absence of adenosine receptor-1 antagonists. [38]

Additional animal studies have shown exercise-induced release of endogenous opioids and axonal regeneration of injured peripheral nerves. [39-41]

Finally, cortical changes observed in brain imaging can be positively impacted by exercise. A discussion of the somatosensory cortex changes seen in CRPS will be discussed in section two. Immobilization, can represent the most polar opposite state to exercise and directed movement training. In a small human study, eight weeks of ankle immobilization was sufficient to slow transmission of indirect corticospinal motor pathways in response to transcranial magnetic stimulation (TMS) without affecting spinal reflexes. [42] Constraint-induced movement therapy in stroke survivors that undertook intense rehabilitation had the opposite effect with functional magnetic resonance imaging (fMRI) changes observed in sensorimotor cortical activation and corticospinal activity following TMS that correlated with clinical progress in hand motor function. [43] Similarly, individuals with upper extremity paresis, following stroke, that were trained with therapeutic exercise for six weeks displayed fMRI activation changes that again correlated with functional ability. [44] Taubert et. al. found motor training initially resulted in greater functional connectivity between frontal and parietal networks. Long-term effects were seen in structural changes and white matter connectivity, which were observed over a six-week course of motor training. These findings are suggestive of lasting benefits due to exercise at a neural network level. [45] Overall stimulation of the motor cortex, via implanted electrodes or exercise training, initiated improved motor function and associated analgesic effects. [46, 47]

Logistic Considerations

Despite physiological evidence to suggest the benefit of exercise and active movement in CRPS, the heterogeneity of this population, time of presentation, necessary concurrent pain and medical therapy, and inconsistent diagnostic evaluation and treatment makes clinical interpretation of efficacy much more convoluted than animal or controlled human studies. The utmost confounding aspect within active treatment studies is the reality that pain often prohibits an individuals' ability to fully participate, regardless of intention. For instance, in a patient with mechanical allodynia or hypersensitivity to temperature simultaneous pharmaceutical analgesia may be required for the patient to tolerate the painful desensitization process. Similarly, greater than 20% of participants in Kemler's randomized control trial (RCT) that were initially within the PT only arm crossed over to inclusion of spinal cord stimulation (SCS) with PT. [48] This may have been due to the intolerance of long-term PT in the absence of adequate concomitant pain control – a notion that is supported by this study's findings, emphasizing that at one year pain was improved in the SCS and PT group but worsened in the PT only group (Change in pain score: SCS + PT= -2.7, PT= 0.4, p<0.001). By nonmaleficence and our empathetic clinical desire to help our patients, pharmaceutical or interventional adjuvant therapies are almost universally offered in conjunction with physical therapy. Ideally this multimodal approach enables full patient participation and optimal attainment of the benefits from activity. [49, 50]

The presence of other, albeit often necessary, concurrent interventions complicate translation of the pure effects of activity and exercise. In the present recommendations for CRPS patient management, physical therapy is a strongly advocated as an adjunct to all other interventions. Therefore pure physiotherapy application is often absent in CRPS studies except in children, wherein invasive or unpleasant therapeutic options are more stringently reserved in lieu of more natural activities, like letting, if not encouraging, a child to actively play.

EFFICACY

Although a more detailed investigation of CPRS in children will be discussed in Chapter 9, the isolated exercise and PT effects evaluated by Sherry et. al. will be reviewed briefly here. This work was a replication and expansion (n=103) of a smaller study of exercise in children by Ruggeri et. al (n=6), both of which showed drastic improvement in pain from activity in this population (initial recovery in 92%). [51, 52] Severely disabled children of a mean age of 13 were weaned off any medicinal therapy and subsequently treated 5 days/week with 4-6 hours a day of exercise training in the form of PT, occupational therapy (OT), and hydrotherapy, as well as 45 minutes to 3 hours of "homework exercise" for weekend and evening hours. Specifically activities included jumping, running stairs, sports drills, weight-bearing functional tasks, bilateral coordinated movements on trampolines or in the pool, and desensitization in children that had allodynia at baseline. Follow-up for more than two years was possible with 49 of the initial participants and within this cohort 88% were asymptomatic despite fifteen (31%) of these having had a least one recurrence, usually within the first 6-months after treatment, that resolved with reinstitution of the exercise program. Five individuals (10% of children) had mild persistent pain that did not interrupt function and one child had persistent incapacitating symptoms at follow-up. This study appeared to support prior trials that found benefits of exercise therapy in this population and outperformed more invasive multimodal programs that reported more than half of subjects had residual pain and dysfunction. [53] Caveats of this apparent success lie in the study limitations and lack of generalizability to adult CRPS. Study dropout rate was greater than 50% by follow-up, which without data may all represent failures of therapy and success was only measured in completers potentially misleading the reader. Secondly, adult CRPS is by nature more traumatic, persistent, and refractory to treatment, perhaps due to less inherent cortical plasticity with aging. Notwithstanding these limitations, by engaging participants in enjoyable activities that were translatable to home and outpatient settings, there was ownership of one's treatment (with family support). This philosophy allowed for individualized up/down-titration of activity with improvements, setbacks, or recurrences, which likely imparted some of the lasting long-term benefits observed in this collective at follow-up and is a worthy point to consider for treatment planning of all chronic pain patients.

Early physiotherapy in adult CRPS was modeled after Watson's active stress loading design for upper extremities. [54] This paradigm consisted of active traction and compression that provided stressful stimulation and weight bearing without movement of the affected joints until pain and swelling were decreased. Active ROM could be added once tolerance to stress loading activities developed with concomitant incrementally improved function. This approach prevented contracture and fibrosis, specifically in the hand, during the interim when pain prohibited more aggressive motion. Two distinct activities formed the framework of this program: "scrub" and "carry." Scrubbing was defined as the act of pretending to scrub the floor or table with simultaneous weight-bearing pressure on the affected arm and repetitive back and forth motions At the beginning, three minutes of steady scrubbing three times a day was recommended then increased to five and seven minute increments as tolerated over the following weeks. Increased weight of a carried bag in the extended affected arm throughout the day constituted the second portion of the individualized, outpatient, and consistent commitment to treatment employed by the stress loading program. Application of this program to 52 subjects, each enrolled between one week to three years following CRPS diagnosis and for an average duration of 3.3 months, resulted in improved pain in 88%, motion in 95%, and grip strength in all participants with 84% of previously employed subjects returning to work at program completion. [54] Recovery at the time of this study was attributed to rapid restoration of normal neurovascular relationships and illustrated in three case reports within the study. Limitations of this study consist of missing or unintentionally overlooked information, including the potential use of medications throughout treatment, influence of typical daily activities outside of therapy, number of return visits to the clinic, overall compliance, previous treatment exposure, and the absence of a study control group that were randomized or opted out of this specific program.

The first prospective RCT analyzing effectiveness of PT or OT, versus a social support control in acute upper extremity CRPS (diagnosed within the year prior to study enrollment) was performed by Oerlemans et. al. All participants (n=135) received medical treatment including free-radical scavengers, peripheral vasodilators (in "cold CRPS"), and the option of trigger point treatment. Despite the conceivable contributions of this therapeutics, and the self-admitted difficulty in truly blinding participants to their treatment arm, this study exceled in their well-designed control study arm with similar clinician interactions and follow-up, thus removing the risk that structured supportive therapy of any kind would provide benefit compared with a veritably ignored cohort. With assessments of pain by VAS, both PT and OT had significant improvement in pain compared to control with more substantial analgesia at one year follow-up in the PT group than in the OT group. Active ROM at the wrist, thumb, and fingers were most improved in the PT group at most time points except for at one year. [55] Additional analyses with respect to impairment ratings and cost-effectiveness in this trial were also done and generally showed consistent benefit of PT greater than OT, both of which were still superior to control treatment. At first application of the American Medical Association's Guide to Evaluation of Permanent Impairment scores showed no significant differences between scores of treatment groups in mean whole body impairments. [56]

The authors discussed the absence of pain perception, the presence of trophic or vasomotor changes, and a patient's subjective feeling of recovery, within this impairment rating scale and looked at the body as a whole instead of just the affected limb. To more thoroughly assess impairment, re-analysis was achieved by compiling collected data into an impairment level score that included pain assessment by VAS, the McGill pain questionnaire, hand temperature changes, hand vasomotor changes, and active ROM for five joints. [57] With this template, PT demonstrated a clinically significant improvement of 6 points over controls. OT patients similarly improved by 4 points, which was also significant versus social work controls. No disability or handicap level, sub-type differences were observed at follow-up. Cost effectiveness relative to the larger improvements in function was dominated by PT. [58]

To address the efficacy of physical therapy in chronic CRPS (>six months duration since diagnosis), few RCT studies exist that were targeted at PT alone and are often designed to test another intervention with PT alone as the control group. Kemler et. al. studied the impact of SCS, with or without permanent implant, (n=36 and 24, respectively) in conjunction with 6-months of PT compared with PT alone (n=18) and followed these individuals for five years. Follow-up assessments at 6-months, one and two years showed significant improvements in pain perception and global perceived effect within the SCS group, however PT alone was non-inferior with respect to functional status and long-term pain, temperature, or pressure thresholds. [59-61] By five years post-treatment there was no difference between the groups with respect to pain.

Although not the intent of the study, pain trended down over time in all groups, albeit more in the dual intervention subjects, suggesting a beneficial role of PT, especially in combination with pain lowering therapies. [48] The non-randomized control study performed by this group that predated SCS intervention, found that PT alone did not improve overall function or patient satisfaction. Subgroup analyses did find that subjects with better baseline function, lower pain, absence of allodynia, and shorter duration of CRPS had the best outcomes, which supports the notion that excessive pain and prolonged pain can be helped by PT but only in the context of effective pain management. [60] Case reports suggest a possible role of PT manipulation following nerve blocks to prevent contracture and work on ROM physiotherapy but eloquent clinical trials are absent and prevent formal recommendations for this permutation of pain control and physiotherapy combinations. [62, 63]

COMPLICATIONS AND IMPLICATIONS FOR TREATMENT

The strength and frequency of clinical evidence for PT in the treatment of CRPS have been assessed by evidence-based review articles that determined the presence of high quality or moderately sized RCTs, non-controlled studies, and expert opinion publications in this realm. Perez et. al. found level two evidence ($\geq$ 2 moderate RCTs) for physiotherapy benefitting upper limb forms of CRPS with respect to function and coping. [64] Less convincing evidence was found for the use of PT in chronic CRPS and the commonly purported statement that PT should be a part of standard therapy was only supported by the opinions of experts (least strongly validated level of evidence). Daly and Bialocerkowski commented on the lack of separate and adequately controlled or designed studies to determine the true efficacy of PT yet "…the very nature of CRPS-I require that multiple disciplines contribute to this painful, disabling, and distressing condition. Therefore, perhaps determining the effect of physiotherapy in isolation is not a helpful exercise." [65] Nevertheless, more recent integrated mind-body targeted physical rehabilitation, such as graded motor imagery, mirror therapy, and graded exposure therapy, have demonstrated evidence of clinical benefit and will be discussed further in the following sections. These additional interventions build upon the idea that getting to a point of increased activity will benefit long-term outcomes in CRPS.

GRADED MOTOR IMAGERY, MIRROR THERAPY, AND FUNCTIONAL IMAGING: COMBATING DISTORTED BODY PERCEPTIONS AT A NEURONAL AND BEHAVIORAL LEVEL

A sense of frustration and denial towards a perceived imperfection in form or function of one's body is a relatable concept, although generally perceived in a transient subjective state of mind. A constant preoccupation with anatomically incongruent thoughts, however, is considered body dysmorphic disorder. Cortical injury to the non-dominant parietal, temporal, or frontal lobes, conversely, may cause hemi-spatial inattention, absent awareness, or visual neglect to an entire side or portion of the body. Pathologically altered perceptions of the body have been observed in chronic pain patients with aspects from both ends of the awareness spectrum. Anger is a prevalent emotion in chronic pain and among targets of this resentment, up to 74% of patients reported that their aggravation was at least partially directed at themselves. [66] Interviewing patients suffering from chronic back pain (CBP) revealed a counterintuitive lack of conscious attention to self until pain was elicited, which then prompted robust attentiveness and a corresponding exclusion of that body area from their ideal imagined self-concept. [67] Similarly, Lewis et. al. identified six recurring thought schemas conveyed by a collection of CRPS patients: hostile feelings towards the affected limb, differing levels of dissociation from that body part, a replicable disparity between stimuli in reality and those reported at the painful extremity, a distorted mental image of the affected limb with decreased awareness of its spatial position, and finally a correspondingly altered conscious attention towards the CRPS site. [68] Analogous anecdotal descriptions are present throughout the literature that have been termed a "Body Perception Disturbance" (BPD) with a prevalence of 54.4 – 84% in CRPS. Potentially important for our discussion, BPD may cause poorer integration of the affected limb into rehabilitation. [69, 70] Research has focused on dissociation, positional awareness abnormalities, somatosensory dysfunction, and identified both anatomical and perceptual size-incongruent manifestations of BPD.

A neglect-like behavior within CRPS was first described by Galer et. al. and divided into the "cognitive" neglect akin to a dissociated sense of their affected limb, defined as "not being a part of them," and the "motor neglect" component that, by definition, required "focused mental and visual attention in order to voluntarily move their limb." [71, 72] In a total of 242 patients, 84% endorsed at least one statement of neglect-like behavior with 47% confirming personal conduct from both cognitive and motor types of neglect. Many wrote in the comments about the embarrassing and negative impact these symptoms were having on their life. [72] Elevated neglect-like symptoms with greater severity have been found in CRPS patients compared to controls. Comparison between CRPS and non-CRPS unilateral limb pain demonstrated neglect-like symptoms in both but the odds of confirming a given symptom were three times higher in CRPS, which also displayed heightened symptom severity and amplified pain. [73] Affirmation of all five symptoms (affected limb is foreign, requires concerted effort to move, lies still in absence of effort, moves involuntarily, and feels dead) resulted in a diagnostic specificity upwards of 90% for CRPS, although this scale had poor sensitivity (21%) with respect to differentiating unilateral pain type. This apparent neglect is notably different than the unilateral or hemi-neglect observed in right-sided parietal strokes. Following strokes early onset visual, spatial, and attentional left-sided deficits are observed that are body-side specific versus the reference frame-specific changes recounted in

CRPS. [74] This difference is perhaps best illuminated by studies evaluating the effects of crossing limbs on somatosensory perception. In normal healthy controls there is a decreased perceived sensation of touch and pain from noxious or non-painful stimuli from the same hand once it crosses to the opposite side of the body, which corresponded to a decreased multimodal processing electroencephalogram (EEG) signal. [75] In CRPS patients, the ability to identify the temporal nature of bilateral hand stimulation was initially prioritized away from the affected limb but reversed towards the affected hand once the arms were crossed. [76] A review of data on motor neglect showed smaller, less frequent or spontaneous movements, also known as hypokinesia, that developed over time in CRPS and may be a consequence of protective immobility from learned non-use. [77] Avoidance of movement contributes to poorer baseline muscle tone with worse functional utility of that limb and paired with increased pain may reinforce non-use. Similarly in 36% of knee arthroplasty patients, neglect scores are tied to greater postoperative pain and feebler motor function. [78, 79] Reinforcement of compensatory upregulated use of the unaffected limb in combination with modified cortical representations may contribute to a lack of accurate positional awareness of the injured area, further strengthening this maladaptive cycle.

Commonly, CRPS patients express feeling as though the affected limb is in one position when in reality it is maintained in another posture altogether. [80] Lewis et. al. found a decreased unilateral awareness was described by 60% of patients, in addition to bilateral disruption of arm localization and positioning that was improved by visual cues. [69] Support of global aberrations in spatial processing, specifically when visual confirmation is lacking, was demonstrated by the relationship between objective and subjective midline in light and dark conditions. Contrasted with a control population, CRPS patients shifted their subjective midline towards the affected limb in dark conditions and this shift was not replicated in other painful syndromes, such as post-herpetic neuralgia. [81, 82] Nerve blockage for the painful site caused a reversal of subjective midline away from the affected limb and towards the midline, while somatosensory stimuli in controls altered the midline perception to a lesser extent. Right hemispheric lateralization of sensory processing could contribute to conflicting findings of universal left-sided shifts in subjective midlines, regardless of the side of the affected limb. [83, 84] Within this study only right-sided injuries showed a significant correlation between midline shift and neglect-like symptoms. In spite of the variance within visual subjective midline shift direction in CRPS, mislocalization has been associated with increased mechanical hyperalgesia. Broadly, the degree of BPD positively correlates with pain intensity, even if the extent of mislocalization does not. [85-87] In a study of CBP patients, evoked magnetic field intensity induced more pain at sites closest to the area of their chronic pain than further away, with greater pain felt at all sites compared with controls. [88]

Positional awareness is noticeably distorted in CRPS and may contribute to transformation of somatosensory interpretation that is alluded to by the inverse relationship between tactile acuity and BPD. [86] A disrupted body image, in both CBP and CRPS, is coupled with an increased area of two point discrimination (TPD) in affected areas, which translates to site-specific decreased tactile acuity. [86, 89, 90] Pioneering work with phantom limb pain patients found that light touch, within expanded reference fields, elicited pain in the missing limb as early as four weeks post-operatively. [91] These fields were always at the border of the amputation and those adjacent to the injury in the somatosensory cortex, the latter of which was likewise substantiated in referred sensations stated by CRPS patients. [87] Agnosia, alluded to by impaired identification of the finger that received tactile stimulation within the CRPS-affected hand, was present within 48% of CRPS patients, irrespective of self-reported knowledge of a stimulus sensation being felt somewhere. [70] Hemisensory insufficiency, predominantly decreased pinprick pain sensation and temperature sense, on the ipsilateral side of the affected arm was reported on the entire half of the body in 33%, within the upper quadrant in 17%, or only within that particular limb in 33%. Quadrant or true unilateral decreased sensory perception predicted a greater likelihood of allodynia and/or motor impairments. [92]

Dampened sensation with poorer localization of stimuli around the injury, coupled with hyperalgesia and allodynia that increase sensory perception within the affected area, may lead to a transformed somatotopic map and alleged mental image of the CRPS-involved site itself. Patients routinely depict their affected extremity as larger than it actually is, even resizing images to approximately 106% of original. Disproportional enlargement is accompanied by longer disease duration, increased TPD area, and neglect-like symptoms scores. [93, 94] An enlarged perceived body image is significantly correlated with decreased tactile acuity, also seen in CBP, and may present as a fallacious sense of swelling in the affected body part. [90, 95] Artificially changing the apparent size of an affected body part, through binoculars (or inverted binoculars) during movement, results in worsened pain, swelling, and recovery period with magnification. Shrinking the visual cues of the painful site conversely ameliorates these symptoms, relative to normal unadulterated vision. [96] The pervasive and crucial element of visual and, therefore, multimodal input has been elucidated as an assistive tactic in BPD and CRPS.

Recurrent themes, gleaned from BPD research, illustrate an innate lack of basal attention to the injury-associated hemifield in CRPS and improved perception and function with visual reinforcement during tasks. Taken together, the data supports visualization as a conceivable target for CRPS intervention with evidence of improved positional orientation, subjective midline approximation, and decreased referred sensations in patients while watching their affected limb. [69, 81, 83, 87] Seeing the injured or painful area of the body during movement, via mirror utilization for example, may actually ameliorate post-task pain and facilitate faster recovery to pre-movement pain level, as noted in a CBP cohort. [97] Meticulously designed studies by the Institute of Cognitive Neuroscience at the University College London evaluated pain, unpleasantness, and thermal pain thresholds in healthy participants when the target site was directly seen, figuratively seen via mirror image, obscured by an object, or replaced by another person's reflected hand. [98, 99] In addition to self-described uncomfortable sensations, EEG early somatosensory-specific wave amplitude (N1) and later peak-to-peak multimodal waves (N2-P2) were recorded. The initial negative deflection, N1 is an evoked potential that occurs within 80-120 milliseconds following a stimulus, which in this case was observed over the temporally placed electrodes representing operculoinsular cortex activity. Intensity or amplitude of a stimulus can be discerned from N1. Later twin peaks on the EEG waveform, such as those within the N2-P2 complex are presumed to be parallel activations within S1, cingulate, and paraslyvian cortices. [98] Consistent with Gallace et. al., changes in awareness of stimuli did not prompt changes in N1 while N2-P2 strongly and significantly correlated with diminished intensity of stimulation perception, implicating alterations in associated S1, cingulate, and paraslyvian cortices. [75, 98] Mirrored image trials were reported to "feel" like participants' real hands, without the visual cues of painful stimuli, and were described asless unpleasant than direct viewing. Diminution of pain was least effective while watching an object or another person's hand.

[98] Moreover, visualization of the body increased thermal pain thresholds by an average of 3.2°C with falsified reduction of body size further alleviating pain while ficticious enlargement of the body exacerbated unpleasantness. [96, 99]

In stark contrast to post-stroke neglect syndromes that are frequently complicated by anosognosia, the sense of self versus other, pseudo-neglect in CRPS has preserved excessive vigilance and self-awareness of their deficit. [100, 101] This is apparent in the lack of pain modification seen when viewing another individual's hand in the study by Longo et. al. [98] A disturbed sense of ownership over one's body can increase susceptibility to incorporation of a foreign object into their body schema. A patient with a localized right sided sensorimotor ischemic stroke had greater incorporation of a rubber hand into their sense of self on the contraleisonal (left) side, based solely on visual cues. [102] Presentation of a rubber hand that is being painfully manipulated may then trigger heightened distress, which was observed in a right hemispheric stroke patient but not CRPS patients. [101, 103] Despite these differences, Van Staelen et. al. demonstrated that touching the affected limb may be a promising intervention to help correct BPD. [102] Visualization of a more extreme modified version of themselves, at the bodily or perceptual level, on the contrary, is especially disconcerting for CRPS patients and may be rooted in increased BPD. Elevated distress was likewise reported when ambiguous visual stimuli, such as bistable duck or rabbit or reversible Necker cube images were presented, which aberrantly engage object identification or spatial cue pathways. [104] Forced attention to these pictorial illusions caused increased pain in 61% of CRPS patients, which precipitated asymmetric vasomotor sympathetic responses, monitored by skin conductance, and dystonia in the affected limb of 33% of patients. [104] Taken together, integration of multimodal stimuli and cortical activity corresponding to the affected limb appear to underlie a part of the pathophysiology of CRPS, distinct from unilateral ischemic brain injury.

PHYSIOLOGY

The overarching premise that cortical reorganization generates the incorrectly interpreted perceptions within CRPS and triggers a feed-forward reinforcement of maladaptive connections has been discussed extensively with the advent of functional neuroimaging. The reactive or causative nature of the observed plasticity has not been unearthed but understanding what aspects of the brain are different in CRPS patients should direct more efficacious interventions. The possibility of a centralized neurological aberration present in CRPS was implied by a study that showed ipsilateral but not contralateral forehead cooling increased pain in CRPS subjects. [105] Animal studies that induced spared nerve injury or lesioned a hindlimb-associated portion of the somatosensory cortex highlighted the influence of cortical plasticity on pain behavior. Spared nerve injury in rats resulted in basal dendritic expansion of medial prefrontal cortex neurons, increased excitatory N-methyl-D-aspartate (NMDA) tone, and a linear relationship between the ratio of NMDA to α-Amino-3-hydroxy-5-methyl-4-isoxazolepropionic acid (AMPA) receptor synaptic current, in response to sensory input, and correlated with pain behavior in the injured paw. [106]

Initial patient analyses using magnetoencephalography (MEG) response to stimuli and MRI overlays, within phantom limb pain, found cortical reorganization was proportional to the magnitude of their phantom pain. [107] This concept had been historically described by neurosurgeons and pioneered by denervation-induced dramatic changes in receptive fields found by Wall and colleagues. [108, 109] Follow-up work by Flor et. al. in CBP patients noted changes in early evoked magnetic field changes with back versus finger stimuli, eliciting more intense pain in patients versus controls. [88] This site-specific heightened pain perception was associated with the chronicity of pain and the maximal cortical response within the primary somatosensory cortex (S1) was shifted more medially compared to controls.

In CRPS patients' responsiveness to fingertip touch in S1, contralateral to the affected limb, elicited 25-55% stronger activation on MEG. [110] Closer MEG-defined proximity between thumb and index finger S1 representations suggested shrinkage of the S1 associated with the affected side. [110] Maihoffner et. al. confirmed that a smaller cortical S1 hand representation of the affected limb existed in CRPS. This somatosensory hand map was shifted towards the homunculus-adjacent lip representation and the contraction of its territory correlated with pain and mechanical hyperalgesia, the latter of which was most highly predictive of plastic changes. [111] Compared to healthy controls or the ipsilateral S1 to the injury in CRPS, contralateral distance between the representation of thumb and little finger were again found to be significantly smaller. [112] Functional MRI (fMRI) assessment of bilateral electrical index finger stimulation exposed decreased cortical activity of S1 and S2 and tactile acuity within CRPS patients compared with controls, both of which were linked to mean sustained but not current pain intensity. [113] Both the S1 and S2 are located within the parietal cortex and this region has been heavily implicated in CRPS pathology with Cohen et. al. discovering 68% of a CRPS patient cohort displayed parietal dysfunction, which was correlated (r= 0.674, p<0.001) with a greater body surface area affected by allodynia. [114]

A lack of ownership over one's body and a sense of foreignness often surround the affected limb in CRPS. During a tactile challenge test, conducted under fMRI investigation, BPD was associated with greater bilateral sensitivity within the somatosensory network of the parietal and insula areas. Alienation of a limb, however, revealed specific dampening of responsiveness in the contralateral ventral premotor cortex, implying that this area may be critical to BPD. [115] Possible disinhibition of S1 has also been proposed to be present within CRPS, as seen in paired pulse suppression experiments in CRPS hand patients, which showed bilaterally reduced inducible suppression similar to that observed in the motor cortex. [116] A top-down approach in a rat model of pain discovered that by creating a targeted lesion within the somatosensory cortex behavioral correlates of altered mechanical stimulation responses were elcitied. This S1 lesion did not abolish inflammation-induced levels of pain, however, suggesting that the pain experience is more widely facilitated throughout the brain. [121]

Reversal of altered somatosensory brain activity was first shown with monkey tactile behavioral training then clinical treatment demonstrated the ability to overturn the shrunken S1 and S2 maps. [117] In two separate studies, behavioral graded sensorimotor training for up to six months or after one year of PT and medical management showed parallel improvements in perceived pain. [118, 119] Lending further credence to the concept of cortical changes as a reactionary development, rather than playing a causal role in CRPS, is the conclusion that immobilization itself results in S1 shrinkage following casting in otherwise healthy individuals, which rebounds upon resumption of use. [120] Perhaps this hints that the cortical reorganization in CRPS, in and of itself, isn't pathological but an inability to psychologically, physically, and molecularly mobilize a return to baseline function.

The involvement of motor cortices in the neurological reorganization identified in CRPS is less well established. Accounts of similar asymmetrical primary motor cortex (M1) representation of the affected limb have been described. [122] Modification of inhibitory input within M1 has also been purported to be present in CRPS, based upon bilateral reductions in intracranial inhibition in response to TMS. [110, 123] The threshold for motor activation was also decreased in patients with allodynia. Strength training, even unilaterally, corresponded to increased bilateral strength, motor-evoked potential amplitude recruitment curves, and decreased intracortical inhibition within the untrained leg, all of which supports the modulation of M1 via coordinated inter-hemispheric changes in response to activity or potentially lack thereof. [126]

Disinhibition or hyperexcitability in corticospinal tracts was only reproducible in upper-limb CRPS with no significant inter-hemispheric asymmetry in TMS response in lower-limb CRPS patients. [124] Similarly conflicting with earlier bilateral accounts of deficits, a reduction of intracranial inhibition was only observed in M1 corresponding to the painful extremity by Lefaucheur et. al., although this disinhibition was significantly related to pain score. [125] Repetitive TMS exposure to the motor cortices caused increased inhibition in the contralateral M1, which correlated with pain relief. Implied disruption in gamma-aminobutyric acid (GABA) inhibitory neurotransmitter signaling began showing up in many discussion sections of manuscripts without molecular animal study correlates. Recent work by Bank et. al. again challenges motor cortex disinhibition in CRPS by revealing normal mirror epochs of electromyography (EMG) activity in the affected arm compared with controls and less activity counterintuitively in the healthy arm. [127] These findings suggest that overpowering inhibition of the associated cortex with the injured extremity may not be the source of motor dysfunction but changes observed in activity may be pain avoidance or learned disuse phenomenon. Further trials are needed to dissect these contradictions in motor cortex activity and function in CRPS.

While the primary motor and somatosensory cortices have been a focus of neuronal reorganization in CRPS, other pain-related areas of the brain also have shown modifications that may lead to greater understanding of the physiology underlying BPD and chronic pain in this population. During pin-prick mechanical hyperalgesia, fMRI revealed significantly increased activation of not only contralateral S1 and bilateral S2, as previously reported, but also bilateral insula, as well as contralateral associative-somatosensory cortices, frontal cortices, and portions of the anterior cingulate cortex (ACC). [128] In another study by Maihofner et. al. fMRI was used to record allodynia responses to gentle brush application on the affected CRPS limb, which led to vastly different activation patterns contrasted with normal proprioception. After pain-rating weighted predictors were accounted for, however, altered activations only included contralateral S1 and parietal association cortices, as well as bilateral S2, insula, and posterior cingulate cortices (PCC). Coinciding appraisal of positron emission tomography (PET) disparities between control and CRPS cerebral glucose metabolism detected bilateral increases in glucose uptake within S2, ACC, PCC, parietal cortex, cerebellum, right posterior insula and right thalamus with subsequent decreased activity in the dorsal prefrontal cortex and M1. [129] This was done at basal conditions and was speculated to echo upregulated sensory perception due to the presence of continuous pain.

Criticism over the obvious difference in perceived sensations to the allodynia and hyperalgesia stimuli in CRPS and controls led to employment of graded painful electrical stimulation. Bilateral simultaneous application of the stimuli with a well-defined temporal character in both left-hand CRPS and control subjects was used by Fruend et. al. In two subsequent studies this group analyzed baseline versus stimulus cortical responses in fMRI, at each tier of intensity, and compared the change in activation relative to sidedness, in addition to between controls and patients. During non-painful stimuli significant suprathreshold differences could not be found, nonetheless, pain caused a comparatively increased activation in the PCC of CRPS patients, when applied to their affected limb, with concurrently decreased posterior operculum or S2 activation. In the context of bilateral operculum activity, stronger activation was uncovered in the left ACC during painful stimulation of the symptomatic hand of patients, which may correspond to the emotional or suffering aspect known to these individuals. [130] In response to the task of suppressing painful feelings with constant stimuli, CRPS patients displayed a decreased periaqueductal gray and cingulate cortex activation, regardless of the hand that was stimulated. [131] Given the role of these anatomically distinct brain regions in the descending endogenous analgesic pathway, one may assume that a ceiling effect is reached in chronic pain patients or that these anatomical differences signify the end result of generalized maladaptation. Alternatively, intrinsic variations in these anatomical regions may exist since neuronal development and predispose an individual to have an increased risk of developing CRPS if exposed to a sufficiently traumatic injury.

A collection of supplementary studies have explored various additional cortical changes or discrepancies in CRPS. Structural connectivity changes in the brain of CRPS patients have been described, specifically selective atrophy or expansion of gray matter within the prefrontal cortex that may relate to pain duration and intensity, while altered white matter tracts have been suggested to represent emotional responses to constant pain. [132, 133] Other pain-related brain structures, such as the dorsal insula, cingulate cortex, orbitofrontal cortex, and hypothalamus display gray matter density differences based on a whole brain voxel-based morphometry MRI study by Barad et al. [134] It is possible that within one of these altered areas of the brain, mirror neurons are affected in CPRS and other pain conditions. Mirror neurons, first found within monkeys and now identified within the human supplementary motor cortex, ventral premotor area, inferior parietal cortex, and S1, have been proposed to fluidly moderate sensorimotor mimicry of actions and related emotions while observing self or others. [69, 135, 136] The usefulness of targeting this area of the brain for rehabilitation has been suggested for stroke recovery. [137] Recent work has supported this suggestion and in response to observational tasks, increased activation of inferior temporal gyrus clustered neurons occurred over post-stroke time and corresponded with clinical recovery. [138]

The ability to activate this mirror neuron center of the brain necessitates visual input. The role of vision in tactile discrimination has also been observed in somatosensory event-related potential activity and improved performance in the presence of visual cues. [139-141] Multi- and cross-modal processing between visual and somatosensory cortices, in similar tasks, has been shown via PET signals and a computational modelling study. [142, 143] Visual enhancement of touch (VET) was even present after viewing a video of a hand being touched compared with a no-touch video followed by tactile stimulation. [144] The parietal component of this VET effect was explored via single pulse TMS to the integrating area near the anterior intraparietal sulcus, which abolished VET if done just after visual stimulation but not during the touch itself. Nearby areas stimulated by TMS did not affect the role of vision to tactile processing. [145] Finally, in healthy subjects and ten brain damaged individuals that had a deficit in somatosensory functioning TPD performance was improved when the stimulated forearm was viewed, suggesting a plausible integration of visual and stimulus paired therapy. [146]

In combination these authors confirmed what had been presumed about abnormal sensory perception in CRPS; a complex cortical network, particularly involving the parietal cortex, is implicated and modified compared with internal or healthy controls. Armed with the hypotheses of where CRPS pathology exists in patients, if not the physiologic cause, targeted integration utilizing visual stimuli with physiotherapy has been applied in the form of mirror therapy, graded motor imagery, prism induced visual alterations, and newly virtual reality therapy.

LOGISTIC CONSIDERATIONS

In order to determine the effectiveness of various interventions on the underlying BPD in CRPS a tool to measure this aspect of the condition and its change is required. In 2010 Lewis and McCabe developed the The Bath CRPS BPD Scale that contains 7 items, 5 of which require individuals to rate from 0-10 the degree of perception abnormality they experience with an additional item for whether a disturbance in size, temperature, pressure, or weight is felt in the affected limb. Perception abnormalities touch on thoughts concerning ownership, positional awareness, attentiveness to limb, emotions toward the limb, and if the desire to amputate permeated their schema. Finally there is a mental imagery and explanation task. [69] Justification of this assessment lies in the hope of understanding patient experiences to guide more relevant corrective input to help normalize the body schema. Internal consistency (Cronbach's alpha was 0.66) in early studies with inter-rater reliability of Cohen's Kappa exceeding 0.85 suggests acceptable reliability of results generated from this assessment. [86] BPD was significantly higher in CRPS patients compared to controls and this correlated ($r > 0.57$, $p < 0.01$) with duration of the condition, pain and TPD.

Anecdotal difficulty of patients' describing their perceptual alterations to doctors, therapists, and support contacts cause great distress, thus creating a barrier in understanding and empathy during rehabilitation. Turton et. al. developed a highly modifiable avatar based digital media application that could not only alter size, shape, and surface-level appearance of the affect area but also incorporate colors and texture to describe painful phenomena at different locations. Ideally this would be a fluid schematic of a patients' body schema that could be tracked over time and facilitate interdisciplinary comprehension during the recovery process. In a proof of concept study ten volunteer patients worked with a trained nurse to create their avatar with powerful representations of their painful reality in a therapeutic cathartic manner. [147] This concept has yet to be broadly applied to CRPS patients and therapy to date but may be a useful tool in future studies and patient management.

In treating CRPS with visual stimuli, breaking down perceptual borders to recovery, and retraining brains with centrally sensitized pain, there is a delicate balance between time and financial investment and accessibility. Unwieldy large and awkward mirror boxes are not conducive to hourly practice for patients at home. Guided attentive therapists on a daily basis improve outcomes in clinical studies but are far too impractical and expensive in the current format of our medical care network. If accessibility is improved by more portable, dynamic, and self-sufficient technology the cost of initiating care will likely increase despite potential long-term fiscally sound benefits.

Along these lines, identifying patients with CRPS early and intervening sooner with the goal of preventing sustained cortical changes is nearly unanimously agreed upon as beneficial from the clinician perspective yet the potentially expensive, time-consuming, specialized, and often painful techniques described in this section are too frequently only considered by "end-stage" patients that have failed medications and traditional PT. Chronic CRPS patients are thus more biased to seek out unconventional treatments and unfortunately have shown less robust recovery responses than those earlier in the chronic pain progression. Hindrances to early treatment implementation must motivate practitioners and researchers to move the field forward to establish a new standard of care at earlier patient time points.

EFFICACY

Building upon the data that suggests both somatosensory and broader cortical alterations are present in CRPS, a variety of tactile, mirror, prism or graded motor imagery therapies have been attempted with varying degrees of efficacy. Given the patient experience of poor touch discrimination and the ability to alter the S1 cortex of owl monkeys with repeated and controlled sensory stimuli, tactile training was explored as a chronic pain or CRPS treatment. [117] In healthy individuals visualization of the back did not improve tactile acuity. [148] Initial case studies on the benefits of sensorimotor retraining in back pain were promising but, when expanded, this therapy did not show significant changes. [97] A sample of 24 CBP patients randomized to tactile acuity training for 21 consecutive days found no significant improvement in pain or function compared to the placebo treatment. [149] Sensory discrimination training in amputees with phantom limb pain, however, resulted in significant reductions in pain with associated cortical reorganization. [150] Although tactile stimulation alone was not sufficient to decrease pain or improve tactile acuity in CRPS patients, tactile discrimination training led to decreased self-reported pain and TPD. [89] Following an additional two to three week phase, in which identical tactile stimulation was provided but the participant was now asked to discriminate between the stimulus site (1 of 5 sites on painful limb) and type (pen point vs. wine cork probes) for each of the 72 stimuli over a 24 minute training period, both pain level and TPD were substantially lower. At three months after the experiment, nine of the thirteen participants reported an overall reduction in their analgesic medication use and stable TPD functional outcomes were present. [89] Recently a case study stressed the significance of tactile training at the initial site of injury for these patients, which decreased severe pain both at that site and secondary painful areas, whereas stimulation at secondary sites did not have this analgesic effect. [151] This distinction may underlie the discrepancy between results in CRPS versus the broad predominantly secondary sites present in CBP. Further and perhaps most intriguingly, when tactile discrimination training was repeated with participants looking towards the stimulated and injured arm but instead seeing the reflection of their unaffected arm, enhanced pain reduction and improvement in TPD were discovered. [152] Unfortunately, after 16 training sessions this effect was not retained after 2-day follow-up.

Mirror therapy capitalized on the multimodal signaling of visual input, which was first explored in phantom limb patients, where a mirror was placed vertically on a table between the amputated limb and the intact limb such that a normal extremity was superimposed where the pain from the missing limb originated. A decrease in painful phantom spasms resulted, as well as emergence of perceived kinesthesia and synesthesia in the missing limb. [153] McCabe et. al. performed the initial mirror therapy pilot study in CRPS patients with stages of pain at rest and on movement with no board, a non-reflective board, and finally a mirrored board between the affected and unaffected limbs. [154] Early analgesia was present in all three participants with less than eight weeks of a CRPS diagnosis, which was transient once the mirror was removed. Six weeks after preliminary testing, with up to 10 minutes per session 4-9 times per day spent training with the mirror, this period of relief was extended by several hours. Intermediate disease (n=2, between five months to one year duration) subjects found mirror-related improvement in the stiffness of their affected limb without changes in analgesia during training, however, upon completion they reported improved function and reported less overall pain. No discernable recuperation was described by any of the three subjects with greater than two years CRPS duration. Case reports soon followed, including the resolution of intractable CRPS pain in a 63-year old woman with 50% reduction in pain reported immediately following mirror box therapy. [155] Two case reports of burning CRPS type 2 pain had split results with one only experiencing less pain fleetingly while the other had substantially decreased overall pain. [156] A combination of mirror and cognitive behavioral therapy (CBT, to be discussed further in last section of this chapter) in a small sample of three individuals found improved strength and decreased allodynia, each in one of the subjects, while all experienced an increased area of hyperalgesia and one still expressed dissociation from their affected limb at trial completion. [157] While this did not replicate the promisingearly findings of McCabe et. al., subsequent use of mirror therapy in a RCT of stroke survivors with upper limb pain (n=48) and disability found that after six months there was an amelioration of pain at rest, during movement, and following brush-induced tactile allodynia, in addition to motor function, none of which were observed in control subjects. [158] Cacchio et. al. went on to repeat this approach in a blinded RCT in 24 CRPS patients with a third condition containing mental imagery. [158] Active mirror training for 30 minutes daily caused 88% to report significantly reduced pain (4-week pain scores vs. controls, p=0.002; vs. mental imagery p < 0.001) compared with 25% of those within mental imagery alone, the latter of which had 75% of participants describing increased pain. Ninety two percent of cross-over patients from control or imagery arms reported analgesic effects of active mirror therapy. Systematic review of the literature on mirror therapy up to 2009 was declared to have a trend toward effective decreases in pain within stroke and CRPS patients but required more thorough methodological quality trials. [159]

In an attempt to bolster the effectiveness of mirror therapy several variants arose, namely the evolution of mirror therapy into graded motor imagery (GMI) developed by Latimer Mosely. He presumed that preceding mirror therapy with imagined movements and thereby priming cortical activation pathways, would reduce pain and swelling in the affected CRPS limb to a greater extent. [160] A case report showed imagined movement caused temporary pain and swelling after the task but returned to baseline by 60 minutes in the absence of detectable muscle activity with EMG and only a slight delayed autonomic arousal measured by galvanic skin response. Since the participant did not report any stress over the task the autonomic effect was attributed to the pain at a low enough level not to affect the monitored heart rate. None of these effects were observed with imagined movement of the unaffected hand. [160] Prior work utilizing PET and fMRI had described activation of the premotor cortex, supplementary motor area, cingulate cortex, and bilateral parietal areas but not primary motor cortex during imagined movements and less activity in these areas in CRPS patients compared with matched controls. [161, 162] In a later study by Moseley et. al. 21 upper limb CRPS patients and 18 non-CRPS unilateral arm pain patients were recruited for a single imagined imagery task and both showed increased pain and swelling that did not differ significantly between groups. [89] The degree of change in pain/swelling was correlated with duration of symptoms, extent of dysfunction on a body schema task, autonomic responses, catastrophic thoughts about pain, and fear of movement (r>0.42, p < 0.03). These experiments posited that the detected increase in pain may be fear-based in a guarding against learned pain responses to movement, disuse, or changed levels of attention toward the affected body part. [96] In all of these theories, repetition and thus removal of fear, normalization of attention, and slow reversal of disuse-related neuronal pathology may result in a longer term integrated therapy approach. To this end, two weeks each of imagined movement and mirror therapy would be preceded by 2 weeks of a hand laterality recognition test phase to ultimately create the GMI paradigm.

Laterality recognition tests were designed to test the internal body schema, wherein differentiating which hand (left or right) is depicted requires mental rotation of one's own hand into that position. Even in healthy individuals body schema affects performance on this task. [163, 164] If awareness of one's body position is altered, potentially as a result of poor integration of body position monitoring, as sometimes reported in patients with parietal damage and established in CRPS patients, then movements that involve the injured limb/brain area will take longer to recognize. [80, 86, 165, 166] Schwoebel et. al. discovered that in chronic unilateral hand pain, response times to determine the laterality of a depicted hand in one of many orientations were slower in the painful arm (1123 miliseconds slower vs. unaffected limb), especially for complex large amplitude imagined movements. [165] Moseley reproduced these experiments and found duration of CRPS significantly impacted response time. Predicted pain of performing a specific movement accounted for 45% of the variance within the delay in recognition of laterality on the same side as their injury, suggesting a possible fear of movement-related pain. [160] Reinersmann found similar delays, irrespective of attentional performance scores, in both phantom limb pain and CRPS compared to controls. Response times improved over a four day training period in CRPS and healthy participants alike but previously reported differences in delay with respect to the injured versus unaffected arm were not validated. [167] Practice, nonetheless, improved hand laterality recognition.

The first trial of GMI with sequential experimental phases of hand laterality recognition training, followed by imagined movement, and finally active movement with the assistance of a mirror box, was conducted by Moseley in 2004. Randomization and control cross-over to GMI, after a 12-week washout period, resulted in 13 total post-wrist fracture CRPS patients, with disease duration < 6 months, that underwent the process and showed a main effect of treatment group on pain and swelling (p < 0.01) with an effect size of 25 points on the Neuropathic Pain Scale (NPS). A number needed to treat (NNT) analysis for a 50% reduction in NPS score was approximately two and heralded this as a very promising multimodal, mind-body integrated physiotherapy approach to CRPS. [160] One major limitation of this and previously designed intensive treatment programs for CRPS was an inability to account for the influence of sustained and focused attention towards the affected limb, with the Oerlemans et. al. traditional PT study as one prominent exception. [55] To address this question with GMI, Moseley compared the outcomes of 20 CRPS subjects randomly assigned to one of three groups, each with a different order of 2 week phases (traditional GMI: recognition-imagined-mirror versus imagined-recognition-imagined or recognition-mirror-recognition). [93] Following six weeks of treatment and after an additional 12 week follow-up timeframe, pain and disability were most improved in traditional GMI (p < 0.05). Each phase type imparted some benefit but order mattered significantly. Imagined movements only improved pain following recognition tasks and mirror movements solely enhanced recovery if it was done after imagined movements. Aside from optimizing the sequential order of treatments for CRPS, this research lent evidence to disprove the therapeutic relevance of nonspecific focused attention since it did not see equal improvements with varied order of affected limb focused tasks. Corroboration of the proposed graded cortical activation and reduction of fear attained during GMI was likewise presented. [93] Supporting evidence was presented in a recent case study describing diminished pain intensity following GMI that paralleled fMRI changes in S1 and S2, with a concomitant 33% reduction of posterior parietal activation intensity following recognition tasks and a paucity of anterior cingulate or insula variations during or after GMI. [168]

Repeated RCT use of GMI in 51 CRPS, phantom limb, or brachial plexus participants (n= 37, 9, 5, respectively) recapitulated significant, albeit smaller, decreases in pain and recuperation of function with a NNT of three and four, respectively post-program for a 50% reduction in the visual analog scale of pain (VAS) and 4 point improvement on a numerical rating scale of ability to perform a movement task (0-unable to perform to 10-performs normally). [169] Positive outcomes were stable 12 weeks after program completion, in which optional continuation of control PT with medications or GMI were offered for participants in each respective arm of the study. The decreased apparent efficacy in this study, compared with prior work by this group, was attributed to increased patient heterogeneity given the less stringent inclusion criteria for enrollment. Application of GMI into clinical practice was not nearly as effective at two centers for chronic pain treatment trial in Australia. Notably, integration of a modified GMI protocol into their existing neurocare specialist hospital with outpatient pain management services (center 1, C1) and the national CRPS inpatient treatment hospital (center 2, C2) was met with poor compliance with only 7 of 48 and 11 of 27 enrolled in the study at each site that completed the program. Some of the discrepancy was due to missing assessments at given time points and dropout by patients over the course of an average of six weeks. Primary outcomes found no significant decrease in a numerical rating of pain score at either center, but seven patients had at least a 2-point or 30% reduction corresponding to a probable clinical benefit. In responsive individuals pain reduction was not correlated with any baseline characteristics or disease duration. Secondary assessment of a patient's worst pain intensity was significantly improved at C1 but not C2 following GMI. C1 also saw improvement in function of pre-post paired differences. Overall this study illustrated many of the obstacles to GMI effectiveness, such as less frequent or available patient-therapist contact and potentially challenging home requirements that were unmonitored over a longer course of treatment. The addition of flexibility for patients to simultaneously participate in concurrent tactile discrimination training and/or pain management programs supported a multimodal approach but was underpowered to differentiate these interventional caveats to GMI, likely due to the large amount of patients lost to follow-up and data collection gaps. Finally the heterogeneity present within the 18 individuals across two centers who finished the program could have undermined the appearance of a more robust effect due to poorly understood characteristics of CRPS patient groups that benefit from GMI, such as those with shorter disease duration. A third research group in Canada found when subjects were limited to acute CRPS (< six months duration) in unilateral upper limb injury and GMI was modified such that the third phase was mirror therapy without affected limb movement and the fourth phase included affected extremity activity, there were significant positive effects on extremity grip strength and pain. Average pain experienced within the past seven days (VAS) was significantly improved by study completion, as well as affected extremity grip force and patients' global impression of change, despite a lack of effect on perceived function. [170] Methodological considerations of GMI must balance the need for practical evidence-based structure and less costly or time consuming approaches that do not require a full-time clinical study staff and site. Further trials with larger numbers of patients completing the study should be conducted using multiple centers to optimize improvements in CRPS from an integrated GMI protocol.

Meanwhile, additional modifications in visual-tactile, mind-body rehabilitation approaches are being explored. Based upon the disillusioned viewpoint from which patients perceive their affected limb in CRPS, beneficial effects on pain and function were explored through intentional alterations in perceptual size, shape or location by prism glasses or virtual reality interventions. Healthy individuals that had their vision reversed for a month via prism glasses became bi-perceptual and were able to switch between old or newly developed representations of their hands. The hand became a "visuomotor transformation device" that reframed space for the rest of an arm-centered viewpoint and fMRI showed that this training engaged left-sided posterior frontal areas, in addition to intraparietal and prefrontal cortices. [171] This extreme study paved the way for use of prism glasses to modify perception of pain and "correct" or minimize the misinformed size of an affected limb. In direct application of the altered visual subjective midline findings within CRPS, prism adaptation was used in five patients to shift line of sight for a daily target-pointing task over two weeks. Twenty degree prism shift towards the unaffected side resulted in significant alleviation of pain for all but one patient at the end of the 14-day course but none experienced analgesia during the task itself. [172] If the prism adaptation was shifted towards the affected side then pain was exacerbated. This work is particularly interesting since it argues against the beneficial effect of focused attention on the injured body part but facilitates an overcompensated neglect of visual attention away from the painful side in order to cope. Willful perceptual change during movement tasks utilizing binoculars for magnification of the affected limb and inverted binoculars to minimize it found least pain in the minimized view with significantly less swelling and faster recovery to pre-test pain levels compared with magnification of the painful site. [96] The physiological explanation for this was postulated to be that when seeing a larger area stimulated there is greater activation of S1 and this may trigger the already upregulated pain system in that patient. Disturbances in perception may in fact be more dependent upon perceived spatial sidedness than the physical location of the injured body part itself. Prism glasses were used to adjust the frame of reference twenty degrees and autonomic effects in temperature were measured in the injured upper limb. Whenever the affected arm appeared to be on the normal healthy side of the body, regardless of this appearance being a true image or a prismatic illusion, there was a significant increase in temperature. Conversely, there was a cooling of the hand when the image of the affected limb appeared to be on the affected side of the body. In both cases, exact midline was considered neutral. [173]

Virtual reality transformations of the mirror and graded imagery paradigms have now undergone pilot studies to streamline and standardize the process and tackle another obstacle to the effective application of this promising style of rehabilitation. In a small open-label case series by Sato et. al., five chronic (1-3 year disease duration) hand-affected CRPS patients participated in target-oriented motor control tasks using a virtual reality rendition of mirror therapy for the first time. [174] To do so a desktop computer, real time position and motion tracker [FASTRAK], and Cyber-glove were required to interact with the virtual environment software. The FASTRAK sensor was mounted on the affected arm, which moves the corresponding forearm onscreen, while the Cyber-glove is on the unaffected hand but controls the movement of the virtual "affected" limb. Together this setup both encourages small movement of the painful limb but trains the brain to see precise movement in a representation of the affected hand without inducing the pain that comes with movement in reality. This is the primary advantage of virtual mirror therapy over the original method. The tasks involved grasping and moving objects of various sizes in a free-form and untimed weekly session. After 5-8 sessions 80% of participants showed at least a 50% reduction in pain on VAS. Two patients decreased their analgesic amitriptyline dose following treatment and case-by-case reports of an improved sense of the affected limb belonging to them again, decreased tremor, ongoing pain relief after cessation of therapy and no adverse effects were noted. The authors posit that the interactive and rewarding virtual experience increased engagement while providing a novel distraction against pain that may have alleviated some anxiety, which may limit repeated focused exercise in chronic pain patients. [174] Alternative use of virtual systems for CRPS over the past four years have included head mounted systems for home use and body swapping exercises, as well as for use in healthy individuals while undergoing fMRI. [175-177] Body swapping is simulated by a head mounted display of an interactive video of a healthy person moving limbs that the patient was told to mentally rehearse. While this did not elicit lower post-treatment pain scores it did improve BPD level on the questionnaire designed by Lewis and McCabe. [69, 176, 177] A different head-mounted display, intended for home therapy, utilized cameras that captured the image of the healthy arm in front of the body and displays a second mirrored image of it, representing the affected arm that sends session data back to the source via the internet. [175] Four training tasks, such as flexing, grasping and moving a ball, driving a simple video game, and moving the hand to fit into a silhouette, were designed for use with CRPS but thus far were tested for technical and methodological issues over the course of ten 15 minute sessions with healthy volunteers. [175] Testing these concepts within an fMRI to check the brain activation was done by Diers et. al. who report that compared with the traditional mirror box setup, virtual representation was equally perceived as life-like and S1 activation contralateral to both the moving and virtual limbs showed stronger activation during virtual training. [175] All of these efforts are laying the foundation for future use of virtual mirror therapy that could be better monitored, controlled, engaging, cost-effective, and home-based than previous iterations on this rehabilitation theme. Success with this type of virtual therapy has already been achieved with motor and balance recovery post-stroke, as well aspain reduction with improved function following spinal cord injury. [178, 179]

COMPLICATIONS AND IMPLICATIONS FOR TREATMENT

Complications and adverse effects of mirror or GMI based therapy are minimal compared to pharmaceutical or interventional treatments. A Delphi study of experts examined the adverse effects reported for mirror therapy in phantom limb pain and found general discomfort, including pain, sweating, dizziness, emotional reaction to these symptoms, and sensory changes were reported by patients. This panel of experts concluded that the main contraindication to use of this therapy was practitioner-dependent confidence and training to guide patients through discomfort to meaningful results. [180] As previously alluded to, cost and inconvenience are possible drawbacks to this type of CRPS treatment. Tactile, GMI, or virtual training all require active participation, daily motivation, commitment to therapy, and acceptance of their condition - one that frequently has no cure. Acceptance may involve a lengthy adaptation period and skew willing participants towards those that have more chronic and persistent cortical changes.

Considering the risks and benefits of this field of visually integrated physiotherapy, it is important to maintain an up-to-date knowledge base of the previous study results and limitations, as well as a healthy skepticism that this is a panacea for CRPS. Systematic and evidence-based reviews, prior to Johnson et. al.'s work in 2011, found greatest strength of evidence to support GMI as a part of CRPS treatment recommendations. [64, 181] In light of the poor transition of GMI to clinical practice, as described by Johnson et. al., McCabe commented on clinical mirror therapy integration and the inherent problem of individualized programs, which has made training therapists more difficult and often has resulted in word of mouth transfer of techniques between facilities. [182] Standardization, perhaps via computer or virtual applications of these concepts, would therefore provide the greatest hope of their reproducibility for practitioner training, research, and ultimately patient pain relief.

The foundation of evidence that these therapies are based upon is not exempt from criticism. Many of the motor and some sensorimotor cortical mapping in CRPS has been scrutinized for poorly blinded study design, small numbers of participants, and the inherent bias of amassing many publications on the efficacy of treatment from very few different research groups and institutions. Pietro et. al. describes many of these potential pitfalls in two consecutive meta-analysis publications, in which he states, *"The evidence for a difference in function of the primary somatosensory cortex in CRPS compared with controls is clouded by high risk of bias and conflicting results, but reduced representation size seems consistent"* [183]. The evidence supporting motor cortex dysfunction is even more convoluted according to the 18 studies included within the second meta-analysis that is reiterated in a systematic review by Deconick et. al. [184, 185] Lastly, in both therapy studies and clinical research trials the predominance of upper limb CRPS makes generalizability of this to lower extremity afflicted individuals more challenging. This unintentional distribution is likely a consequence of less frequent lower extremity development of CRPS and an effort to control some aspects of the extraordinarily heterogeneous patient population.

In summary, the critiques of mirror, GMI, prism, and virtual reality therapy, are not intended to dissuade further work in this field or minimize the sometimes exceptionally strong positive outcomes that have been published, but to accurately portray the data and convey the importance of future, multi-center collaborative work in this field.

PAIN EXPOSURE PHYSICAL THERAPY, COGNITIVE BEHAVIORAL THERAPY, AND AN INTERDISCIPLINARY APPROACH

Awareness of the mind-body connection in chronic pain has guided the development of rehabilitation programs yet all too often it is the mind we must work hardest to overcome. The way in which focused and specialized interventions can trigger anatomical changes and neuronal plasticity has been discussed throughout this chapter. Engagement in treatment and acceptance of pathophysiological aspects of CRPS is not easy for patients and perhaps this apprehension is rooted in a primal emotion that predates cortical oversight; fear. Anxiety and fearfulness are emotional aspects of the pain experience and contribute to the "motivational-affective" component of pain described by Melzack and Dennis that compliments the intuitive "sensory-discriminative" portion of human interactions with noxious stimuli. [186] In recent years the presumed entanglement of affect and pain has been substantiated through animal studies, functional brain imaging, and clinical research. [152] Together this has contributed to acceptance of a biopsychosocial understanding of pain, which in and of itself is a vast topic beyond the scope of this chapter.

In chronic pain fear is commonly described as fear of pain and/or fear of (re)injury. The fear avoidance model of exaggerated pain by Lethem et. al. was developed out of anecdotal reports of these phenomena. [187] Interpretation of pain as something to avoid, since it signifies bodily harm, is a survival instinct. A desynchronous overrepresentation of pain behavior without correspondingly severe organic pathology or nociceptive sources has been deemed exaggerated pain. This "exaggeration" is not a conscious choice, as in malingering, but a neuropychological effect of pain. According to Lethem et. al., fear of pain leads individuals to respond along a spectrum between avoidance and confrontation. The latter allows for resumption of normal activity as pain resolves with "a minimal psychological overlay", whereas avoidance of pain experiences or activities initiates inactivity with physical disadvantages (discussed in section 1) and psychological consequences. Persistence of an invalid state or sick role further exacerbates the operant conditioning of pain behavior explained by Fordyce et al. Initially pain positively reinforces avoidance behaviors while learned evasion reduces experienced pain, serving as negative reinforcement. Experimentally this theory was translated into identification of "avoiders" and "confronters" among CBP patients based upon back movement exercise avoidance scores. Greater fear was reported and lower maximal effort in performance of back exercises was observed, signifying avoidance in the former group of individuals. [188] Fordyce ultimately states that since avoidance is based on anticipated outcomes, very little reinforcement is required to cause endurance of these behaviors. [189] Practically since avoidance occurs prior to pain instead of in response to it, more avoidance and inactivity provides fewer opportunities to calibrate actual pain with a given task, such that fear of pain may eventually be uncoupled from recent or actual pain experiences. [190] This was corroborated by the presence of more features of the fear avoidance model found within chronic pain patients compared with those who had recovered in a small pilot study of post-herpetic neuralgia, CBP, and CRPS patients. [191] Rose et. al. was able to correctly predict up to 82% of patients with chronic pain from a retrospective analysis based on this model. A prospective larger scale (n=300) study by Klenerman et. al. followed acute back injury patients and fear avoidance measures held the highest predictive value for development of CBP. [192]

Avoidance, secondary to fear of pain and/or fear of (re)injury, may encompass or lead to a fear of movement thus further hindering rehabilitation. Kori et. al. defined kinesiophobia as "an excessive, irrational, and debilitating fear of physical movement and activity resulting from a feeling of vulnerability to painful injury or re-injury." [193] The Tampa Scale of Kinesiophobia (TSK), a 17-item questionnaire, is frequently used to measure this fear. The TSK has been validated in a heterogeneous chronic pain population and principal component analysis showed four components; harm, fear of (re)injury, importance of exercise, and avoidance of activity. [193-195] Waddell et. al. developed a similar Fear-Avoidance Beliefs Questionnaire (FABQ) based on work-related and physical activity-related fear beliefs. In a sample of 184 CBP patients regression analyses showed FABQ accounted for a greater proportion of variance in work loss and disability than time, anatomical, or pain intensity patterns. [196] Kinesiophobia, measured by TSK or FABQ in CBP patient studies, likewise demonstrated that this measure was not correlated with pain intensity but predicted scores on the Roland disability questionnaire, was associated with higher levels of pain catastrophizing, negative affect, and more traumatic acute onset of injury. [190, 195, 197] Higher self-reported anxiety or fear of pain/(re)injury corresponds to patient over-prediction of pain and this expectation, independent of experienced pain in a previous repetition, leads to poorer behavioral performance and lower maximal effort on subsequent potentially painful tasks [188, 190, 198, 199] A meta-analysis with 41 studies, comprised of 46 independent datasets. found a reliable and stable relationship between pain-related fear and disability with a moderate to large effect size across diverse demographic and pain characteristics. [200] Diminished engagement in activity-based physiotherapy undermines its effectiveness, as discussed in the previous sections, leading to a disabled state. The presence of poor therapy effort, partially due to fear of pain or injury from movement, presents another therapeutic target for recovery.

In order to provide targeted treatments, differentiating between the fear of experiencing pain and fear of (re)injuring or harming oneself is advantageous. Crombez et. al. found that there is a strong correlation (r=0.87, p < 0.001) between fear of pain and fear of injury in 49 CBP patients and both were separately associated with increased variability in behavioral task performance. [188] Chronic pain sufferers (n=39) were asked to define their expected level of pain tolerance and expected danger associated with cold water immersion of their hand prior to two cold pressor trials. After completion of the first two trials participants rated how willing they were to participate in a third trial, testing avoidance. Actual tolerance was only significantly predicted by expected tolerance, suggesting patients can accurately determine their experiential pain in this setting. In addition, avoidance was significantly affected by expected danger in the task, irrespective of the pain they expected to endure during it. [201] In CRPS it appears that the fear of harm is the root of inactivity and pain-related fear. Marinus et. al. found within 238 leg-affected patients the passive, arguably avoidant, coping method of "resting" contributed significantly to the Rising and Walking and social functioning tests, while the fear of harm component of TSK affected walking. [202] In the absence of the pain coping inventory, the activity avoidance component of TSK affected social functioning. Taken together this implied that kinesiophobia and associated fear of pain did not dominate outcomes within CRPS. In a similar study with recently diagnosed CRPS (less than six months), TSK was not predictive. Using a focused assessment of perceived harmfulness with a photograph series of daily activities (PHODA), however, significantly predicted functional limitations beyond pain intensity alone. [203] In comparison to CBP patients, CRPS participants displayed greater influence of psychological distress on pain intensity and disability in a multivariate analysis. Although kinesiophobia contributed to pain intensity prediction in both cohorts, anxiety uniquely contributed in CRPS. [204]

Affective aspects appear to be more salient in CRPS pain and disability, notably focused on fear or anxiety surrounding inflicting additional self-harm. Given the usual sudden traumatic onset of injury and an as yet unidentified trigger that divides these patients from those that follow a normal recovery post-fracture/injury, there is a high amount of uncertainty that surrounds the development of disabling pain in CRPS. Logically it is unsurprising that CRPS patients fear accidentally endangering themselves further. While this outlook may be medically unfounded, people fear what they do not understand and avoid what may cause them harm. To better treat CRPS we must acknowledge these concerns and structure therapy to both address and safely overcome fear avoidance behavior. Graded in vivo exposure (GivE) and graded activity exposure (GA) are variations of CBT that use activity, potentially via PT and OT, to gradually help chronic pain individuals face their fears and recalibrate their activity responses. Acceptance commitment therapy (ACT), although not based purely on CBT, attempts to utilize mindfulness and shifted attention to minimize cognitive negativity associated with pain-related fear.

Conventional exposure treatment of specific fears, also known as phobias, is broadly structured to expose an individual to variations of their fear in a safe and gradual environment to aid in extinguishing unfounded or disproportionate anxiety. Building self-efficacy is a fundamental conceptual construct of this process and Bandura et al. postulates and proves that the more dependable the source of fear opposing information the greater the positive effect on self-efficacy. [205] Performing the task or experiencing the exposure (in vivo) influences behavior more strongly than imagining scenarios of desensitization or observing someone else perform them. GivE therefore aims to have the patient perform greater levels of activity, since that is the source of fear in chronic pain. This may be due to fear of post-activity lingering discomfort or disability, negative affect associated with pain, or fear of harm or (re)injury. The process begins by patient education of the neuroscience behind their pain, physiological consequences of continued avoidance behavior, and established safety with monitoring for all proposed activities. Then an individualized hierarchy of feared behaviors and activities are generated. Over time these are reenacted with increasing intensity up the hierarchy as tolerated. Initially this process engages classical learning theory where the associations between actions and outcomes are learned and anticipated. In the case of fear upon movement, specific exercises may activate a fear response but catastrophic expectations are challenged and disproved through inhibitory learning, uncoupling fear from those tasks. [206] This is not unlike extinction of the operant pain avoidance behavior or altering pain memories by integrating the "exposure without danger" principle during exercise therapy. [207]

Operant behavior is likewise employed during GA therapy with similar incremental increases in movement or exercise. GA encourages individuals to meet predefined activity quotas by engaging in their individualized functional activity plan, initially at 70-80% of their acceptable pain capacity and increasing as tolerated. Instead of focusing on learning to invalidate the catastrophic expectations of a given task by reenacting them without consequence, GA utilizes continuous check-ins with positive encouragement and feedback to reinforce the behavior. Notably, GA differs from GivE, since it progresses regardless of increasing pain with escalating activity. [206, 208]

Pain exposure PT (PEPT) has been described as an analogous functional outcome focused activity-based treatment design that incorporates classical CBT reinforcement, as well as acknowledges and discusses all ongoing incidences of pain catastrophizing or kinesiophobic behavior without an overt educational stage. [120] Particularly important is the forthright and repetitive therapist-patient communication that PEPT differs from traditional PT and may cause transient increased pain but that pain is not an indication of injury or harm.

ACT has been considered an extension of CBT and according the theory behind this treatment approach "…avoidance occurs primarily when negative thoughts and emotions have excessive or inappropriate impact on behavior (denoted as cognitive fusion)." [209] The three elements of ACT, presented by Hayes et. al. are mindfulness, acceptance, and "value-based action." [210] These aspects are centered at changing the function but not the content of an individual's cognitions, thus distinguishing ACT from CBT. Within the context of chronic pain, acceptance refers to a willingness to observe the pain experienced without attempting to control it. Further value-based action is the concept of clarifying personal and hierarchical goals and values while taking targeted actions to achieve those targets. Engaging in previously enjoyable or rewarding activities, in the midst of pain, should shift thoughts away from a preoccupation with pain and thereby help alleviate avoidance. [208]

PHYSIOLOGY

Mechanisms underlying pain-related fear avoidance are complex and interconnected, including ACC and amygdala-associated stimulation, as well as activation of the hypothalamus-pituitary-adrenal (HPA) and sympathetic-adrenal-medullary axes. The amygdala, located deep within the medial temporal lobe of mammals integrates emotions within the limbic system and has been established as the focal brain area encoding conditioned fear experiences and memories. [211-213] Afferent nociceptive input converges onto the amygdala from the spinothalamic tract via direct and indirect projections through the hypothalamus, thalamus, ACC, and insula, in addition to pontine pathways involved in stress, pain, and attention, as reviewed by Stroebel et al. [214] Together the ACC, amygdala, and bed nucleus of the stria terminalis have been shown to be pivotal in emotional pain experiences. Electrophysiological activity, transneuronal nociceptive pathway tracing, activation-induced gene expression levels, and neuroimaging (PET, fMRI) studies have demonstrated ACC and amygdala neurons respond to noxious stimuli. [215-220] Conditioned place aversion (CPA), an experimental approximation of pain induced avoidance in rodent laboratory studies, has also been used to investigate links between pain and fear. In CPA noxious stimuli, such as foot shock or formalin-induced footpad inflammatory pain, are given in a specific and identifiably distinct location, which leads to future avoidance of that place. Selective lesions of either the ACC or amygdala decrease the magnitude of formalin-induced CPA, whereas only excitotoxic destruction of the amygdala decreases shock-induced CPA behavior. [221] Glutamate and norepinephrine (NE) are the predominant neurotransmitters driving pain circuits in these brain regions. [214, 215, 222] The primary source of NE to the rest of the neuraxis is a pontine nucleus, the locus coeruleus (LC). [223, 224] Environmental and emotional stressors, such as pain, are also integrated at the LC by prominent reciprocal innervations from the medial prefrontal cortex, cingulate cortex, and amygdala. [225-228]

Efferent LC projections to the hippocampus and amygdala encode the anxiety associated memory formation and retrieval from a given experience, such as a traumatic painful event. [229] Further, bidirectional connections between the LC and hypothalamus modulate the HPA axis stress networks. [230]

Cortisol (CORT) is the systemically circulating glucocorticoid hormone that is released from the adrenal cortices in a diurnal cycle as part of the HPA axis and serves as the biological messenger of stress to target organs throughout the body. [231, 232] CORT, as well as, upstream neuroendocrine signals adrenocorticotropic hormone (ACTH) and corticotropin releasing hormone (CRH), have widespread physiological functions including feedback onto the HPA axis, hippocampus, and amygdala. Behaviorally the HPA system reacts to the fear and stress of a mortal threat to mobilize an animal for escape and survival through heightened awareness, epinephrine spurred quickness, blood flow reprioritization, and muscle activation. Return to homeostasis from acute stress is crucial and diseases or conditions that perpetuate extended maladaptive HPA activation with resultant down-regulation negatively impact health. Inasmuch as chronic pain stimuli and fear-induced activation of the sympathetic nervous system can be viewed as potent stressors, it is expected that aberrations in this stress system would be found in chronic pain syndromes. In a rat model of repetitive (20 day) exposure to conditioned fear tests *in vivo* biotelemetry showed sympathetic activation, stably increased mean arterial pressure, and flattened diurnal rhythms, paralleling loss of circadian CORT variation or blunted basal levels observed in chronic pain. [233-235] In healthy volunteers in response to acute experimental pain an individual's CORT was associated with fear-avoidance pain responses and inversely proportional to endurance related pain responses, such as active coping and pain persistence behavior. [236] Amygdala activation in response to fear conditioning in healthy individuals, likewise was found to be positively correlated with basal cortisol levels. [237] The relationship between CORT and the amygdala has been shown to facilitate encoding of fear-based memories and interestingly higher CORT during exposure therapy and awakening response on therapy days was predictive of a better response to treatment in panic disorder patients. [238, 239]

Despite the seemingly obvious involvement of HPA in chronic pain, interpretation of animal or patient chronic pain HPA studies are complicated by the presence of gender dimorphic responses, overlaid affective disorder influences, and the complexities of analgesic effects from opioid pain-killers or non-steroidal anti-inflammatory drugs on the axis. [233, 240-243] Tempered by these limitations, only studies specifically within CRPS animals or patients are discussed. Animal models displayed peripheral NE sensitivity, behavioral changes, and central structural modifications within the limbic system. A tibia fracture immobilization mouse model demonstrated anxiety and fear of new areas in a zero maze, poor working memory with novel object or location recognition, and synaptic plasticity changes within the perirhinal cortex, hippocampus, and amygdala. [244] A chronic constriction injury model similarly found limbic system CRH mRNA increases. [245] Observed nociceptive sensitization was reduced with application of epidermal beta-2-adrenergic receptor antagonist, whereas a persistent tissue ischemia model found amplified vasoconstriction responses to NE at the site of injury in the paw. [246, 247]

Within patients systemically elevated NE was noted in one study while inhibitory control of pain during sympathetic arousal appeared to be compromised in another patient sample. [248, 249] The potential role of the sympathetic nervous system and HPA axis in CRPS, discussed in more detail in Chapter__, suggests a possible role of pathology within the LC.

[250] Cortical reorganization and maladaptive neural circuitry changes have been suggested to underlie a great deal of CRPS pathophysiology and In reference to the brain areas implicated in pain-related fear avoidance, evidence of chronic pain induced gray mater or connectivity changes in the amygdala, ACC, and hypothalamus. [130, 134, 251] Finally, Park et. al. ascertained that in CRPS patients with more frequent spontaneous pain, the CORT response on awakening was lower along with a blunted slope of CORT decline throughout the day, implying poorly controlled patients had greater dysregulation of the HPA axis. [252]

Recurrent activation of stress responses in CRPS patients appears to culminate in dysregulation of the HPA axis, regardless of whether it is due to more frequent perseveration on fear of self-harm, or the recurrent pain, in and of itself. Over time, homeostasis may be harder to achieve and a compensatory, albeit maladaptive, dampening of baseline cyclical stress hormone levels and reactivity that bolsters fear extinction learning may be compromised. Additional studies within this specific population are required to discern long-term effects and critical therapeutic targets. Reversibility of CRPS pathophysiology may be attainable similar to the rebound in gray matter density observed in the pain-free post-operative state of chronic hip pain suffers. [253] Amelioration of pain-related fear through behavioral and cognitive interventions may therefore serve as an additive benefit in CRPS patients.

LOGISTIC CONSIDERATIONS

Training and certification to practice CBT, if not always mandatory, is strongly suggestive for safe and effective treatment. Training programs exist across the country but require time, money, and personnel. The psychological backlash of fear and pain exposure in some patients could potentially be dangerous and support from well-trained psychologists and psychiatrists may be beneficial. In a safe well-supported environment, the addition of this type of therapy would likely increase the time commitment of patients and staff alike. Complicating matters is the insurance coverage that is oftentimes different for medical treatment (PT) versus mental health therapy, under which CBT would fall. This is not to say that integrated multidisciplinary programs, requiring patient pre-approval, cannot integrate CBT, exposure therapy, or ACT seamlessly into a patient rehabilitation program. At this point in its development for CRPS patients it may not be readily available to interested patients.

EFFICACY

Fear, whether focused on pain, movement, or danger, will parallel functional outcomes and amelioration of fear has been shown to coincide with recuperation of normal activities. A Swedish full-time multidisciplinary rehabilitation program including physical training, physiological pain management education, and relaxation techniques, over a one month time period, found that in 265 CBP patients a decrease in TSK by at least eight points (34% of subjects) corresponded to significantly greater improvements in disability. [254] A review of exposure therapy by Craske et al. found no predictive value on outcomes of fear level changes within a session and only moderately across sessions. The authors advocate that fear reduction is not an ideal marker of inhibitory learning, which is necessary for extinction and optimization of exposure therapy. Exposure therapy should integrate timing and context of re-exposure, as well as fear toleration training with performance of feared activities as an indicator of progress. [255]

GivE, as described by Vlaeyen et al., was compared with graded activity (GA) in a prospective study (n=6) alternating the order of therapy type, each given for four weeks with results at baseline, completion, and 12-month follow-up. [206] Pain-related fear and catastrophizing only decreased following the GivE treatment, regardless of therapy order. Disability scores decreased and physical activity, measured by a wearable ambulatory monitor, increased significantly following GivE compared with baseline or GA levels. [206] Findings were stable in all five of the responding participants at one year; however this was an extremely small sample of CBP patients without substantial power to fully assess interventional effectiveness. In order to assess the possible contribution of education-based insight on outcomes, randomization to GivE or operant GA after unanimous education exposure was compared in six patients. [256] Utilizing a daily pain diary, pre-, post-, and follow-up standardized questionnaires, as well as activity monitors, this study found that education alone resulted in improvements in pain catastrophizing and pain-related fear, which were further enhanced by subsequent GivE but not operant GA. Ease executing daily activities and pain intensity uniquely improved with GivE at study completion and six month follow up, respectively. [256] A multicenter RCT, including 85 CBP patients treated with either GivE or GA, found no group difference in pain intensity or daily activity levels. [257] Decreased pain catastrophizing and perceived harmfulness of activities was observed following GivE in an intention to treat analysis. Approximately half of all participants reported clinically relevant improvements in the difficulty of their worst three physical activity tasks and related overall functional disability with a nearly significant (p= 0.08 to 0.09) influence of GivE over GA. Predictive regression analyses similarly displayed borderline (p=0.07) contribution of treatment group, favoring GivE. This study observed beneficial effects of both forms of CBT based activity therapy without conclusive benefit of GivE over GA. [257]

The first study of potential GivE effects on disability in a subset of CRPS patients, expressing substantial pain-related fear, was explored by de Jong et. al. Similar to the authors' previous studies with CBP, a single-case experimental ABCD design with random determination of interventional timing was used, in which daily pain, catastrophizing, pain-related fear, and activity goal achievements were kept in a diary. Additionally structured questionnaires on disability, fear, and CRPS symptoms administered prior to and following each intervention, as well as at follow up. GivE, over a 10-week course of 20 sessions, successfully and significantly decreased pain-related fear (TSK and PHODA scores), disability, and CRPS signs and symptoms with an average lag in effects of 4-8 weeks after exposure therapy initiation. [20] In a related, veritable hybrid CBT approach to CRPS, up to five PEPT sessions were performed in case series on 106 chronic (mean duration disease 55 months) arm or leg CRPS patients. Four participants dropped out early due to intolerable increases in pain. [258] Outcomes were measured by Radboud Skills test and walking or stair climbing duration and speed for upper or lower limb affected patients, respectively. Nearly all patients had some recovery of function, full greater than partial in upper limb patients (46.2% full, 48.7% partial) with the opposite trend in lower extremity patients (49.2% full, 42.9% partial). Pain improved in the majority of patients (71.7%) although 13.2% had increased pain and 11.3% had no change in pain. Partial to full functional recovery was documented in 88.5% or 23 individuals despite increased or unchanged pain intensity following PEPT. [258] Safety of PEPT in CRPS with comparison of pre-, post-, and follow-up functional outcomes were examined in 20 adult CRPS patients, which were no more than 18 months past diagnosis, using a multiple single-case design. [259] Without a control cohort it is difficult to assess the generalizability and efficacy adequately from this study, however, significant improvements in several pain assessments, disability, TSK score, and overall perceived health were observed compared to baseline levels of each in this patient subset. [259]

A preliminary study on the effect of 3-4 weeks of ACT on 108 patients with long-standing complex and intractable pain found immediate decreased pain, depression, pain-related anxiety, and daytime resting scores. [260] Follow-up three months post-treatment displayed less pain-related doctor visits and less work loss with sustained lower pain scores. The validity of the ACT theory was strengthened by correlation of acceptance change scores, including those related to activity engagement and pain willingness, with depression, pain-related anxiety, and disability but not pain intensity. [260] Comparable benefits were observed with ACT in a pediatric chronic pain study. [209] In a sample of whiplash induced chronic pain patients (n=20), the difference between pre to post-therapy pain-related disability and life satisfaction were uniquely predicted by psychological inflexibility, not anxiety, depression, kinesiophobia, or self-efficacy self-reports. [261] ACT based interventions are targeted at mediating psychological reframing of pain and thus may provide benefits above and beyond PT or CBT alone. RCTs studying ACT efficacy in chronic pain have had mixed conclusions. In a recent systemic review and meta-analysis of ACT, including ten RCT focused on chronic pain, Ost found mixed conclusions: a 50/50 split (n=4 studies) of improved outcomes compared with treatment as usual, a 3:1 ratio of studies finding ACT efficacy was greater than waiting-list controls, and one study each finding no benefit of ACT versus CBT or relaxation training. [233] Overall Ost found ACT to have a mean effect size of 0.42 across 60 RCTs but empirical support within this analysis lead to Ost's statement that ACT is "probably efficacious" in chronic pain. [233] To date no studies have tested efficacy of ACT specifically in an isolated CRPS chronic pain patient cohort, nevertheless, utilization of acceptance-based coping strategies on a self-regulated basis have been reported to benefit CRPS patients. Advice from 21 interviewed CRPS patients for other CRPS patients stressed that a sense of control was crucial for effective self-management. Recommendations of becoming educated in the disease, attaining a sense of acceptance, and finding a supportive environment, were central to patient-centered and individually driven rehabilitation. [262] Through daily diaries, Cho et. al. found that by engaging more in acceptance-based coping, measured by the brief pain response inventory, same-day activity increased, moods were more positive, pain was reported to be less, and next-day activity levels were augmented. An association with pain intensity was found for poorer mood, activity, and acceptance based coping levels but pain intensity was not predictive of outcome levels. [263] Acceptance could potentially normalize pain expectations and build self-efficacy, both of which may decrease fear of injury or harm.

COMPLICATIONS AND IMPLICATIONS FOR TREATMENT

As with all the other forms of PT discussed in this chapter, CBT, GivE, and ACT are treatments for CRPS that are not as effectively employed in isolation. Integration of psychological and physiological training in chronic pain multidisciplinary programs has been demonstrated in chronic pain for over 30 years. [264] Combined treatment with CBT and traditional PT has resulted in functional improvements in pediatric patients and adult CRPS samples. [265-267]

CONCLUSION

In the clinical setting, CRPS has always provided many challenges for the practitioner treating this entity. Patients who are finally diagnosed with CRPS often already went through multiple diagnostic procedures, treatment modalities, and therapeutic failures, before they arrived at the conclusion that they had CRPS. In essence, these patients usually are in a late and continuous stage of chronic pain when they are diagnosed. Often, physical therapy and other rehab modalities had already been employed prior to obtaining this diagnosis. With a much more appreciated understanding of the disease process affecting them, more specifically defined rehabilitation can then be initiated and tailored to the patient's needs. Functional improvement through the initiation of physical therapy modalities has been seen in patients who present with CRPS, but the outcomes depend on a multitude of factors which are difficult to specifically characterize. The disease process itself presents in various stages and degrees, with no clear endpoint. A multidisciplinary approach, including physical therapy and rehabilitation, continues to be the mainstay of treatment and management for these patients.

REFERENCES

[1]   Frazer F. Persistent post-sympathetic pain treated by connective tissue massage. *Physiotherapy.* 1978;64(7):211.

[2]   Goats G, Keir K. Connective tissue massage. *British journal of sports medicine.* 1991;25(3):131-3.

[3]   Lampen-Smith R. Complex Regional Pain Syndrome I (RSD) & The Physiotherapeutic Intervention. *New Zealand Journal of Physiotherapy.* 1997;25:19-23.

[4]   Chase T, Jha A, Brooks C, Allshouse A. A pilot feasibility study of massage to reduce pain in people with spinal cord injury during acute rehabilitation. *Spinal Cord.* 2013;51(11):847-51.

[5]   Reed BV, Held JM. Effects of sequential connective tissue massage on autonomic nervous system of middle-aged and elderly adults. *Phys Ther.* 1988;68(8):1231-4.

[6]   Robaina FJ, Dominguez M, Diaz M, Rodriguez JL, de Vera JA. Spinal cord stimulation for relief of chronic pain in vasospastic disorders of the upper limbs. *Neurosurgery.* 1989;24(1):63-7.

[7] Bodenheim R, Bennett JH. Reversal of a Sudeck's Atrophy by the Adjunctive Use of Transcutaneous Electrical Nerve Stimulation A Case Report. *Phys Ther.* 1983;63(8):1287-8.

[8] Kesler RW, Saulsbury FT, Miller LT, Rowlingson JC. Reflex sympathetic dystrophy in children: treatment with transcutaneous electric nerve stimulation. *Pediatrics.* 1988;82(5):728-32.

[9] Hardy MA, Hardy S. Reflex sympathetic dystrophy: the clinician's perspective. *Journal of Hand Therapy.* 1997;10(2):137-50.

[10] Thacker M, Gifford L. A Review of the Physiotherapy Management of Complex Regional Pain Syndrome. In: Gifford L, editor. Topical Issues in Pain 3 Sympathetic Nervous System and Pain Pain Management Clinical effectiveness. Falmouth, MA: *CNS Press;* 2002. p. 119-42.

[11] De Mos M, Sturkenboom MC, Huygen FJ. Current understandings on complex regional pain syndrome. *Pain Practice.* 2009;9(2):86-99.

[12] Coderre TJ, Xanthos DN, Francis L, Bennett GJ. Chronic post-ischemia pain (CPIP): a novel animal model of complex regional pain syndrome-type I (CRPS-I; reflex sympathetic dystrophy) produced by prolonged hindpaw ischemia and reperfusion in the rat. *Pain.* 2004;112(1):94-105.

[13] Koban M, Leis S, Schultze-Mosgau S, Birklein F. Tissue hypoxia in complex regional pain syndrome. *Pain.* 2003;104(1):149-57.

[14] Terkelsen AJ, Bach FW, Jensen TS. Experimental forearm immobilization in humans induces cold and mechanical hyperalgesia. *Anesthesiology.* 2008;109(2):297-307.

[15] Ota H, Arai T, Iwatsuki K, Urano H, Kurahashi T, Kato S, et al. Pathological mechanism of musculoskeletal manifestations associated with CRPS type II: An animal study. *PAIN®.* 2014;155(10):1976-85.

[16] Pepper A, Li W, Kingery WS, Angst MS, Curtin CM, Clark JD. Changes resembling complex regional pain syndrome following surgery and immobilization. *The Journal of Pain.* 2013;14(5):516-24.

[17] Rho RH, Brewer RP, Lamer TJ, Wilson PR, editors. Complex regional pain syndrome. *Mayo Clinic proceedings;* 2002: Elsevier.

[18] Stanton-Hicks M, Baron R, Boas R, Gordh T, Harden N, Hendler N, et al. Complex regional pain syndromes: guidelines for therapy. *The Clinical journal of pain.* 1998;14(2):155-66.

[19] Harden NR. A clinical approach to complex regional pain syndrome. *The Clinical journal of pain.* 2000;16(2):S26-S32.

[20] de Jong JR, Vlaeyen JW, Onghena P, Cuypers C, Hollander Md, Ruijgrok J. Reduction of pain-related fear in complex regional pain syndrome type I: the application of graded exposure in vivo. *Pain.* 2005;116(3):264-75.

[21] van Eijs F, Smits H, Geurts JW, Kessels AG, Kemler MA, van Kleef M, et al. Brush-evoked allodynia predicts outcome of spinal cord stimulation in complex regional pain syndrome type 1. *Eur J Pain.* 2010;14(2):164-9.

[22] Sandroni P, Benrud-Larson LM, McClelland RL, Low PA. Complex regional pain syndrome type I: incidence and prevalence in Olmsted county, a population-based study. *Pain.* 2003;103(1):199-207.

[23] de Mos M, De Bruijn A, Huygen F, Dieleman J, Stricker B, Sturkenboom M. The incidence of complex regional pain syndrome: a population-based study. *Pain.* 2007;129(1):12-20.

[24] Wang YC, Li HY, Lin FS, Cheng YJ, Huang CH, Chou WH, et al. Injury Location and Mechanism for Complex Regional Pain Syndrome: A Nationwide Population-Based Case–Control Study in Taiwan. *Pain* Practice. 2014.

[25] Guo T-Z, Offley SC, Boyd EA, Jacobs CR, Kingery WS. Substance P signaling contributes to the vascular and nociceptive abnormalities observed in a tibial fracture rat model of complex regional pain syndrome type I. *Pain.* 2004;108(1):95-107.

[26] Aguiar GC, Do Nascimento MR, De Miranda AS, Rocha NP, Teixeira AL, Scalzo PL. Effects of an exercise therapy protocol on inflammatory markers, perception of pain, and physical performance in individuals with knee osteoarthritis. *Rheumatol Int.* 2014:1-7.

[27] Helmark IC, Mikkelsen UR, Børglum J, Rothe A, Petersen MC, Andersen O, et al. Research article Exercise increases interleukin-10 levels both intraarticularly and peri-synovially in patients with knee osteoarthritis: a randomized controlled trial. 2010.

[28] Nunes RB, Alves JP, Kessler LP, Lago PD. Aerobic exercise improves the inflammatory profile correlated with cardiac remodeling and function in chronic heart failure rats. *Clinics.* 2013;68(6):876-82.

[29] Chen Y-W, Tzeng J-I, Lin M-F, Hung C-H, Wang J-J. Forced treadmill running suppresses postincisional pain and inhibits upregulation of substance P and cytokines in rat DRG. *The Journal of Pain.* 2014.

[30] Tan EC, Janssen AJ, Roestenberg P, van den Heuvel LP, Goris RJA, Rodenburg RJ. Mitochondrial dysfunction in muscle tissue of complex regional pain syndrome type I patients. *European Journal of Pain.* 2011;15(7):708-15.

[31] Eisenberg E, Shtahl S, Geller R, Reznick AZ, Sharf O, Ravbinovich M, et al. Serum and salivary oxidative analysis in Complex Regional Pain Syndrome. *Pain.* 2008;138(1):226-32.

[32] Radak Z, Zhao Z, Koltai E, Ohno H, Atalay M. Oxygen consumption and usage during physical exercise: the balance between oxidative stress and ROS-dependent adaptive signaling. *Antioxid Redox Signal.* 2013;18(10):1208-46.

[33] Lash JM, Bohlen HG. Functional adaptations of rat skeletal muscle arterioles to aerobic exercise training. *J Appl Physiol.* 1992;72(6):2052-62.

[34] Shi Y, Ku DD, Man RY, Vanhoutte PM. Augmented endothelium-derived hyperpolarizing factor-mediated relaxations attenuate endothelial dysfunction in femoral and mesenteric, but not in carotid arteries from type I diabetic rats. *Journal of Pharmacology and Experimental Therapeutics.* 2006;318(1):276-81.

[35] Kurvers HA. Reflex sympathetic dystrophy: facts and hypotheses. *Vascular Medicine.* 1998;3(3):207-14.

[36] de Souza GG, Duarte ID, de Castro Perez A. Differential Involvement of Central and Peripheral α2 Adrenoreceptors in the Antinociception Induced by Aerobic and Resistance Exercise. *Anesthesia & Analgesia.* 2013;116(3):703-11.

[37] Sawynok J. Adenosine receptor activation and nociception. *European journal of pharmacology.* 1998;347(1):1-11.

[38] Martins D, Mazzardo-Martins L, Soldi F, Stramosk J, Piovezan A, Santos A. High-intensity swimming exercise reduces neuropathic pain in an animal model of complex

regional pain syndrome type I: evidence for a role of the adenosinergic system. *Neuroscience.* 2013;234:69-76.

[39] Cobianchi S, Marinelli S, Florenzano F, Pavone F, Luvisetto S. Short-but not long-lasting treadmill running reduces allodynia and improves functional recovery after peripheral nerve injury. *Neuroscience.* 2010;168(1):273-87.

[40] Sabatier MJ, Redmon N, Schwartz G, English AW. Treadmill training promotes axon regeneration in injured peripheral nerves. *Experimental neurology.* 2008;211(2):489-93.

[41] Stagg NJ, Mata HP, Ibrahim MM, Henriksen EJ, Porreca F, Vanderah TW, et al. Regular exercise reverses sensory hypersensitivity in a rat neuropathic pain model: role of endogenous opioids. *Anesthesiology.* 2011;114(4):940-8.

[42] Leukel C, Taube W, Rittweger J, Gollhofer A, Ducos M, Weber T, et al. Changes in corticospinal transmission following 8weeks of ankle joint immobilization. *Clinical Neurophysiology.* 2014.

[43] Könönen M, Tarkka I, Niskanen E, Pihlajamäki M, Mervaala E, Pitkänen K, et al. Functional MRI and motor behavioral changes obtained with constraint-induced movement therapy in chronic stroke. *European Journal of Neurology.* 2012;19(4):578-86.

[44] Whitall J, Waller SM, Sorkin JD, Forrester LW, Macko RF, Hanley DF, et al. Bilateral and Unilateral Arm Training Improve Motor Function Through Differing Neuroplastic Mechanisms A Single-Blinded Randomized Controlled Trial. *Neurorehabilitation and neural repair.* 2011;25(2):118-29.

[45] Taubert M, Lohmann G, Margulies DS, Villringer A, Ragert P. Long-term effects of motor training on resting-state networks and underlying brain structure. *Neuroimage.* 2011;57(4):1492-8.

[46] Fonoff ET, Hamani C, Ciampi de Andrade D, Yeng LT, Marcolin MA, Jacobsen Teixeira M. Pain relief and functional recovery in patients with complex regional pain syndrome after motor cortex stimulation. *Stereotact Funct Neurosurg.* 2011;89(3):167-72.

[47] Schilder J, Sigtermans MJ, Schouten AC, Putter H, Dahan A, Noldus LP, et al. Pain relief is associated with improvement in motor function in complex regional pain syndrome type 1: secondary analysis of a placebo-controlled study on the effects of ketamine. *The Journal of Pain.* 2013;14(11):1514-21.

[48] Kemler MA, de Vet HC, Barendse GA, van den Wildenberg FA, van Kleef M. Effect of spinal cord stimulation for chronic complex regional pain syndrome Type I: five-year final follow-up of patients in a randomized controlled trial. *Journal of neurosurgery.* 2008;108(2):292-8.

[49] Veizi IE, Chelimsky TC, Janata JW. Chronic Regional Pain Syndrome: What Specialized Rehabilitation Services Do Patients Require? *Curr Pain Headache Rep.* 2012;16(2):139-46.

[50] Desai MJ, Ingraham MJ. Rehabilitation Perspectives of Neuromodulation. *Curr Pain Headache Rep.* 2014;18(2):1-7.

[51] Sherry DD, Wallace CA, Kelley C, Kidder M, Sapp L. Short-and long-term outcomes of children with complex regional pain syndrome type I treated with exercise therapy. *The Clinical journal of pain.* 1999;15(3):218-23.

[52]   RuggerI SB, Athreya BH, Doughty R, Gregg JR, Das MM. Reflex sympathetic dystrophy in children. *Clin Orthop Relat Res.* 1982;163:225-30.

[53]   Wilder RT, Vieyra MA. Reflex Sympathetic Dystrophy in Children. *Bone Joint Surg Am.* 1992;74:910-9.

[54]   Watson HK, Carlson L. Treatment of reflex sympathetic dystrophy of the hand with an active "stress loading" program. *The Journal of hand surgery.* 1987;12(5):779-85.

[55]   Oerlemans HM, Oostendorp RA, de Boo T, Goris RJ. Pain and reduced mobility in complex regional pain syndrome I: outcome of a prospective randomised controlled clinical trial of adjuvant physical therapy versus occupational therapy. *Pain.* 1999;83(1):77-83.

[56]   Oerlemans HM, Oostendorp RA, de Boo T, Perez RS, Goris RJ. Signs and symptoms in complex regional pain syndrome type I/reflex sympathetic dystrophy: judgment of the physician versus objective measurement. *The Clinical journal of pain.* 1999;15(3):224-32.

[57]   Oerlemans HM, Oostendorp RA, de Boo T, van der Laan L, Severens JL, Goris RJA. Adjuvant physical therapy versus occupational therapy in patients with reflex sympathetic dystrophy/complex regional pain syndrome type I. *Arch Phys Med Rehabil.* 2000;81(1):49-56.

[58]   Severens JL, Oerlemans HM, Weegels AJ, van't Hof MA, Oostendorp RA, Goris RJA. Cost-effectiveness analysis of adjuvant physical or occupational therapy for patients with reflex sympathetic dystrophy. *Arch Phys Med Rehabil.* 1999;80(9):1038-43.

[59]   Kemler MA, Reulen JP, van Kleef M, Barendse GA, van den Wildenberg FA, Spaans F. Thermal thresholds in complex regional pain syndrome type I: sensitivity and repeatability of the methods of limits and levels. *Clinical neurophysiology: official journal of the International Federation of Clinical Neurophysiology.* 2000; 111(9): 1561-8.

[60]   van de Vusse AC, Goossens VJ, Kemler MA, Weber WE. Screening of patients with complex regional pain syndrome for antecedent infections. *The Clinical journal of pain.* 2001;17(2):110-4.

[61]   Kemler MA, De Vet HC, Barendse GA, Van Den Wildenberg FA, Van Kleef M. The effect of spinal cord stimulation in patients with chronic reflex sympathetic dystrophy: Two years' follow-up of the randomized controlled trial. *Ann Neurol.* 2004;55(1):13-8.

[62]   Çelik D, Demirhan M. Physical therapy and rehabilitation of complex regional pain syndrome in shoulder prosthesis. *The Korean journal of pain.* 2010;23(4):258-61.

[63]   Muhl C, Isner-Horobeti M-E, Laalou F-Z, Vautravers P, Lecocq J. The value of nerve blocks in the diagnoses and treatment of complex regional pain syndrome type 1: A series of 14 cases. *Annals of Physical and Rehabilitation Medicine.* 2014.

[64]   Perez RS, Zollinger PE, Dijkstra PU, Thomassen-Hilgersom IL, Zuurmond WW, Rosenbrand KC, et al. Evidence based guidelines for complex regional pain syndrome type 1. *BMC Neurol.* 2010;10(1):20.

[65]   Daly AE, Bialocerkowski AE. Does evidence support physiotherapy management of adult Complex Regional Pain Syndrome Type One? A systematic review. *European Journal of Pain.* 2009;13(4):339-53.

[66]   Okifuji A, Turk DC, Curran SL. Anger in chronic pain: investigations of anger targets and intensity. *J Psychosom Res.* 1999;47(1):1-12.

[67] Osborn M, Smith JA. Living with a body separate from the self. The experience of the body in chronic benign low back pain: an interpretative phenomenological analysis. *Scand J Caring Sci.* 2006;20(2):216-22.

[68] Lewis JS, Kersten P, McCabe CS, McPherson KM, Blake DR. Body perception disturbance: a contribution to pain in complex regional pain syndrome (CRPS). *Pain.* 2007;133(1-3):111-9.

[69] Lewis JS, Kersten P, McPherson KM, Taylor GJ, Harris N, McCabe CS, et al. Wherever is my arm? Impaired upper limb position accuracy in complex regional pain syndrome. *Pain.* 2010;149(3):463-9.

[70] Förderreuther S, Sailer U, Straube A. Impaired self-perception of the hand in complex regional pain syndrome (CRPS). *Pain.* 2004;110(3):756-61.

[71] Galer BS, Bruehl S, Harden RN. IASP diagnostic criteria for complex regional pain syndrome: a preliminary empirical validation study. International Association for the Study of Pain. *The Clinical journal of pain.* 1998;14(1):48-54.

[72] Harden RN, Bruehl S, Galer BS, Saltz S, Bertram M, Backonja M, et al. Complex regional pain syndrome: are the IASP diagnostic criteria valid and sufficiently comprehensive? *Pain.* 1999;83(2):211-9.

[73] Frettlöh J, Hüppe M, Maier C. Severity and specificity of neglect-like symptoms in patients with complex regional pain syndrome (CRPS) compared to chronic limb pain of other origins. *Pain.* 2006;124(1):184-9.

[74] Legrain V, Bultitude JH, De Paepe A, Rossetti Y. Pain, body, and space: What do patients with complex regional pain syndrome really neglect? *Pain.* 2012;153(5):948-51.

[75] Gallace A, Torta DM, Moseley GL, Iannetti G. The analgesic effect of crossing the arms. *Pain.* 2011;152(6):1418-23.

[76] Moseley GL, Gallace A, Spence C. Space-based, but not arm-based, shift in tactile processing in complex regional pain syndrome and its relationship to cooling of the affected limb. *Brain: a journal of neurology.* 2009;132(Pt 11):3142-51.

[77] Punt TD, Cooper L, Hey M, Johnson MI. Neglect-like symptoms in complex regional pain syndrome: learned nonuse by another name. *Pain.* 2013;154(2):200-3.

[78] Kolb L, Lang C, Seifert F, Maihofner C. Cognitive correlates of "neglect-like syndrome" in patients with complex regional pain syndrome. *Pain.* 2012;153(5):1063-73.

[79] Hirakawa Y, Hara M, Fujiwara A, Hanada H, Morioka S. The relationship among psychological factors, neglect-like symptoms and postoperative pain after total knee arthroplasty. Pain Research & Management: *The Journal of the Canadian Pain Society.* 2014;19(5):251.

[80] McCabe CS, Shenker N, Lewis J, Blake DR. Impaired self-perception of the hand in complex regional pain syndrome (CRPS) [S. Förderreuther, U. Sailer, A. Straube, Pain 2004; 110:756-761]. *Pain.* 2005;114(3):518; author reply 9.

[81] Sumitani M, Shibata M, Iwakura T, Matsuda Y, Sakaue G, Inoue T, et al. Pathologic pain distorts visuospatial perception. *Neurology.* 2007;68(2):152-4.

[82] Uematsu H, Sumitani M, Yozu A, Otake Y, Shibata M, Mashimo T, et al. Complex regional pain syndrome (CRPS) impairs visuospatial perception, whereas post-herpetic neuralgia does not: possible implications for supraspinal mechanism of CRPS. *Annals Academy of Medicine Singapore.* 2009;38(11):931.

[83] Reinersmann A, Landwehrt J, Krumova EK, Ocklenburg S, Gunturkun O, Maier C. Impaired spatial body representation in complex regional pain syndrome type 1 (CRPS I). *Pain.* 2012;153(11):2174-81.

[84] Coghill RC, Gilron I, Iadarola MJ. Hemispheric lateralization of somatosensory processing. *Journal of neurophysiology.* 2001;85(6):2602-12.

[85] Maihofner C, Neundorfer B, Birklein F, Handwerker HO. Mislocalization of tactile stimulation in patients with complex regional pain syndrome. *Journal of neurology.* 2006;253(6):772-9.

[86] Lewis JS, Schweinhardt P. Perceptions of the painful body: the relationship between body perception disturbance, pain and tactile discrimination in complex regional pain syndrome. *Eur J Pain.* 2012;16(9):1320-30.

[87] McCabe CS, Haigh RC, Halligan PW, Blake DR. Referred sensations in patients with complex regional pain syndrome type 1. *Rheumatology* (Oxford). 2003;42(9):1067-73.

[88] Flor H, Braun C, Elbert T, Birbaumer N. Extensive reorganization of primary somatosensory cortex in chronic back pain patients. *Neuroscience letters.* 1997;224(1):5-8.

[89] Moseley GL, Zalucki NM, Wiech K. Tactile discrimination, but not tactile stimulation alone, reduces chronic limb pain. *Pain.* 2008;137(3):600-8.

[90] Nishigami T, Mibu A, Osumi M, Son K, Yamamoto S, Kajiwara S, et al. Are tactile acuity and clinical symptoms related to differences in perceived body image in patients with chronic nonspecific lower back pain? *Manual therapy.* 2014.

[91] Ramachandran VS, Stewart M, Rogers-Ramachandran D. Perceptual correlates of massive cortical reorganization. *Neuroreport.* 1992;3(7):583-6.

[92] Rommel O, Gehling M, Dertwinkel R, Witscher K, Zenz M, Malin J-P, et al. Hemisensory impairment in patients with complex regional pain syndrome. *Pain.* 1999;80(1):95-101.

[93] Moseley GL. Is successful rehabilitation of complex regional pain syndrome due to sustained attention to the affected limb? A randomised clinical trial. *Pain.* 2005;114(1):54-61.

[94] Peltz E, Seifert F, Lanz S, Muller R, Maihofner C. Impaired hand size estimation in CRPS. *The journal of pain: official journal of the American Pain Society.* 2011;12(10):1095-101.

[95] Lotze M, Moseley GL. Role of distorted body image in pain. *Current rheumatology reports.* 2007;9(6):488-96.

[96] Moseley GL, Zalucki N, Birklein F, Marinus J, van Hilten JJ, Luomajoki H. Thinking about movement hurts: the effect of motor imagery on pain and swelling in people with chronic arm pain. *Arthritis and rheumatism.* 2008;59(5):623-31.

[97] Wand BM, Tulloch VM, George PJ, Smith AJ, Goucke R, O'Connell NE, et al. Seeing it helps: movement-related back pain is reduced by visualization of the back during movement. *The Clinical journal of pain.* 2012;28(7):602-8.

[98] Longo MR, Betti V, Aglioti SM, Haggard P. Visually induced analgesia: seeing the body reduces pain. *The Journal of neuroscience.* 2009;29(39):12125-30.

[99] Mancini F, Longo MR, Kammers MP, Haggard P. Visual distortion of body size modulates pain perception. *Psychol Sci.* 2011;22(3):325-30.

[100] Kortte K, Hillis AE. Recent advances in the understanding of neglect and anosognosia following right hemisphere stroke. *Current neurology and neuroscience reports.* 2009;9(6):459-65.

[101] Reinersmann A, Landwehrt J, Krumova EK, Peterburs J, Ocklenburg S, Gunturkun O, et al. The rubber hand illusion in complex regional pain syndrome: preserved ability to integrate a rubber hand indicates intact multisensory integration. *Pain.* 2013;154(9):1519-27.

[102] van Stralen HE, van Zandvoort MJ, Kappelle LJ, Dijkerman HC. The Rubber Hand Illusion in a patient with hand disownership. *Perception.* 2013;42(9):991-3.

[103] Van Stralen H, Van Zandvoort M, Dijkerman H. The role of self-touch in somatosensory and body representation disorders after stroke. *Philosophical Transactions of the Royal Society B: Biological Sciences.* 2011;366(1581):3142-52.

[104] Hall J, Harrison S, Cohen H, McCabe CS, Harris N, Blake DR. Pain and other symptoms of CRPS can be increased by ambiguous visual stimuli--an exploratory study. *Eur J Pain.* 2011;15(1):17-22.

[105] Drummond PD. Sensory disturbances in complex regional pain syndrome: clinical observations, autonomic interactions, and possible mechanisms. *Pain medicine.* 2010;11(8):1257-66.

[106] Metz AE, Yau H-J, Centeno MV, Apkarian AV, Martina M. Morphological and functional reorganization of rat medial prefrontal cortex in neuropathic pain. *Proceedings of the National Academy of Sciences.* 2009;106(7):2423-8.

[107] Flor H, Elbert T, Knecht S, Wienbruch C, Pantev C, Birbaumer N, et al. Phantom-limb pain as a perceptual correlate of cortical reorganization following arm amputation. *Nature.* 1995;375(6531):482-4.

[108] Ramachandran VS, Hirstein W. The perception of phantom limbs. The DO Hebb lecture. *Brain: a journal of neurology.* 1998;121(9):1603-30.

[109] Melzack R, Wall PD. Pain mechanisms: a new theory. *Science.* 1965;150(3699):971-9.

[110] Juottonen K, Gockel M, Silén T, Hurri H, Hari R, Forss N. Altered central sensorimotor processing in patients with complex regional pain syndrome. *Pain.* 2002;98(3):315-23.

[111] Maihofner C, Handwerker HO, Neundorfer B, Birklein F. Patterns of cortical reorganization in complex regional pain syndrome. *Neurology.* 2003;61(12):1707-15.

[112] Vartiainen N, Kirveskari E, Kallio-Laine K, Kalso E, Forss N. Cortical reorganization in primary somatosensory cortex in patients with unilateral chronic pain. *The Journal of Pain.* 2009;10(8):854-9.

[113] Pleger B, Ragert P, Schwenkreis P, Forster AF, Wilimzig C, Dinse H, et al. Patterns of cortical reorganization parallel impaired tactile discrimination and pain intensity in complex regional pain syndrome. *Neuroimage.* 2006;32(2):503-10.

[114] Cohen H, McCabe C, Harris N, Hall J, Lewis J, Blake D. Clinical evidence of parietal cortex dysfunction and correlation with extent of allodynia in CRPS type 1. *European Journal of Pain.* 2013;17(4):527-38.

[115] van Dijk MT, van Wingen GA, van Lammeren A, Blom RM, de Kwaasteniet BP, Scholte HS, et al. Neural basis of limb ownership in individuals with body integrity identity disorder. *PLoS One.* 2013;8(8):e72212.

[116] Lenz M, Hoffken O, Stude P, Lissek S, Schwenkreis P, Reinersmann A, et al. Bilateral somatosensory cortex disinhibition in complex regional pain syndrome type I. *Neurology.* 2011;77(11):1096-101.

[117] Jenkins WM, Merzenich MM, Recanzone G. Neocortical representational dynamics in adult primates: implications for neuropsychology. *Neuropsychologia.* 1990;28(6):573-84.

[118] Pleger B, Tegenthoff M, Ragert P, Forster AF, Dinse HR, Schwenkreis P, et al. Sensorimotor retuning [corrected] in complex regional pain syndrome parallels pain reduction. *Ann Neurol.* 2005;57(3):425-9.

[119] Maihofner C, Handwerker HO, Neundorfer B, Birklein F. Cortical reorganization during recovery from complex regional pain syndrome. *Neurology.* 2004;63(4):693-701.

[120] Lissek S, Wilimzig C, Stude P, Pleger B, Kalisch T, Maier C, et al. Immobilization impairs tactile perception and shrinks somatosensory cortical maps. *Current Biology.* 2009;19(10):837-42.

[121] Uhelski ML, Davis MA, Fuchs PN. Pain affect in the absence of pain sensation: evidence of asomaesthesia after somatosensory cortex lesions in the rat. *Pain.* 2012;153(4):885-92.

[122] Krause P, Förderreuther S, Straube A. TMS motor cortical brain mapping in patients with complex regional pain syndrome type I. *Clinical Neurophysiology.* 2006;117(1):169-76.

[123] Schwenkreis P, Janssen F, Rommel O, Pleger B, Volker B, Hosbach I, et al. Bilateral motor cortex disinhibition in complex regional pain syndrome (CRPS) type I of the hand. *Neurology.* 2003;61(4):515-9.

[124] Eisenberg E, Chistyakov AV, Yudashkin M, Kaplan B, Hafner H, Feinsod M. Evidence for cortical hyperexcitability of the affected limb representation area in CRPS: a psychophysical and transcranial magnetic stimulation study. *Pain.* 2005;113(1):99-105.

[125] Lefaucheur J, Drouot X, Menard-Lefaucheur I, Keravel Y, Nguyen J. Motor cortex rTMS restores defective intracortical inhibition in chronic neuropathic pain. *Neurology.* 2006;67(9):1568-74.

[126] Goodwill AM, Pearce AJ, Kidgell DJ. Corticomotor plasticity following unilateral strength training. *Muscle Nerve.* 2012;46(3):384-93.

[127] Bank PJ, Peper CLE, Marinus J, Beek PJ, van Hilten JJ. Evaluation of mirrored muscle activity in patients with Complex Regional Pain Syndrome. *Clinical Neurophysiology.* 2014.

[128] Maihofner C, Forster C, Birklein F, Neundorfer B, Handwerker HO. Brain processing during mechanical hyperalgesia in complex regional pain syndrome: a functional MRI study. *Pain.* 2005;114(1-2):93-103.

[129] Shiraishi S, Kobayashi H, Nihashi T, Kato K, Iwano S, Nishino M, et al. Cerebral glucose metabolism change in patients with complex regional pain syndrome: a PET study. *Radiation medicine.* 2006;24(5):335-44.

[130] Freund W, Wunderlich AP, Stuber G, Mayer F, Steffen P, Mentzel M, et al. Different activation of opercular and posterior cingulate cortex (PCC) in patients with complex regional pain syndrome (CRPS I) compared with healthy controls during perception of

electrically induced pain: a functional MRI study. *The Clinical journal of pain.* 2010;26(4):339-47.

[131] Freund W, Wunderlich AP, Stuber G, Mayer F, Steffen P, Mentzel M, et al. The role of periaqueductal gray and cingulate cortex during suppression of pain in complex regional pain syndrome. *The Clinical journal of pain.* 2011;27(9):796-804.

[132] Geha PY, Baliki MN, Harden RN, Bauer WR, Parrish TB, Apkarian AV. The brain in chronic CRPS pain: abnormal gray-white matter interactions in emotional and autonomic regions. *Neuron.* 2008;60(4):570-81.

[133] Pleger B, Draganski B, Schwenkreis P, Lenz M, Nicolas V, Maier C, et al. Complex regional pain syndrome type I affects brain structure in prefrontal and motor cortex. *PLoS One.* 2014;9(1):e85372.

[134] Barad MJ, Ueno T, Younger J, Chatterjee N, Mackey S. Complex Regional Pain Syndrome Is Associated With Structural Abnormalities in Pain-Related Regions of the Human Brain. *The Journal of Pain.* 2014;15(2):197-203.

[135] Acharya S, Shukla S. Mirror neurons: enigma of the metaphysical modular brain. *Journal of natural science, biology, and medicine.* 2012;3(2):118.

[136] Gallese V, Fadiga L, Fogassi L, Rizzolatti G. Action recognition in the premotor cortex. *Brain: a journal of neurology.* 1996;119(2):593-609.

[137] Pomeroy VM, Clark CA, Miller JSG, Baron J-C, Markus HS, Tallis RC. The potential for utilizing the "mirror neurone system" to enhance recovery of the severely affected upper limb early after stroke: a review and hypothesis. *Neurorehabilitation and neural repair.* 2005;19(1):4-13.

[138] Brunner IC, Skouen JS, Ersland L, Grüner R. Plasticity and Response to Action Observation A Longitudinal fMRI Study of Potential Mirror Neurons in Patients With Subacute Stroke. *Neurorehabilitation and neural repair.* 2014:1545968314527350.

[139] Kennett S, Taylor-Clarke M, Haggard P. Noninformative vision improves the spatial resolution of touch in humans. *Current Biology.* 2001;11(15):1188-91.

[140] Taylor-Clarke M, Kennett S, Haggard P. Vision modulates somatosensory cortical processing. *Current Biology.* 2002;12(3):233-6.

[141] Taylor-Clarke M, Jacobsen P, Haggard P. Keeping the world a constant size: object constancy in human touch. *Nat Neurosci.* 2004;7(3):219-20.

[142] Macaluso E, Frith C, Driver J. Selective spatial attention in vision and touch: unimodal and multimodal mechanisms revealed by PET. *Journal of neurophysiology.* 2000;83(5):3062-75.

[143] Magosso E, Serino A, Di Pellegrino G, Ursino M. Crossmodal links between vision and touch in spatial attention: a computational modelling study. *Computational intelligence and neuroscience.* 2010;2010:2.

[144] Schaefer M, Heinze H-J, Rotte M. Seeing the hand being touched modulates the primary somatosensory cortex. *Neuroreport.* 2005;16(10):1101-5.

[145] Konen CS, Haggard P. Multisensory Parietal Cortex contributes to Visual Enhancement of Touch in Humans: A Single-Pulse TMS Study. *Cerebral Cortex.* 2014;24(2):501-7.

[146] Serino A, Farnè A, Rinaldesi ML, Haggard P, Làdavas E. Can vision of the body ameliorate impaired somatosensory function? *Neuropsychologia.* 2007;45(5):1101-7.

[147] Turton AJ, Palmer M, Grieve S, Moss TP, Lewis J, McCabe CS. Evaluation of a prototype tool for communicating body perception disturbances in complex regional pain syndrome. *Frontiers in human neuroscience.* 2013;7:517.

[148] Catley MJ, Tabor A, Miegel RG, Wand BM, Spence C, Moseley GL. Show me the skin! Does seeing the back enhance tactile acuity at the back? *Manual therapy.* 2014.

[149] Ryan C, Harland N, Drew BT, Martin D. Tactile acuity training for patients with chronic low back pain: a pilot randomised controlled trial. *BMC Musculoskelet Disord.* 2014;15(1):59.

[150] Flor H, Denke C, Schaefer M, Grüsser S. Effect of sensory discrimination training on cortical reorganisation and phantom limb pain. *The Lancet.* 2001;357(9270):1763-4.

[151] Osumi M, Imai R, Ueta K, Nakano H, Nobusako S, Morioka S. Factors associated with the modulation of pain by visual distortion of body size. *Frontiers in human neuroscience.* 2014;8.

[152] Moseley GL, Wiech K. The effect of tactile discrimination training is enhanced when patients watch the reflected image of their unaffected limb during training. *Pain.* 2009;144(3):314-9.

[153] Ramachandran VS, Rogers-Ramachandran D. Synaesthesia in phantom limbs induced with mirrors. *Proceedings of the Royal Society of London Series B: Biological Sciences.* 1996;263(1369):377-86.

[154] McCabe CS, Haigh RC, Ring EF, Halligan PW, Wall PD, Blake DR. A controlled pilot study of the utility of mirror visual feedback in the treatment of complex regional pain syndrome (type 1). *Rheumatology* (Oxford). 2003;42(1):97-101.

[155] Karmarkar A, Lieberman I. Mirror box therapy for complex regional pain syndrome. *Anaesthesia.* 2006;61(4):412-3.

[156] Selles RW, Schreuders TA, Stam HJ. Mirror therapy in patients with causalgia (complex regional pain syndrome type II) following peripheral nerve injury: two cases. *Journal of rehabilitation medicine.* 2008;40(4):312-4.

[157] Tichelaar YV, Geertzen JH, Keizer D, Van Wilgen CP. Mirror box therapy added to cognitive behavioural therapy in three chronic complex regional pain syndrome type I patients: a pilot study. *International Journal of Rehabilitation Research.* 2007;30(2):181-8.

[158] Cacchio A, De Blasis E, Necozione S, Orio Fd, Santilli V. Mirror therapy for chronic complex regional pain syndrome type 1 and stroke. *New England Journal of Medicine.* 2009;361(6):634-6.

[159] Ezendam D, Bongers RM, Jannink MJ. Systematic review of the effectiveness of mirror therapy in upper extremity function. *Disability & Rehabilitation.* 2009;31(26):2135-49.

[160] Moseley GL. Why do people with complex regional pain syndrome take longer to recognize their affected hand? *Neurology.* 2004;62(12):2182-6.

[161] Decety J. Do imagined and executed actions share the same neural substrate? *Cognitive brain research.* 1996;3(2):87-93.

[162] Gieteling EW, van Rijn MA, de Jong BM, Hoogduin JM, Renken R, van Hilten JJ, et al. Cerebral activation during motor imagery in complex regional pain syndrome type 1 with dystonia. *Pain.* 2008;134(3):302-9.

[163] Parsons LM. Temporal and kinematic properties of motor behavior reflected in mentally simulated action. *Journal of Experimental Psychology: Human Perception and Performance.* 1994;20(4):709.

[164] Parsons LM, Fox P. The neural basis of implicit movements used in recognising hand shape. *Cognitive Neuropsychology.* 1998;15:583-616.

[165] Schwoebel J, Friedman R, Duda N, Coslett HB. Pain and the body schema evidence for peripheral effects on mental representations of movement. *Brain: a journal of neurology.* 2001;124(10):2098-104.

[166] Sirigu A, Daprati E, Pradat-Diehl P, Franck N, Jeannerod M. Perception of self-generated movement following left parietal lesion. *Brain: a journal of neurology.* 1999;122(10):1867-74.

[167] Reinersmann A, Haarmeyer GS, Blankenburg M, Frettloh J, Krumova EK, Ocklenburg S, et al. Left is where the L is right. Significantly delayed reaction time in limb laterality recognition in both CRPS and phantom limb pain patients. *Neuroscience letters.* 2010;486(3):240-5.

[168] Walz AD, Usichenko T, Moseley GL, Lotze M. Graded motor imagery and the impact on pain processing in a case of CRPS. *The Clinical journal of pain.* 2013;29(3):276-9.

[169] Moseley GL. Graded motor imagery for pathologic pain A randomized controlled trial. *Neurology.* 2006;67(12):2129-34.

[170] Lagueux E, Charest J, Lefrancois-Caron E, Mauger M-E, Mercier E, Savard K, et al. Modified graded motor imagery for complex regional pain syndrome type 1 of the upper extremity in the acute phase: a patient series. *International Journal of Rehabilitation Research.* 2012;35 (2):138-45.

[171] Sekiyama K, Miyauchi S, Imaruoka T, Egusa H, Tashiro T. Body image as a visuomotor transformation device revealed in adaptation to reversed vision. *Nature.* 2000;407(6802):374-7.

[172] Sumitani M, Rossetti Y, Shibata M, Matsuda Y, Sakaue G, Inoue T, et al. Prism adaptation to optical deviation alleviates pathologic pain. *Neurology.* 2007;68(2):128-33.

[173] Moseley GL, Gallace A, Di Pietro F, Spence C, Iannetti GD. Limb-specific autonomic dysfunction in complex regional pain syndrome modulated by wearing prism glasses. *Pain.* 2013,154(11):2463-8.

[174] Sato K, Fukumori S, Matsusaki T, Maruo T, Ishikawa S, Nishie H, et al. Nonimmersive Virtual Reality Mirror Visual Feedback Therapy and Its Application for the Treatment of Complex Regional Pain Syndrome: An Open-Label Pilot Study. *Pain medicine.* 2010;11(4):622-9.

[175] Diers M, Kamping S, Kirsch P, Rance M, Bekrater-Bodmann R, Foell J, et al. Illusion-related brain activations: A new virtual reality mirror box system for use during functional magnetic resonance imaging. *Brain* research. 2014.

[176] Hwang H, Cho S, Lee J-H. The effect of virtual body swapping with mental rehearsal on pain intensity and body perception disturbance in complex regional pain syndrome. *International Journal of Rehabilitation Research.* 2014;37(2):167-72.

[177] Jeon B, Cho S, Lee J-H. Application of Virtual Body Swapping to Patients with Complex Regional Pain Syndrome: A Pilot Study. *Cyberpsychology, Behavior, and Social Networking.* 2014;17(6):366-70.

[178] Villiger M, Estévez N, Hepp-Reymond M-C, Kiper D, Kollias SS, Eng K, et al. Enhanced activation of motor execution networks using action observation combined with imagination of lower limb movements. *PLoS One.* 2013;8(8):e72403.

[179] Lloréns R, Noé E, Colomer C, Alcañiz M. Effectiveness, usability, and cost-benefit of a virtual reality-based telerehabilitation program for balance recovery after stroke: a randomized controlled trial. *Archives of physical medicine and rehabilitation.* 2014.

[180] Hagenberg A, Carpenter C. Mirror Visual Feedback for Phantom Pain: International Experience on Modalities and Adverse Effects Discussed by an Expert Panel: A Delphi Study. *PM&R.* 2014.

[181] Tran DQ, Duong S, Bertini P, Finlayson RJ. Treatment of complex regional pain syndrome: a review of the evidence. *Canadian Journal of Anesthesia/Journal canadien d'anesthésie.* 2010;57(2):149-66.

[182] McCabe C. Mirror visual feedback therapy. A practical approach. *Journal of Hand Therapy.* 2011;24(2):170-9.

[183] Di Pietro F, McAuley JH, Parkitny L, Lotze M, Wand BM, Moseley GL, et al. Primary somatosensory cortex function in complex regional pain syndrome: a systematic review and meta-analysis. *The journal of pain: official journal of the American Pain Society.* 2013;14(10):1001-18.

[184] Di Pietro F, McAuley JH, Parkitny L, Lotze M, Wand BM, Moseley GL, et al. Primary motor cortex function in complex regional pain syndrome: a systematic review and meta-analysis. *The journal of pain: official journal of the American Pain Society.* 2013;14(11):1270-88.

[185] Deconinck FJ, Smorenburg AR, Benham A, Ledebt A, Feltham MG, Savelsbergh GJ. Reflections on Mirror Therapy A Systematic Review of the Effect of Mirror Visual Feedback on the Brain. *Neurorehabilitation and neural repair.* 2014:1545968314546134.

[186] Melzack R, Dennis S. Neurophysiological foundations of pain. *The psychology of pain.* 1986:1-24.

[187] Lethem J, Slade P, Troup J, Bentley G. Outline of a fear-avoidance model of exaggerated pain perception—I. *Behaviour research and therapy.* 1983;21(4):401-8.

[188] Crombez G, Vervaet L, Lysens R, Baeyens F, Eelen P. Avoidance and confrontation of painful, back-straining movements in chronic back pain patients. *Behavior Modification.* 1998;22(1):62-77.

[189] Fordyce WE, Shelton JL, Dundore DE. The modification of avoidance learning pain behaviors. *Journal of Behavioral Medicine.* 1982;5(4):405-14.

[190] Crombez G, Vlaeyen JW, Heuts PH, Lysens R. Pain-related fear is more disabling than pain itself: evidence on the role of pain-related fear in chronic back pain disability. *Pain.* 1999;80(1):329-39.

[191] Rose MJ, Klenerman L, Atchison L, Slade PD. An application of the fear avoidance model to three chronic pain problems. *Behaviour research and therapy.* 1992;30(4):359-65.

[192] Klenerman L, Slade P, Stanley I, Pennie B, Reilly J, Atchison L, et al. The prediction of chronicity in patients with an acute attack of low back pain in a general practice setting. *Spine.* 1995;20(4):478-84.

[193] Kori S, Miller R, Todd D. Kinesiophobia: a new view of chronic pain behavior. *Pain Manag.* 1990;3(1):35-43.

[194] Hapidou EG, O'Brien MA, Pierrynowski MR, de las Heras E, Patel M, Patla T. Fear and Avoidance of Movement in People with Chronic Pain: Psychometric Properties of the 11-Item Tampa Scale for Kinesiophobia (TSK-11). *Physiotherapy Canada.* 2012;64(3):235-41.

[195] Vlaeyen JW, Kole-Snijders AM, Rotteveel AM, Ruesink R, Heuts PH. The role of fear of movement/(re) injury in pain disability. *Journal of occupational rehabilitation.* 1995;5(4):235-52.

[196] Waddell G, Newton M, Henderson I, Somerville D, Main CJ. A Fear-Avoidance Beliefs Questionnaire (FABQ) and the role of fear-avoidance beliefs in chronic low back pain and disability. *Pain.* 1993;52(2):157-68.

[197] Vlaeyen JW, Kole-Snijders AM, Boeren RG, Van Eek H. Fear of movement/(re) injury in chronic low back pain and its relation to behavioral performance. *Pain.* 1995;62(3):363-72.

[198] Crombez G, Vervaet L, Baeyens F, Lysens R, Eelen P. Do pain expectancies cause pain in chronic low back patients? A clinical investigation. *Behaviour research and therapy.* 1996;34(11):919-25.

[199] McCracken LM, Gross RT, Sorg P, Edmands TA. Prediction of pain in patients with chronic low back pain: effects of inaccurate prediction and pain-related anxiety. *Behaviour research and therapy.* 1993;31(7):647-52.

[200] Zale EL, Lange KL, Fields SA, Ditre JW. The relation between pain-related fear and disability: a meta-analysis. *The Journal of Pain.* 2013;14(10):1019-30.

[201] Cipher DJ, Fernandez E. Expectancy variables predicting tolerance and avoidance of pain in chronic pain patients. *Behaviour research and therapy.* 1997;35(5):437-44.

[202] Marinus J, Perez RS, van Eijs F, van Gestel MA, Geurts JW, Huygen FJ, et al. The role of pain coping and kinesiophobia in patients with complex regional pain syndrome type 1 of the legs. *The Clinical journal of pain.* 2013;29(7):563-9.

[203] de Jong JR, Vlaeyen JW, de Gelder JM, Patijn J. Pain-related fear, perceived harmfulness of activities, and functional limitations in complex regional pain syndrome type I. *The Journal of Pain.* 2011;12(12):1209-18.

[204] Bean DJ, Johnson MH, Kydd RR. Relationships Between Psychological Factors, Pain and Disability in Complex Regional Pain Syndrome and Low Back Pain. *The Clinical journal of pain.* 2013.

[205] Bandura A. Self-efficacy: toward a unifying theory of behavioral change. *Psychological review.* 1977;84(2):191.

[206] Vlaeyen JW, de Jong J, Geilen M, Heuts PH, van Breukelen G. The treatment of fear of movement/(re) injury in chronic low back pain: further evidence on the effectiveness of exposure in vivo. *The Clinical journal of pain.* 2002;18(4):251-61.

[207] Nijs J, Girbés EL, Lundberg M, Malfliet A, Sterling M. Exercise therapy for chronic musculoskeletal pain: Innovation by altering pain memories. *Manual therapy.* 2014.

[208] Bailey KM, Carleton RN, Vlaeyen JW, Asmundson GJ. Treatments addressing pain-related fear and anxiety in patients with chronic musculoskeletal pain: a preliminary review. *Cognitive behaviour therapy.* 2010;39(1):46-63.

[209] Wicksell RK, Melin L, Lekander M, Olsson GL. Evaluating the effectiveness of exposure and acceptance strategies to improve functioning and quality of life in longstanding pediatric pain–a randomized controlled trial. *Pain.* 2009;141(3):248-57.

[210] Hayes SC, Strosahl KD, Wilson KG. Acceptance and commitment therapy: An experiential approach to behavior change: *Guilford Press;* 1999.

[211] LeDoux JE, Cicchetti P, Xagoraris A, Romanski LM. The lateral amygdaloid nucleus: sensory interface of the amygdala in fear conditioning. *The Journal of neuroscience.* 1990;10(4):1062-9.

[212] Kwon J-T, Nakajima R, Kim H-S, Jeong Y, Augustine GJ, Han J-H. Optogenetic activation of presynaptic inputs in lateral amygdala forms associative fear memory. *Learning & Memory.* 2014;21(11):627-33.

[213] Duvarci S, Pare D. Amygdala Microcircuits Controlling Learned Fear. *Neuron.* 2014;82(5):966-80.

[214] Strobel C, Hunt S, Sullivan R, Sun J, Sah P. Emotional regulation of pain: the role of noradrenaline in the amygdala. *Science China Life Sciences.* 2014;57(4):384-90.

[215] Minami M. Neuronal Mechanisms for Pain-Induced Aversion: Behavioral Studies Using a Conditioned Place Aversion Test. *International review of neurobiology.* 2009;85:135-44.

[216] Jasmin L, Burkey AR, Card JP, Basbaum AI. Transneuronal labeling of a nociceptive pathway, the spino-(trigemino-) parabrachio-amygdaloid, in the rat. *The Journal of neuroscience.* 1997;17(10):3751-65.

[217] Lei L-G, Zhang Y-Q, Zhao Z-Q. Pain-related aversion and Fos expression in the central nervous system in rats. *Neuroreport.* 2004;15(1):67-71.

[218] Neugebauer V, Li W, Bird GC, Han JS. The amygdala and persistent pain. *The Neuroscientist.* 2004;10(3):221-34.

[219] Sehlmeyer C, Schöning S, Zwitserlood P, Pfleiderer B, Kircher T, Arolt V, et al. Human fear conditioning and extinction in neuroimaging: a systematic review. *PLoS One.* 2009;4(6):e5865.

[220] Simons LE, Moulton EA, Linnman C, Carpino E, Becerra L, Borsook D. The human amygdala and pain: Evidence from neuroimaging. *Hum Brain Mapp.* 2014;35(2):527-38.

[221] Gao Y-J, Ren W-H, Zhang Y-Q, Zhao Z-Q. Contributions of the anterior cingulate cortex and amygdala to pain-and fear-conditioned place avoidance in rats. *Pain.* 2004;110(1):343-53.

[222] Maren S, Aharonov G, Stote DL, Fanselow MS. < em> N-methyl-D-aspartate receptors in the basolateral amygdala are required for both acquisition and expression of conditional fear in rats. *Behavioral neuroscience.* 1996;110(6):1365.

[223] Dahlström A, Fuxe K. Localization of monoamines in the lower brain stem. *Cellular and Molecular Life Sciences.* 1964;20(7):398-9.

[224] Berridge CW, Waterhouse BD. The locus coeruleus–noradrenergic system: modulation of behavioral state and state-dependent cognitive processes. *Brain research reviews.* 2003;42(1):33-84.

[225] Cedarbaum JM, Aghajanian GK. Afferent projections to the rat locus coeruleus as determined by a retrograde tracing technique. *Journal of Comparative Neurology.* 1978;178(1):1-15.

[226] Jodo E, Aston-Jones G. Activation of locus coeruleus by prefrontal cortex is mediated by excitatory amino acid inputs. *Brain research.* 1997;768(1):327-32.

[227] Jodoj E, Chiang C, Aston-Jones G. Potent excitatory influence of prefrontal cortex activity on noradrenergic locus coeruleus neurons. *Neuroscience.* 1998;83(1):63-79.

[228] Van Bockstaele E, Chan J, Pickel V. Input from central nucleus of the amygdala efferents to pericoerulear dendrites, some of which contain tyrosine hydroxylase immunoreactivity. *Journal of neuroscience research*. 1996;45(3):289-302.

[229] Samuels ER, Szabadi E. Functional neuroanatomy of the noradrenergic locus coeruleus: its roles in the regulation of arousal and autonomic function part I: principles of functional organisation. *Current neuropharmacology*. 2008;6(3):235-53.

[230] Reyes BA, Valentino RJ, Xu G, Van Bockstaele EJ. Hypothalamic projections to locus coeruleus neurons in rat brain. *European Journal of Neuroscience*. 2005;22(1):93-106.

[231] Hellhammer DH, Wust S, Kudielka BM. Salivary cortisol as a biomarker in stress research. *Psychoneuroendocrinology*. 2009;34(2):163-71.

[232] Kirschbaum C, Hellhammer DH. Salivary cortisol. *Encyclopedia of stress*. 2000;3(379-383).

[233] Generaal E, Vogelzangs N, Macfarlane GJ, Geenen R, Smit JH, Penninx BW, et al. Reduced hypothalamic-pituitary-adrenal axis activity in chronic multi-site musculoskeletal pain: partly masked by depressive and anxiety disorders. *BMC musculoskeletal disorders*. 2014;15(1):227.

[234] Johansson AC, Gunnarsson LG, Linton SJ, Bergkvist L, Stridsberg M, Nilsson O, et al. Pain, disability and coping reflected in the diurnal cortisol variability in patients scheduled for lumbar disc surgery. *European Journal of Pain*. 2008;12(5):633-40.

[235] Muhtz C, Rodriguez-Raecke R, Hinkelmann K, Moeller-Bertram T, Kiefer F, Wiedemann K, et al. Cortisol response to experimental pain in patients with chronic low back pain and patients with major depression. *Pain medicine*. 2013;14(4):498-503.

[236] Sudhaus S, Held S, Schoofs D, Bültmann J, Dück I, Wolf OT, et al. Associations between fear-avoidance and endurance responses to pain and salivary cortisol in the context of experimental pain induction. *Psychoneuroendocrinology*. 2014.

[237] Merz CJ, Stark R, Vaitl D, Tabbert K, Wolf OT. Stress hormones are associated with the neuronal correlates of instructed fear conditioning. *Biological psychology*. 2013;92(1):82-9.

[238] Hannibal KE, Bishop MD. Chronic Stress, Cortisol Dysfunction, and Pain: A Psychoneuroendocrine Rationale for Stress Management in Pain Rehabilitation. *Physical therapy*. 2014;94(12):1816-25.

[239] Meuret AE, Trueba AF, Abelson JL, Liberzon I, Auchus R, Bhaskara L, et al. High cortisol awakening response and cortisol levels moderate exposure-based psychotherapy success. *Psychoneuroendocrinology*. 2015;51:331-40.

[240] Bomholt SF, Harbuz MS, Blackburn-Munro G, Blackburn-Munro RE. Involvement and role of the hypothalamo-pituitary-adrenal (HPA) stress axis in animal models of chronic pain and inflammation. *Stress: The International Journal on the Biology of Stress*. 2004;7(1):1-14.

[241] Wang Q, Verweij E, Krugers H, Joels M, Swaab D, Lucassen P. Distribution of the glucocorticoid receptor in the human amygdala; changes in mood disorder patients. *Brain Structure and Function*. 2013:1-12.

[242] Turner-Cobb JM, Osborn M, da Silva L, Keogh E, Jessop DS. Sex differences in hypothalamic-pituitary-adrenal axis function in patients with chronic pain syndrome. *Stress: The International Journal on the Biology of Stress*. 2010;13(4):293-301.

[243] Aloisi AM, Buonocore M, Merlo L, Galandra C, Sotgiu A, Bacchella L, et al. Chronic pain therapy and hypothalamic-pituitary-adrenal axis impairment. *Psychoneuroendocrinology.* 2011;36(7):1032-9.

[244] Tajerian M, Leu D, Zou Y, Sahbaie P, Li W, Khan H, et al. Brain neuroplastic changes accompany anxiety and memory deficits in a model of complex regional pain syndrome. *Anesthesiology.* 2014;121(4):852-65.

[245] Ulrich-Lai YM, Xie W, Meij JT, Dolgas CM, Yu L, Herman JP. Limbic and HPA axis function in an animal model of chronic neuropathic pain. *Physiology & behavior.* 2006;88(1):67-76.

[246] Li W, Shi X, Wang L, Guo T, Wei T, Cheng K, et al. Epidermal adrenergic signaling contributes to inflammation and pain sensitization in a rat model of complex regional pain syndrome. *Pain.* 2013;154(8):1224-36.

[247] Xanthos DN, Bennett GJ, Coderre TJ. Norepinephrine-induced nociception and vasoconstrictor hypersensitivity in rats with chronic post-ischemia pain. *Pain.* 2008;137(3):640-51.

[248] Harden RN, Rudin NJ, Bruehl S, Kee W, Parikh DK, Kooch J, et al. Increased systemic catecholamines in complex regional pain syndrome and relationship to psychological factors: a pilot study. *Anesthesia & Analgesia.* 2004;99(5):1478-85.

[249] Drummond PD, Finch PM, Skipworth S, Blockey P. Pain increases during sympathetic arousal in patients with complex regional pain syndrome. *Neurology.* 2001;57(7):1296-303.

[250] Drummond PD. A possible role of the locus coeruleus in complex regional pain syndrome. *Frontiers in integrative neuroscience.* 2012;6.

[251] Linnman C, Becerra L, Lebel A, Berde C, Grant PE, Borsook D. Transient and persistent pain induced connectivity alterations in pediatric complex regional pain syndrome. *PLoS One.* 2013;8(3):e57205.

[252] Park JY, Ahn RS. Hypothalamic–pituitary–adrenal axis function in patients with complex regional pain syndrome type 1. *Psychoneuroendocrinology.* 2012;37(9):1557-68.

[253] Rodriguez-Raecke R, Niemeier A, Ihle K, Ruether W, May A. Brain gray matter decrease in chronic pain is the consequence and not the cause of pain. *The Journal of neuroscience.* 2009;29(44):13746-50.

[254] Lüning Bergsten C, Lundberg M, Lindberg P, Elfving B. Change in kinesiophobia and its relation to activity limitation after multidisciplinary rehabilitation in patients with chronic back pain. *Disabil Rehabil.* 2012;34(10):852-8.

[255] Craske MG, Kircanski K, Zelikowsky M, Mystkowski J, Chowdhury N, Baker A. Optimizing inhibitory learning during exposure therapy. *Behaviour research and therapy.* 2008;46(1):5-27.

[256] de Jong JR, Vlaeyen JW, Onghena P, Goossens ME, Geilen M, Mulder H. Fear of movement/(re) injury in chronic low back pain: education or exposure in vivo as mediator to fear reduction? *The Clinical journal of pain.* 2005;21(1):9-17.

[257] Leeuw M, Goossens ME, van Breukelen GJ, de Jong JR, Heuts PH, Smeets RJ, et al. Exposure in vivo versus operant graded activity in chronic low back pain patients: results of a randomized controlled trial. *Pain.* 2008;138(1):192-207.

[258] Ek J-W, Van Gijn JC, Samwel H, Van Egmond J, Klomp FP, van Dongen RT. Pain exposure physical therapy may be a safe and effective treatment for longstanding

complex regional pain syndrome type 1: a case series. *Clin Rehabil.* 2009;23(12):1059-66.

[259] van de Meent H, Oerlemans M, Bruggeman A, Klomp F, van Dongen R, Oostendorp R, et al. Safety of "pain exposure" physical therapy in patients with complex regional pain syndrome type 1. *Pain.* 2011;152(6):1431-8.

[260] McCracken LM, Eccleston C. A prospective study of acceptance of pain and patient functioning with chronic pain. *Pain.* 2005;118(1):164-9.

[261] Wicksell RK, Olsson GL, Hayes SC. Psychological flexibility as a mediator of improvement in Acceptance and Commitment Therapy for patients with chronic pain following whiplash. *European Journal of Pain.* 2010;14(10):1059. e1-. e11.

[262] Rodham K, Boxell E, McCabe C, Cockburn M, Waller E. Transitioning from a hospital rehabilitation programme to home: exploring the experiences of people with complex regional pain syndrome. *Psychology & health.* 2012;27(10):1150-65.

[263] Cho S, McCracken LM, Heiby EM, Moon D-E, Lee J-H. Pain acceptance-based coping in complex regional pain syndrome Type I: daily relations with pain intensity, activity, and mood. *Journal of Behavioral Medicine.* 2013;36(5):531-8.

[264] Smith GT, Hughes LB, Duvall RD, Rothman S. Treatment outcome of a multidisciplinary center for management of chronic pain: a long-term follow-up. *The Clinical journal of pain.* 1988;4(1):47-50.

[265] Lee BH, Scharff L, Sethna NF, McCarthy CF, Scott-Sutherland J, Shea AM, et al. Physical therapy and cognitive-behavioral treatment for complex regional pain syndromes. *The Journal of pediatrics.* 2002;141(1):135-40.

[266] Monticone M, Ambrosini E, Rocca B, Magni S, Brivio F, Ferrante S. A multidisciplinary rehabilitation programme improves disability, kinesiophobia and walking ability in subjects with chronic low back pain: results of a randomised controlled pilot study. *European Spine Journal.* 2014;23(10):2105-13.

[267] Bliokas VV, Cartmill TK, Nagy BJ. Does systematic graded exposure in vivo enhance outcomes in multidisciplinary chronic pain management groups? *The Clinical journal of pain.* 2007;23(4):361-74.

In: Complex Regional Pain Syndrome
Editors: Nader D. Nader and Ognjen Visnjevac

ISBN: 978-1-63483-130-7
© 2015 Nova Science Publishers, Inc.

Chapter 8

COMPLEMENTARY AND ALTERNATIVE MEDICINE

Delano Ramsoomair[1,], MD and Arvinder Gill, MD*
[1]Director, Pain Center, Veterans Affairs Hospital of Western New York,
Buffalo, NY, US
[2]Clinical Pain Fellow, University at Buffalo, Buffalo, NY, US

INTRODUCTION

Complex regional pain syndrome (CRPS) is an umbrella term for a variety of clinical presentations characterized by chronic persistent pain that is disproportionate to any proceeding injury and that is not restricted anatomically to distribution for specific peripheral nerve. [1] CRPS is characterized by continuing pain, allodynia, or hyperalgesia disproportionate to the inciting event. CRPS is not limited to distribution of a single peripheral nerve and is associated with sudomotor activity. The precise cause of complex regional pain syndrome has not been established. Multidisciplinary approach is recommended for the treatment of CRPS. [2]

After CRPS is diagnosed, treatment should start as early as possible. Multimodal approach that includes rehabilitation pathway and psychological pathway is recommended. [2] Rehabilitation pathway includes pain management with anticonvulsants, antidepressants, opioids and topical agents. Physiotherapy, occupational therapy and interventional pain management are also part of the pathway that focuses on rehabilitation. Treatment could be based on severity of CRPS divided into severe, moderate and mild classification. Severe CRPS includes intense pain at rest and during movements and treatment should be focused on intense pain management, functional rehabilitation, physiotherapy and sympathetic blocks. Moderate CRPS is classified as no pain at rest but pain during movements and therapy should focus on pain management and physiotherapy. Occupational therapy should also be a part of the treatment for moderate CRPS. Mild CRPS is classified as no pain at rest and no pain during movement and intense physiotherapy and occupational therapy are recommended. If CRPS is refractory then neuromodulation, epidural clonidine and intrathecal baclofen could be considered. The psychological pathway for treatment of CRPS includes focusing on pain-

---

* Director, Pain Center, Veterans Affairs Hospital of Western New York, Buffalo, NY dramsoomai@aol.com.

coping skills, biofeedback, relaxation training and cognitive-behavioral therapy. Psychological therapy frequency and intensity should be increase if patient has inadequate or partial response to psychological therapy.

The central theme of treatment is functional restoration with introduction of multiple treatment aspects to achieve remission and rehabilitation. [3] Also, an individual approach should be the mainstay of treatment. The therapy should include motivation, mobilization and desensitization along with pharmacologic and interventional treatment options. Nociceptive stimulation using heat, massage, pressure, cold, vibration and movement could be used to help restore normal sensory processing. It is also recommended that the patient overcome movement phobia to actually move and allow the limb to be touched. Maintenance of gentle active range of motion is the goal and aggressive or passive range of motion tests should be avoided. Therapy should be guided to achieve postural normalization, stabilization and balanced use of limb. Cutaneous allodynia may be a limiting factor and might require specific additional therapies including massage, medications, regional interventions, or one or more of several complementary and alternative therapies.

Various treatment modalities including pharmacologic and minimally invasive interventional pain techniques have been described in detail in other chapters of this book. In this chapter, focus will be placed on complementary and alternative medicine (CAM) treatment modalities including acupuncture, mirror therapy, lymphatic drainage, and various other uncommon alternative techniques that have been evaluated and tried in the treatment of complex regional pain syndrome.

ACUPUNCTURE

Acupuncture has been used in the treatment of medical illness and pain in a continuous fashion for over 2000 years. It is the most frequently used complimentary medical therapy worldwide. Acupuncture was first described in the 1st century BC and early 1st century AD in the yellow Emperor's inner classic, now known as the Huang Di Nei Jing. This body of work formed the nucleus of understanding of the then known natural sciences. The text reflected the organizing principal that the body was a reflection of the Cosmos and that healing came about from reestablishing balance with the internal and external environment. [4, 5]

Acupuncture from its agrarian roots has undergone several incarnations. The French became exposed to the traditions of Chinese medicine, including acupuncture, as a result of colonization of Indochina. Acupuncture practice and theory were imported and refined in France by a returning French physician acupuncturist. Acupuncture in the United States was not practiced except in perhaps isolated fashion in Asian communities until popularized by the newspaper article in 1971, describing James Reston's experience of surgical analgesia from acupuncture during an emergency appendectomy, which was published in the New York Times. [6] Confirmation of this report by a US team of physicians 3 months later observing surgical anesthesia and Chinese hospitals was then published in The Journal of the American medical Association. [7]

The potential benefits of acupuncture were later embodied into 1997 NIH consensus statement, which articulated documented results indicating efficacy in treating pain, drug and nicotine addiction, stroke, asthma, surgical analgesia, and control of nausea and vomiting induced by chemotherapy. [8] NIH funded research has also provided evidence of acupuncture's utility in the treatment of knee pain secondary to osteoarthritis. This was demonstrated in the NIH funded trial in 2005 conducted at the University of Maryland at the Center of integrated medicine. [9] Recent acupuncture efficacy in the treatment of acute pain from Battlefield injuries via auricular acupuncture therapy has led to the development of acupuncture protocols for the treatment of acute pain. [10]

The worldwide collective contributions from clinical trials and international forums of practicing acupuncture physicians have enhanced the public awareness and acceptance of acupuncture in its role as a valued treatment modality. As a consequence, millions of Americans benefit from acupuncture on a yearly basis. The American Academy of medical acupuncture has been influential in defining standards of practice and appropriate training pathways. Physician champions such as Joseph Helms have provided stewardship in areas of training and to date have been responsible for the training of greater than 5000 physician acupuncturists.

MECHANISMS UNDERLYING ACUPUNCTURE ANALGESIA

The mechanisms underlying the clinical effects observed from acupuncture have been the subject of debate and controversy. The People's Republic of China has compiled a body of work dating back to the 1950s. Acupuncture's effects on the body can best be summarized as having a regulatory function. This function is able to modulate hypoactive states by activating regulatory functions or, conversely, by increasing inhibitory activity in cases of hyperactivity. Several publications have examined the regulatory physiologic role of acupuncture in metabolism, endocrine function, neuronal transmissions, as well as immune function and visceral organ systems.

Acupuncture analgesia can also be applied to attain surgical anesthesia. Surgical pain signals are transmitted cephalad generally via thinly myelinated nerve fibers. Acupuncture, needling, and electrical stimulation of the needles generate afferent signals with conduction via both thick and thinly myelinated nerve fibers. Both these fiber types share ascending pathways in the spinal cord on their way to the cerebral cortex, the site of final pain perception. The gate theory proposed by Melzack and Wall in 1965 postulates that thick fiber conduction is able to modulate and reduce afferent signal transmission from thinly myelinated fibers. The gate theory might explain that sensory receptive activation from needling of muscle spindles can result in inhibition of pain signal transmission in the thinly myelinated fibers at the level of the dorsal horn of the spinal cord.

Acupuncture analgesia has been reported to exceed the duration of an induction period, during which acupuncture needling is applied, with this analgesic effect persisting without further needling. In 1959, it was first proposed that these effects were the result of humoral factors. Evidence for this has been elegantly demonstrated in cross-circulatory animal studies. Cortical evoked potentials were used as an indicator for pain perception. Research has from the Medical Academia Sinica, connected the circulation of 2 cats via their cervical arteries. Electrical stimulation was applied to needles at specific acupoints in one of the cats. The cortical evoked potentials caused by stimulation of the greater splanchnic nerve were inhibited in the cat, as well as the recipient cat, with various levels of intensity correlating with the duration of pain modulation.

The factors involved in acupunctutre analgesia have been further elucidated and include endogenous opioid-like substances and several neurotransmitters, including serotonin, dopamine, and acetylcholine. Amongst the various humeral factors, endorphins, and enkephalins appear to be most important in facilitating acupuncture-mediated analgesia. The ability of naloxone, and antiserum against endorphins, to inhibit the analgesic effects of acupuncture is further confirmation of humeral involvement in electroacupuncture-induced analgesia.

Central nervous system activation has been demonstrated by the use of functional MRI studies in acupuncture analgesia. Hui et al. of Harvard Medical School demonstrated that needling of the specific acupuncture points such as Li4 with the experience of needling sensations produced decreased FMRI signals in areas such as the nucleus accumbens, amygdala with deactivation of the rostral portion of the anterior cingulate cortex, amygdala, and hippocampal complex. This was in marked contrast to increases in signals seen in the somatosensory cortex. This observation implies that acupuncture with needle manipulation may modulate limbic and subcortical gray structures. [11] The role of the central nervous system in acupuncture analgesia is believed to operate at various levels. Afferent signals from painful stimuli and needling are transmitted via sensory nerves in the spinal cord. Initial pain modulation probably occurs at the level of the dorsal horn. Afferent transmission of pain signals is primarily via the spinothalamic track to the thalamus and then to the cerebral cortex for conscious pain perception. Although it is known that integration of signals occurs at almost every level of the central nervous system, major integration occurs at the level of the thalamus. It has been proposed that needling more easily inhibits nonspecific sensory signals, whereas specific sensory signals require selection of specific acupoints and greater stimulation at each acupoint to achieve adequate pain modulation.

Diffuse noxious inhibitory control (DNIC) is yet another proposed mechanism involved in pain modulation and surgical anesthesia. DNIC, described by Le Bars, produces generalized nociceptive inhibition by application of a noxious stimulus in a seemingly unrelated part of the body or acupoint. In DNIC theory, the neuroanatomical model lacks somatotopic organization and analgesia may be produced by intense stimulation of any part of the body. The mechanism appears to involve wide dynamic range neurons in the dorsal horn as well as complex neural loops within the spinal cord not directly involving the spinothalamic fibers. Neurotransmitters such as endorphins, epinephrine, and serotonin are involved at the level of the brainstem. [12, 13]

The above mechanisms portray a basic outline of the complex physiologic response to electroacupuncture. The totality of the clinical response to electroacupuncture seems to be a confluence of neuronal and neurotransmitter responses at various levels of the central and peripheral nervous system. The information reviewed is but a brief overview of human and animal studies in acute pain settings, application to chronic pain models, and specific pain syndromes requires further research and further trials to be validated.

CLINICAL EVIDENCE FOR THE USE OF ACUPUNCTURE

A large study conducted to assess the therapeutic effect of acupuncture combined with rehabilitation therapy on post-stroke shoulder-hand syndrome concluded that acupuncture combined with rehabilitation therapy could significantly improve upper limb motor function, pain and joint activity. [14] Patients with post-stroke shoulder-hand syndrome were randomly divided into one of three groups: an acupuncture-rehabilitation group, an acupuncture-only group, and a rehabilitation-only group. The acupuncture-rehabilitation group was treated with acupuncture in combination with motor therapy (rehabilitation training); the acupuncture-only group was treated with simple acupuncture therapy; and the rehabilitation-only group was treated with simple motor therapy. Upper extremity motor function, pain, and joint range of motion were used for assessment of therapeutic effects. The study pointed out that functional status was significantly better in acupuncture-rehabilitation group compared to both the acupuncture-only group and the rehabilitation-only group.

Another case control study identified increases in blood volume flow in CPRS-affected limbs with the use of acupuncture treatment. [15] The study included patients with unilateral CRPS and compared them to healthy sex and age-matched controls. The study investigated whether acupuncture has an effect in blood volume flow and correlated this with a clinical assessment. Blood volume flow was measured by duplex sonography before, during, and after acupuncture. During acupuncture, blood volume flow increased significantly in the patients' effected limbs compared with the patients' untreated limb. Blood volume flow was also elevated compared with the controls' treated limb. All patients reported improved symptoms, except for one. Subjective improvement in function correlated positively with this increase in blood volume flow, but improvements in pain were not found to correlate similarly. Thus, this study concluded that a significant acupuncture-mediated increase in blood volume flow was correlated to CRPS patients' functional improvement.

Ernst et al. conducted a randomized, double-blind controlled trial to evaluate traditional acupuncture for treatment of CRPS. [16] Patients with CRPS of the upper or lower limb of one to four months duration were included, whether diagnosed clinically or with scintigraphically. Patients were randomly assigned to one of two groups: traditional acupuncture or sham acupuncture. The primary outcome was pain (measure by visual analog scale). At baseline, pain was similar in both groups, but patients in the active acupuncture group demonstrated a greater reduction in pain scores compared to those in the sham group. Unfortunately, these results were not statistically significant.

Acupuncture has repeatedly been suggested as an effective control for CRPS pain. Brief, intense and low frequency electroacupuncture for two CRPS patients showed encouraging clinical results. [17] Chan and Chow reported on 20 patients with established RSD, of whom 14 were successfully treated by electroacupuncture. [18] Leo also described a child suffering from CRPS treated successfully with electroacupuncture. [19]

MANUAL LYMPH DRAINAGE

Manual lymphatic drainage (MLD) has also been studied as a treatment modality for CRPS. MLD is a type of gentle massage which is intended to encourage the natural drainage of the lymph. Manual lymph drainage uses a specific amount of pressure and rhythmic circular movements to stimulate lymph flow. Prospective and randomized studies performed for MLD are few but informative about the role of MLD as a potential treatment for CRPS. It has been postulated that MLD and physical therapy should be instituted as early as possible in order to avoid major functional limitations. [20] Exercise in combination with manual lymph drainage, when compared to exercise alone, applied over six weeks showed no significant improvement in clinical parameters (pain, swelling, temperature, and range of motion). Significant improvements in clinical parameters were observed in both groups, but the study pointed out that manual lymph drainage provided no additional benefit when applied in conjunction with an intensive exercise program. [20]

Another randomized study compared efficacy of MLD therapy on management of limb edema in CRPS. A control group received three treatment modalities (non-steroidal anti-inflammatory drugs, physical therapy, and a regimented exercise program), while the intervention group received the same plus MLD. Edema improved significantly in the short term for the intervention group only, but this improvement was no longer evident through follow-up visits. [21]

MIRROR THERAPY

Mirror therapy is discussed to a greater extent in Chapter 7 (*Physical Therapy & Functional Rehabilitation*), but is also briefly noted here as it is viewed by some as falling under the realm of complementary and alternative therapy.

In mirror therapy, patients perform movements of the unaffected limb while watching its mirror reflection superimposed over the affected limb. This creates a visual illusion (and therefore positive feedback for the motor cortex) of the affected limb movement. The visual illusion of the affected limb movement generates positive feedback to the motor cortex, which is intended to in turn interrupt the cycle of chronic pain. [22]

Although initially applied to other patient populations, like phantom limb pain, mirror therapy now has established evidence in CRPS care. In a 2009 study, stroke patients with upper limb CRPS were randomly allocated to undertake the conventional stroke rehabilitation program plus mirror therapy or conventional stroke rehabilitation program alone. Primary outcomes (visual analogue scale score of pain at rest, with movement, and with brush-induced tactile allodynia) and secondary end points (motor function) significantly improved in the mirror group. No statistically significant improvement was observed in any of the control group values. The results indicate that mirror therapy can effectively reduce pain and enhance upper limb motor function in stroke patients with upper limb CRPS I. [23]

GRADED MOTOR IMAGERY

Similar to mirror therapy, graded motor imagery (GMI) is described in greater detail in Chapter 7 (*Physical Therapy & Functional Rehabilitation*) and is briefly noted in this chapter as it may also fall under the auspices of complementary and alternative medicine. GMI follows the primary principle of mirror therapy. It involves activating cortical networks including pre-motor cortex in a manner that does not initially involve movement of the affected limb. Thus, GMI treatment involves motor imagery, which activates similar cortical networks to executed movements but does not involve physical movement. In patients with chronic CRPS I, the efficacy of GMI was evaluated in a randomized fashion with results favoring its use for care of CRPS I patients. [24]

ELECTROMAGNETIC FIELD THERAPY

Electromagnetic field therapy (EFT) has also been studied as a treatment option in CRPS. EFT uses directed magnetic fields through affected tissue. Magnetic fields are created by electrical energy and there are various devices in the market that could be used. A randomized double-blind, placebo-controlled study was conducted to evaluate the benefit of EFT in patients with CRPS I, but did not find a significant statistical improvement with EFT over control therapy. [25] While all participants received calcitonin and followed an exercise regimen for 6 weeks, the intervention and control groups differed in that the intervention group also received EFT and the control group received placebo treatment. No statistically significant additional benefit was observed with EFT over calcitonin and exercise.

CONCLUSION

Physical and psychological therapy, along with medications, interventional pain procedures, and surgical options, have been the mainstay in the treatment of CRPS. CAM strategies, including acupuncture as well as other therapies, are gaining recognition as available treatment options for CRPS. A treatment algorithm for CRPS should include a plethora of therapeutic strategies for effective management. Physical and rehabilitation techniques have been effective in restoring range of motion in patients suffering from CRPS. Acupuncture has been effective in lessening the burden of severe allodynia and restoring functional status. Lymph drainage may be acutely helpful to decrease edema in the effected limb.

Despite this evidence for application of CAM therapies, further studies are needed for each type of treatment in order to elucidate its effectiveness as both a single as well as a combination treatment. It should also be noted that acupuncture and other modalities described herein also have the added property of being operator dependent.

CAM modalities have the potential of being beneficial when used in combination with medication management, minimally invasive procedures, and surgical interventions. Functional MRI and other emerging imaging technologies (See Chapter 9: Future Research and Advances in Technology) will help to guide the application of CAM interventions and evaluate their efficacy for patients affected by CRPS.

REFERENCES

[1]   Bruehl S, Harden RN, Galer BS, Saltz S, Bertram M, Backonja M, et al. External validation of IASP diagnostic criteria for Complex Regional Pain Syndrome and

proposed research diagnostic criteria. International Association for the Study of Pain. *Pain.* 1999;81(1-2):147-54.

[2]   Stanton-Hicks MD, Burton AW, Bruehl SP, Carr DB, Harden RN, Hassenbusch SJ, et al. An updated interdisciplinary clinical pathway for CRPS: report of an expert panel. *Pain practice: the official journal of World Institute of Pain.* 2002;2(1):1-16.

[3]   Stanton-Hicks M, Baron R, Boas R, Gordh T, Harden N, Hendler N, et al. Complex Regional Pain Syndromes: guidelines for therapy. *The Clinical journal of pain.* 1998;14(2):155-66.

[4]   Yang LM. [Medico-psychology in Huang di nei jing (Yellow Emperor's Inner Canon)]. *Zhonghua yi shi za zhi.* 2004;34(1):21-6.

[5]   Liao SJ. Acupuncture for low back pain in huang di nei jing su wen. (Yellow Emperor's Classic of Internal Medicine Book of Common Questions). *Acupuncture & electro-therapeutics research.* 1992;17 (4):249-58.

[6]   Reston J. Now about my operation in Peking. *New York Times.* 1971 July 26,1971.

[7]   Bonica JJ. Acupuncture anesthesia in the People's Republic of China Implications for American medicine. *JAMA.* 1974;229(10):1317-25.

[8]   NIH Consensus Conference. Acupuncture. *JAMA.* 1998;280(17):1518-24.

[9]   Berman BM, Singh BB, Lao L, Langenberg P, Li H, Hadhazy V, et al. A randomized trial of acupuncture as an adjunctive therapy in osteoarthritis of the knee. *Rheumatology* (Oxford). 1999;38(4):346-54.

[10]   Niemtzow RC. Battlefield Acupuncture. *Medical acupuncture.* 2007;19(4):225-8.

[11]   Hui KK, Liu J, Makris N, Gollub RL, Chen AJ, Moore CI, et al. Acupuncture modulates the limbic system and subcortical gray structures of the human brain: evidence from fMRI studies in normal subjects. *Human brain mapping.* 2000;9(1):13-25.

[12]   Pud D, Granovsky Y, Yarnitsky D. The methodology of experimentally induced diffuse noxious inhibitory control (DNIC)-like effect in humans. *Pain.* 2009;144(1-2):16-9.

[13]   Le Bars D, Villanueva L, Bouhassira D, Willer JC. Diffuse noxious inhibitory controls (DNIC) in animals and in man. *Patologicheskaia fiziologiia i eksperimental'naia terapiia.* 1992(4):55-65.

[14]   Shang YJ, Ma CC, Cai YY, Wang DS, Kong LL. [Clinical study on acupuncture combined with rehabilitation therapy for treatment of poststroke shoulder-hand syndrome]. *Zhongguo zhen jiu = Chinese acupuncture & moxibustion.* 2008;28(5):331-3.

[15]   Bar A, Li Y, Eichlisberger R, Angst F, Aeschlimann A. Acupuncture improves peripheral perfusion in patients with reflex sympathetic dystrophy. *Journal of clinical rheumatology: practical reports on rheumatic & musculoskeletal diseases.* 2002;8(1):6-12.

[16]   Ernst E, Resch K, Fialka V, Ritter-Dittrich D, Alcamioglu Y, Chen O, et al. Traditional acupuncture for reflex sympathetic dystrophy: a randomised, sham-controlled, double-blind trial. *Acupunct Med.* 1995;13(2):78-80.

[17]   Melzack R. Prolonged relief of pain by brief, intense transcutaneous somatic stimulation. *Pain.* 1975;1(4):357-73.

[18]   Chan CS, Chow SP. Electroacupuncture in the treatment of post-traumatic sympathetic dystrophy (Sudeck's atrophy). *British journal of anaesthesia.* 1981;53(8):899-902.

[19] Leo KC. Use of electrical stimulation at acupuncture points for the treatment of reflex sympathetic dystrophy in a child. *A case report. Physical therapy.* 1983;63(6):957-9.

[20] Uher EM, Vacariu G, Schneider B, Fialka V. [Comparison of manual lymph drainage with physical therapy in complex regional pain syndrome, type I. A comparative randomized controlled therapy study]. *Wiener klinische Wochenschrift.* 2000; 112(3):133-7.

[21] Duman I, Ozdemir A, Tan AK, Dincer K. The efficacy of manual lymphatic drainage therapy in the management of limb edema secondary to reflex sympathetic dystrophy. *Rheumatology international.* 2009;29(7):759-63.

[22] McCabe CS, Haigh RC, Ring EF, Halligan PW, Wall PD, Blake DR. A controlled pilot study of the utility of mirror visual feedback in the treatment of complex regional pain syndrome (type 1). *Rheumatology* (Oxford). 2003;42(1):97-101.

[23] Cacchio A, De Blasis E, Necozione S, di Orio F, Santilli V. Mirror therapy for chronic complex regional pain syndrome type 1 and stroke. *The New England journal of medicine.* 2009; 361(6):634-6.

[24] Moseley GL. Graded motor imagery is effective for long-standing complex regional pain syndrome: a randomised controlled trial. *Pain.* 2004;108(1-2):192-8.

[25] Durmus A, Cakmak A, Disci R, Muslumanoglu L. The efficiency of electromagnetic field treatment in Complex Regional Pain Syndrome Type I. *Disability and rehabilitation.* 2004;26(9):537-45.

In: Complex Regional Pain Syndrome
Editors: Nader D. Nader and Ognjen Visnjevac

ISBN: 978-1-63483-130-7
© 2015 Nova Science Publishers, Inc.

Chapter 9

FUTURE RESEARCH AND ADVANCES IN TECHNOLOGY

Ognjen Visnjevac, MD[*]

Department of Anesthesiology and Pain Medicine,
University at Buffalo, Buffalo, NY, US

INTRODUCTION

The next several of decades hold immeasurable promise in many areas of future research for CRPS. This chapter is designed to educate the reader about the limitations of current evidence while encouraging new investigations in all aspects of CRPS and CRPS-related fields of research. At the same time, in an effort to inspire original investigations in management of CRPS, this chapter was written to provide the readership with an introduction to some new technologies, potential pharmaceutical agents, and emerging cellular and molecular evidence from other fields of research not directly related to CRPS or pain management. Lastly, this chapter is meant to stir some discussion about gaps in current evidence, potential directions of future research, and to encourage collaboration between clinicians from multiple disciplines. The readership must recognize, however, that this chapter is current as of early 2015 and its contents should be taken in this context.

SURGICALLY IMPLANTED SUPRASPINAL STIMULATORS

Overview

Neuromodulation encompasses a broad range of interventions, including supraspinal neurostimulation. At its core, all neurostimulatory devices are developed with the intent to manipulate the basic principles of gate-control theory, initially described in 1965, but several additional physiologic mechanisms have since been elucidated and will be described herein.

---

[*] Corresponding author: Clinical Instructor, Department of Anesthesiology and Pain Medicine, University at Buffalo, Buffalo, NY, USA ovisnjevac@yahoo.com.

[1] Essentially any neuronal structure can become the target of neurostimulatory devices, from peripheral nerves, to dorsal root ganglia, to spinal cord, cranial nerves, and both cortical and deep brain structures.

The utility of neurostimulatory devices is not limited to analgesia, however, and has in fact been arguably more widely accepted in other medical and surgical specialties. Since the 1970s, spinal cord stimulation was used for treatment of neurogenic bladder and deep brain stimulation (DBS) has been used for the treatment of Parkinson's disease. [2, 3] Transcutaneous nerve stimulation has been utilized for more than 40 years with various pain-related indications and is broadly accepted. Both peripheral and spinal cord stimulation have been the topic of numerous investigations throughout the latter half of the 20th century, but have just recently become expansively popularized by increasing media attention and a growing mass of evidence, despite a disparity in research funding. [4]

Although DBS was first described 60 years ago, initially reported to result in successful analgesia in patients with psychiatric disease with an expansive array of indications for which it was utilized since its inception, the FDA rescinded its approval status in 1986. [5] In 1996, the FDA allowed for the re-introduction of these devices for movement disorders, shortly thereafter followed by off-label implantation of DBS for a variety of refractory pain syndromes. Unfortunately, for chronic pain indications, DBS remains under the auspices of off-label investigational use at present. Another supraspinal neurostimulatory modality, motor cortex stimulation, has been FDA approved, however, and together these are currently the only two implantable supraspinal modalities available for treatment of pain.

Despite evidence for their use in other chronic pain syndromes, these deep brain and MCS interventions have only sparingly been used in the CRPS and represent a youthful frontier of potential therapeutic targets for analgesia and functional improvements.

DEEP BRAIN STIMULATION (DBS)

Neuroanatomical Targets

Conventional targets for DBS seek to stimulate neuroanatomical areas of sensory discrimination. [6-15] Thus, targets like the periaqueductal grey and periventricular grey, along with the ventroposterolateral and ventroposteromedial nuclei of the thalamus, have classically been investigated as analgesic targets for DBS. The periaqueductal grey and periventricular grey are involved in inhibition of nociception through descending pathways, but may also facilitate ascending analgesic activity in the thalamus and frontal lobe. [9, 16, 17] It appears clear that implantation of a neurostimulatory device into the periaqueductal or periventricular grey leads to naloxone-reversible endorphin production and release. [7, 9, 16, 18-20] Although, the ventroposterolateral and ventroposteromedial nuclei of the thalamus are classic targets for pain relief with DBS, the thalamic nucleus ventralis caudalis has more recently been described as an effective target site as well. [21]

Surgical Technique

Electrode placement and implantation for DBS is performed stereotactically through a parasagittal frontal burr hole. Once the stereotactic frame is in place, thin-cut MRI imaging is done to identify the target area(s) and plan the procedure. Local anesthesia is utilized with additional as-needed intravenous sedation. Target sites are deep by definition and thorough planning must be undertaken to avoid blood vessels and damage to other neurological structures while performing this highly invasive procedure. [6] It is important to recognize that stereotactic localization is preliminary only and must be confirmed intraoperatively by physiological microelectrode and/or macroelectrode recording and stimulation for more precise localization. [13, 22] It is also important to consider that some facilities will have the capability to perform a stereotactic MRI on the day of surgery, but others will not, necessitating the MRI to be done preoperatively, followed by a CT with the frame in place on the day of surgery for merging of images.

Once intraoperative physiologic localization has been confirmed, permanent electrodes are placed and the leads are externalized for trial stimulation. A postoperative CT or MRI Is often performed both to identify possible intracranial hemorrhage and to confirm electrode placement. Stimulation trials follow after the patient has recovered postoperatively and typically last 5 to 9 days. Subsequently, patients with successful trials typically return to the OR for the leads to be connected to a permanent pulse generator, while those with unsuccessful trials have their leads removed. [5]

Efficacy

DBS efficacy has been variable in relation to both pain indication and neuroanatomical target for stimulator lead placement. Target sites include the sensory thalamic nuclei (ventroposterolateral, ventroposteromedial, ventralis caudalis) along with the periaqueductal and periventricular grey, and, in the case of treating chronic cluster headaches, the posterior hypothalamus. Indications have varied widely across reports, with broad inclusive descriptions like nociceptive and neuropathic pain, along with more narrowly defined pain syndromes like phantom limb pain, thalamic pain syndrome, and post-stroke pain. To date, DBS has not been used to treat CRPS pain or other CRPS symptomatology. Thus, the evidence presented herein is intended to act as a conglomerated set of data upon which CRPS-focused DBS trials may be designed.

A review of DBS found that 50% (561 of 1,114) of DBS patients experienced long-term analgesia, but that the results varied widely (19% to 79%) based on population studied and neuroanatomical site of stimulation. [5] Stimulation of the thalamus directly, for example, specifically the ventroposterolateral nucleus, does not always result in analgesia. 56% of patient (228 of 409) with neuropathic pain who received ventroposterolateral stimulation were reported to have long term success, while zero of the 51 patients experiencing chronic nociceptive pain experiencing lasting relief. Conversely, when the periventricular grey was stimulated, only 23% of patients (35 of 155) suffering neuropathic pain experienced lasting relief, but 59% of nociceptive pain patients (172 of 291) had long-term success. It is important to recognize that some pain syndromes, like failed back surgery syndrome, are not comprised of isolated pathophysiology and have components of both nociceptive (i.e., lumbar pain) and neuropathic (radicular) pain. For these patients, deep brain implants into both sensory thalamic nuclei and the periaqueductal or periventricular grey may be necessary for optimal results, but additional research will be needed prior to establishing evidence-based recommendations for this interventional technique.

Phantom limb pain has been treated by DBS implantation with report of 55-70% pain relief in one study, but a mean of 39% in another at 1-year follow-up. [23, 24] Interestingly, one study recruited only phantom limb patients who had persistent pain despite spinal cord stimulator placement for this indication and these patients received DBS, MCS, or both. Of the patients receiving DBS, 60% reported long term pain relief. [25]

In a meta-analysis of post-stroke pain, DBS was found to be less effective than it has been shown for some other syndromes, with 50% of patients having a successful trial and 29% retaining lasting relief. [23] A subsequent study reported that post-stroke pain patients only had successful DBS trials 33% of the time. [26] In what is currently the largest prospective study in this body of evidence, a 12-year prospective study of DBS for neuropathic pain, post-stroke pain patients reported a mean 44% pain relief at 1-year follow-up. [24]

DBS has not been effective in treating central pain syndromes like, thalamic pain syndrome, with few having successful trials and rare long-term success. [42, 28] This may in part be due to the post-infarction encephalomalacia associated with thalamic pain syndrome resulting in a futile attempt to place leads at damaged thalamic targets. [6] Similarly, pain post-spinal cord injury has also shown modest results with treatment by DBS, with reports of 6 of 22 patients receiving lasting relief. [24, 28] Generally, DBS is not thought to be effective for central pain syndromes. [5, 6]

Chronic cluster headaches may arguably be the most consistent indication for which DBS is effective. 60.5% of patients had complete resolution or "almost pain free" at 12-23 month follow-up and pain-free days increased from 2% to 71% at 5-year follow-up. [29-31] These findings include data from a randomized, double-blind, sham-controlled DBS trial, presenting the highest level of evidence for DBS in pain therapy among any of the pain syndromes mentioned herein. [30] Several interesting findings are to be highlighted in regard to this subset of studies. For one, in this randomized controlled trial, when patients were assessed at 1-month follow-up, there were no differences between DBS and sham stimulation groups, yet differences became highly evident in the subsequent 1-year follow-up with the intervention group showing marked improvement. Secondly, the target site for stimulation was different than all other studies: the posterior hypothalamus. Together, these two observations provide a slew of questions for future research relating not only to the target site and the best measure of outcomes in relation to timing of follow-up, but to investigations of neurophysiology and pathophysiology with potential for identifying broader and more diverse indications for this therapy, including CRPS.

Complications

Intracranial hemorrhage is the most significant complication with DBS placement and has been reported at both the time of insertion and the time of removal of the electrode. Of the 4 deaths associated with DBS placement for pain, 3 were the result of intracranial hemorrhage. Although the incidence has been reported between 1.9% and 4.1%, the use of contemporary coaxial DBS electrodes may have resulted in a decreased incidence. Of 649 patients assessed, 14 patients suffered permanent neurological injury, the majority of which were attributed to intracranial hemorrhage. [5] Most intracranial hemorrhage occurs at the cortical entry site and is asymptomatic, with few symptomatic cases requiring evacuation or devise removal. [6] Infectious complications are more common related to hardware, rarely being intracranial, and are reported at 2.4%. [32]

Headache is the most common minor complication (51.5%) and adverse effects from periaqueductal or periventricular grey stimulation have mostly been confined to transient visual phenomena with the following distribution: diplopia (14.2%), nausea (10.6%), vertical gaze palsies (9.9%), blurred vision (9.2%), horizontal nystagmus (4.3%), and persistent oscillopsia (3.5%). [5]

Future Research

Herein, many pain indications for DBS, including their efficacies and complications, have been described but there have been no studies or reports of DBS for CRPS. Future DBS research for CRPS can be broadly, but not exclusively, separated by neuroanatomical target site, types of studies, safety, efficacy, and ethical considerations.

Neuroanatomical target sites and their relative efficacies for nociceptive pain (periaqueductal and periventricular grey) and neuropathic pain (ventroposterolateral and ventroposteromedial nuclei of the thalamus) have been identified. Both of these pain types are major components of CRPS and show promise for future research with DBS. Although success has been specific to chronic cluster headaches for another neuroanatomical target site, the posterior hypothalamus, the lasting analgesic effects are consistent across chronic cluster headache studies and this represents a potential target area for CRPS therapy as well. As with failed back surgery syndrome, research with DBS for CRPS may yield more favorable results when multiple target sites are trialed and implanted concurrently. [5]

In regard to types of studies, several considerations should be taken into account. Although the easiest strategy would be to publish a retrospective report of a case or series, it would not be overly cumbersome to perform a prospective observational trial. As DBS is currently still in off-label investigational use per the FDA, whether a DBS is to be placed for research or non-research purposes, informed patient consent would necessitate a thorough discussion of risks, benefits, and follow-up, with focus on the experimental or investigational nature of this treatment modality for CRPS. Having discussed the experimental nature already, it would take minimal extra effort to obtain consent to retain data for research purposes and continue procuring data postoperatively during preset follow-up times. Such prospective observational studies would yield data of higher value than a retrospective case report or series.

To address safety and efficacy, such data could be utilized to obtain high-level evidence by providing the basis to design and conduct a robust randomized controlled trial. It is worth noting, however, that sham controls will likely be ethically controversial both due to the invasive nature of this therapy and due to questions of vulnerability in this patient population. More than likely, a crossover design with stimulator "on" and "off" periods would need to be utilized. Well-documented transient adverse effects experienced by non-CRPS patient populations with periaqueductal and periventricular grey stimulation may complicate safety assessments, confound the blinded nature necessary to maintain validity in a randomized controlled trial, and increase risk of patients choosing to remove themselves from the active arm of the study or being lost to follow-up.

Thus, like other pain states, patient selection must play a primary role for choice of intervention. As DBS has the potential for highly morbid complications, along with transient unpleasant symptoms, it may be wise to recruit patients with CRPS refractory to physical therapy, psychotherapy, medical management, and other interventional techniques. As was done in a study of DBS therapy for phantom limb pain patients, where recruitment was limited to those who failed spinal cord stimulator therapy, a similar recruitment strategy may select for CRPS patients with a better risk-benefit profile, given that they may have exhausted other potential therapies without relief prior to undergoing a DBS trial. This refractory subset of CRPS patients may indeed provide the first evidence of CRPS-specific DBS safety and efficacy.

MOTOR CORTEX STIMULATION

Neuroanatomical Targets

In contrast to DBS, motor cortex stimulation (MCS) is thought to function primarily by increasing blood flow to the brainstem and thalamus, while upregulating endogenous opioid production in the periaqueductal grey. [33-35] There is some evidence of MCS leading to dorsal horn inhibition by activation of descending inhibitory pathways, but the degree to which this contributes to analgesia is controversial. [6, 36] MCS has also been implicated to affect the emotional interpretation of pain by inducing hypermetabolism in the anterior cingulate cortex and insula. [34, 37-40]

Although seemingly off mark when compared to the sensory cortex, the motor cortex has been shown to be more effective target area than the sensory cortex. [41-46] Considering that the motor cortex coverage of body parts is represented by the classic homunculus, one must recognize that targeting different structures will involve varying degrees of difficulty. Although surgical techniques for MCS are discussed in greater detail in Chapter 6 (Interventional Techniques and Neuromodulation), it is important to note that structures like the interhemispheric fissure present surgical and logistical difficulties for targeting lower extremity pain that clinicians would not be faced with when stimulating the cortical convexity to target facial or upper extremity pain. To combat anatomical barriers to optimal lead placement, some surgeons choose increased stimulation intensities with midline epidural leads to indirectly drive current deeper into the motor cortex of the lower extremity, while others choose a subdural approach in the interhemispheric fissure for direct stimulation. [5, 47]

Future Research

Herein, preliminary reports of MCS for treatment of CRPS have been described. In fact, despite the first report of MCS for a pain syndrome published more than 2 decades ago, there is a lack of high-level evidence to implement MCS for pain indications. [5, 48, 49] Future MCS research for CRPS can be separated into studies regarding neuroanatomy and physiology, equipment, and efficacy.

Compared to DBS, neuroanatomical targeting differs for MCS in one major facet: the motor cortex is the only available target site. Thus, the neuroanatomical targeting questions yet to be elucidated are not a question of where, but how to be most effective at stimulating specific desired regions of the homunculus. Part of this dilemma stems from difficulties of anatomical approach (i.e., targeting the interhemispheric fissure for lower extremity CRPS), but another part is electrode design, while another still is stimulator or pulse generator programming and optimization. MCS was first performed using paddle electrodes designed for spinal cord stimulators, which did not have the ideal anatomical design or discrimination for motor cortex implantation. Recently, an octopolar lead has been trialed, but lead design and optimization remain a broad area of research and development. [50] Together, neuroanatomical targeting and electrode development represent a vast and expansive field of inquiry, spanning questions of neurophysiology or disease-specific pathophysiology, therapeutic efficacy, and complications. Neuroanatomical investigations are not limited to the empirical, however, and can be expanded to involve positron emission tomography (PET), as was done in a recent CRPS case series and in studies of other patient populations. [34, 37] In fact, PET-integrated studies may yield prognostic data to objectively measure outcomes beyond clinical observations, potentially improving therapeutic efficacy for all therapies used in CRPS.

As with DBS, a higher level of evidence is required before any recommendations can be made regarding MCS for treatment of CRPS. Although 2 of the 4 published reports are randomized, double-blinded crossover trials with evidence that MCS for CRPS is an effective therapy, the sample size remains small with a total of 7 patients. Future studies are not limited to larger sample sizes, but open to a variety of topics like optimization of outcomes, defining predictive values for success from a slew of patient or equipment parameters, and further elucidating the pathophysiological and/or surgical mechanisms involved in MCS as it pertains to CRPS.

In designing larger trials, MCS has one distinct advantage over DBS: the lack of paresthesia or other symptoms that are more commonly associated with DBS. The only effect of stimulator activation experienced by the patient is pain relief, or lack thereof, with associated improvement in function and, in the case of treating CRPS, sympathetic signs. Hence, potential CRPS patients treated with sham versus active MCS remain blind to their therapy. Although a crossover design remains ideal to show efficacy, larger, multicenter, long-term studies along with safety trials are needed before this therapy can be recommended for use in CRPS.

Lastly, even if efficacy is proven in larger future trials, this remains a highly invasive intervention and should not be first line therapy. The patients described in the current literature failed medical management, physiotherapy, psychotherapy, and in many cases spinal cord stimulator placement, or other interventional techniques and were, thus, felt to be refractory CRPS patients for whom MCS was to be considered.

Summary

- Supraspinal stimulation is an option for CRPS therapy, especially for those CRPS patients with disease refractory to all other therapies, but both DBS and MCS remain investigational or "off-label" for this indication.
- DBS has shown efficacy for neuropathic pain and nociceptive pain states, both of which are components of CRPS, but this intervention has not yet been applied to CRPS patients.
- MCS has been consistently effective for the treatment of CRPS, but equipment optimization and larger clinical trials are needed before recommendation can be made to use this therapy.
- For optimal management of chronic pain states, whether CRPS or otherwise, patient selection and technical considerations must play a primary role in the decision to undergo implantation of deep brain or motor cortex neuromodulatory devices.

TRANSCRANIAL MAGNETIC STIMULATION

Overview

As mentioned previously in this chapter, DBS and MCS can be effective for managing a variety of otherwise treatment-resistant chronic pain syndromes, but these invasive strategies require careful perioperative care and carry the risk of significant complications, including death. [5, 6] Transcranial magnetic stimulation (TMS) offers a potential alternative approach to achieve similar neuromodulatory results as deep brain or MCS without surgical intervention. TMS is a non-invasive, magnetic field-driven, neuromodulatory technology used for inducing electrical currents (depolarization or hyperpolarization) in targeted areas of the brain for the purpose of modulating the activity of underlying neuronal networks. [51-53] It has been used both prognostically (for predicting success of surgically implanted MCSs) and therapeutically. Therapeutic approaches have differed in many ways, however, including neuroanatomical target sites, type of magnetic coil used, frequency and intensity of stimulation, number of pulses applied, orientation of induced current, number of therapeutic sessions, and patient pathophysiology. Unsurprisingly, this heterogeneity of therapeutic protocols has produced a wide spectrum of results.

TMS mechanisms of action are similarly multifactorial, pertaining not only to site of stimulation but to technical parameters and patient pathophysiology as well. It is important to recognize that the body of knowledge regarding TMS mechanisms of action is evolving with much of the data limited to animal studies or human studies integrating other technologies to target the same neuroanatomical areas. Targeting the primary motor cortex is thought to inhibit hyperactive thalamic nuclei by activation of inhibitory gamma-aminobutyric acid (GABA)-responsive neurons within corticothalamic pathways, thereby attenuating nociception. In healthy patients, unilateral TMS of the primary motor cortex induces a bilateral increase in pain thresholds in a naloxone-reversible manner, suggesting involvement of opiate-mediated signaling within this set of pain pathways. [54, 55] Although stimulation of the dorsolateral prefrontal cortex has also been reported to induce analgesia in some studies, others have found that has a more profound effect on the emotional aspects of pain perception with only modest effects on analgesia directly. [54, 56, 57] Stimulation of either locus appears to induce activity in distant brain areas to modulate pathways involved in integration and processing of pain, with evidence of activity in lateral and medial thalami, anterior cingulate cortex, brain stem, and insula. [55-61] Interestingly, there is evidence that NMDA activation plays a role in anti-nociceptive modulation of spinal pain inputs, with findings that ketamine reduces the analgesic efficacy of TMS at both the motor cortex and the dorsolateral prefrontal cortex. [62]

TMS was not developed solely for the treatment of pain, however, with the initial 1985 report focusing on this technology's ability to obtain motor evoked potentials. [53] Subsequent technological advancements in the early 1990s resulted in the capacity to provide repetitive stimulations, or pulses, of TMS (repetitive TMS or rTMS). Early clinical applications focused on stimulation of the dorsolateral prefrontal cortex for treatment of depressive disorders after observation that rTMS was able to induce neuromodulatory changes that exceeded the duration of rTMS treatment. [51, 63-65] A decade after the first report of surgical implantation of a MCS for treatment of pain, rTMS was investigated as a non-invasive alternative with the added finding that it had potential as a prognosticative modality to be used for patient selection of candidates prior to surgical MCS implants. [49, 66, 67]

Since its inception, TMS has been used for neurophysiological investigations, adopted as a therapeutic modality for treatment of major depressive disorder, and is actively being pursued for its potential as an tool for management of both acute and chronic pain. [52, 53, 68-71] It has been shown to be effective for treatment of various types of depression, often by targeting stimulation of the dorsolateral prefrontal cortex. [71-75] More recently, it has been investigated as a therapeutic modality for the treatment of pain, including CRPS, but varied results and methodological concerns have limited generalizability of results. [68, 69, 76-81]

TMS Evidence in CRPS

There has been a paucity of evidence for the use of TMS in CRPS, specifically. [81-87] The majority of studies have focused on identifying changes in cortical excitability. [81, 83-85] To date, only two randomized trials have been conducted with this technology, collectively involving a total of 33 treatment-resistant CRPS patients. [82, 87] Given this lack of CRPS-specific TMS data, there are many avenues for future research, ranging from investigations of neural network activity in various subsets of CRPS patients or animal models to optimizing TMS parameters to meet specific treatment goals (i.e., modulation of anti-nociceptive, anti-anxiety or anti-depressive pathways).

The first sham-controlled randomized crossover trial of rTMS for treatment of CRPS was conducted in 2004 and had positive results in 7 of 10 patients receiving real rTMS, with findings of discernable analgesia beginning within 30 seconds after treatment and peak effect at 15 minutes. The duration of analgesia was limited, however, with recession of analgesia starting at 45 minutes post-treatment for some. The sham-rTMS did not result in any positive findings. Side effects were minor. The treatment arm received rTMS through a figure-of-eight magnetic stimulation coil targeting the primary motor cortex in a single session with the following parameters: 10 rTMS administrations of pulses at 10 Hz, each applied over a duration of 1.2 seconds, at an intensity of 110% of motor threshold with 10-second breaks between trains of pulses. This study's inclusion and exclusion criteria limited recruitment to patients with CRPS I affecting a unilateral hand and the duration of symptomatology for those recruited ranged from 24 to 72 months. [87]

In the second sham-controlled randomized trial of rTMS for treatment of CRPS, rTMS was implemented as an adjunct therapy to patients already following a protocol of pharmacologic management. This study's authors also used a figure-of-eight coil with a 10 Hz frequency for stimulation of the homuncular portion of the primary motor cortex representing the affected hand, but differed in their other parameters. Rather than one session, each participant received 10 consecutive rTMS sessions over a two week period. Each session consisted of 25 10-second trains of rTMS pulses at 10 Hz, with 60-second breaks between trains of pulses, for a total of 2500 pulses per session (significantly greater than the 120 total pulses applied in the first trial) at an intensity of 100% of motor threshold. [82] Pain ratings and quality-of-life measures improved over the course of rTMS sessions, with peak reduction in pain rating (50.9%) immediately following the last treatment session. These positive findings were unfortunately no longer evident at 1 week and 3 month follow-up assessments. This study also included an internal control for placebo-effect among sham-controls in that patients were asked to discern their sham versus real rTMS sessions, which showed effective patient blinding. Questions of blinding efficacy due to adverse events of real treatment (skin irritation) have come up in TMS-depression studies as well, but a meta-analysis of sham-placebo controlled studies of TMS for depression also showed effective blinding between active and sham TMS groups. [88]

TMS for Other Chronic Pain Conditions

A recent meta-analysis of rTMS for neuropathic pain established several associations with success of therapy, including intensities below 100% of motor threshold, using a figure-of-eight coil over the hand or face area of the primary motor cortex (reflecting the difficulty of motor cortex targeting for lower extremity CRPS), frequencies of 10-20Hz, application of more than 1000 total pulses, and a posterior-anterior, rather than medial-lateral, coil orientation. [78]

In the only randomized sham-controlled trial of long-term maintenance of rTMS, sustained analgesic efficacy was reported even at 1-month intervals between treatments, but this study was limited by a 6-month follow-up period and included only fibromyalgia. Active rTMS participants received stimulation to the right primary motor cortex and showed long-term improvements in quality of life (fatigue, morning tiredness, general activity, walking, and sleep) in addition to analgesia. [89] In a 10-week randomized sham-controlled trial of rTMS to the left primary motor cortex, there was no analgesic benefit, but PET imaging showed increased right-sided limbic activity, which correlated with quality of life improvements, as measured by the Fibromyalgia Impact Questionnaire, as well as improvements in the mental component of the SF-36. [90, 91]

There have been failures with the use of rTMS as well. For example, postoperative rTMS was not effective in mitigating pain or morphine consumption with patient-controlled analgesia following lumbar spine surgery. [92] rTMS was similarly found to be ineffective at mitigating central pain after spinal cord injury. [76]

Future Research

Future research for rTMS in CRPS may fall into one or more of three broad categories:

- Pathophysiological and mechanism-focused investigations
- Technological advancements and parameter optimization in rTMS
- CRPS-specific clinical applications and development of goal-specific protocols

Pathophysiological and mechanism-focused investigations will likely entail investigations of neural network activity and modulation. These studies may be designed to assess pain or functional outcomes in animal models or humans. These studies may further be paired with other imaging technologies (i.e., PET or functional MRI) to elucidate regional neural network activity. Animal studies may further allow for cellular, neurophysiological, and neuropharmacologic investigations to be paired with rTMS to identify a variety of mechanisms that can lead to new basic science data that can then be applied through translational research to CRPS management. Examples of potential findings include changes in gene-expression, receptor and substrate regulation and signaling, along with data regarding medication-rTMS synergy or antagonism.

Much early research is expected to focus on technological advancements and parameter optimization in rTMS. Targets for research may include magnetic coil type used, frequency and intensity of stimulation, continuous versus intermittent stimulation, number of pulses applied, and number of therapeutic sessions.

For example, although rTMS appears to show consistent efficacy in treatment of depression, variable efficacy in pain has been theorized to coil design and its inability to target deeper structures of the brain. Thus, a newer design, the H-Coil, was proposed and trialed to target deeper structures in a population of patients with diabetic neuropathy. [70] Other coil designs are being investigated with promise for a broad spectrum of applications.

Frequencies of rTMS have varied greatly, from 1 Hz to 20 Hz, and optimization of intensities may be related to the pathophysiological target structures. The majority of investigations have used intermittent rTMS, as emphasized by a set frequency, but continuous TMS has emerged as a potential alternative. Theta-burst continuous TMS may be more effective than high-frequency rTMS, but investigations regarding its use are limited. [93, 94] One randomized trial of healthy volunteers compared three groups: theta-burst rTMS, high-frequency rTMS, and sham-rTMS as a control. They found that both active rTMS groups provided significantly greater analgesia and that theta-burst rTMS was superior to high-frequency rTMS both in patient outcomes and ease of administration of this technique. [95] Clinical outcomes and safety analyses will most likely drive research regarding the optimal number of pulses and therapeutic sessions. Although rTMS has generally been found to be safe, investigations are likely to be needed identify modifying factors that may limit unpleasant side effects of therapy. [71, 96]

CRPS-specific clinical applications will likely focus on individual patient symptomatology and studies may be designed to target multiple specific pathologies (i.e., pain, depression, self-perception, motor limitations). Thus, good quality research will require a high degree of care to minimize confounding factors during the patient selection process. Pathophysiological mechanisms of pain, functional impairment, and psychiatric symptoms may also guide optimization attempts and have an impact on efficacy of choice of neuroanatomical targeting in rTMS. [97] As the dorsolateral prefrontal cortex has been used for treatment of both pain and depression, it may become an increasingly investigated neuroanatomical target site. To date, the two randomized sham-controlled trials investigating rTMS efficacy in CRPS have targeted the primary motor cortex, which is more strongly associated with analgesia. [82, 87] Studies in fibromyalgia have shown variability in analgesia between left and right MCS, but there were also several methodological differences in the design of these studies. [89, 90] As careful targeting specific to the affected region of the homunculus on the motor cortex is a standard-of-care when MCSs are surgically implanted, neuronavigation strategies may become increasingly useful for optimizing outcomes in TMS therapy. [98] Of course, with the only study of maintenance rTMS, which was done in fibromyalgia patients, long-term studies will be needed to establish the long-term efficacy of rTMS in CRPS and investigations regarding optimal treatment protocols for maintenance therapy will need to be investigated.

Summary

- rTMS has shown promise in treatment of chronic pain of various etiologies, but methodologies and concurrent results have varied greatly
- There have been two randomized sham-controlled trials in CRPS patients with unilateral upper limb pathology with evidence of analgesic benefit and potential for long-term relief, but additional data is needed to optimize long-term efficacy and safety. These data may not be applicable to CRPS patients with other phenotypic presentations, as the efficacy of rTMS appears to be target-site dependent.
- rTMS may have implications for improvement in psychiatric symptoms and functional pathology as well, but CRPS-specific research is needed to evaluate the translatability of findings derived from studies done in other patient populations.
- TMS technology is rapidly evolving, with active investigation into optimization of coil types, parameters, and types of stimulation.

Functional Pain Imaging

Overview

Many forms or research investigate a single mechanism, tool, or therapy, and functional pain imaging research has the promise to become an integrative modality with many such investigations. It can also be used to substantiate the data obtained using other mechanisms. Furthermore, as imaging rarely presents itself as a confounding variable, it would unlikely hamper experimental designs and it has the potential to be more easily integrated into a wide variety of studies. This is especially true in an age when information processing is rapidly becoming more efficient and cost-effective, data sharing is becoming increasingly seamless, and powerful image-computing algorithms require perpetually smaller hardware installation. While some evidence exists to guide the roles of functional pain imaging in CRPS, additional investigation will be necessary. The following are broad areas of potential future research in functional pain imaging.

Understanding Neurological Mechanisms of CRPS-Specific Pathophysiology

Many investigations, while rooted in past pathophysiological or animal evidence, may not be able to provide cause-and-effect relationships or establish mechanisms of action, limiting their results to empirically obtained findings. Furthermore, central nervous system pathophysiological mechanisms often remain unaddressed, or alluded to without substantiated evidence of real-time activity. With the introduction of newer imaging technologies, real-time assessments are possible and have yielded some preliminary CRPS-specific data.

Changes in the prefrontal and motor cortex have been implicated in CRPS pathophysiology as assessed by functional MRI (fMRI). [99, 100] fMRI has also been used to identify insular activity corresponding to patients' central distributions of pain and corroborate data from neuroinflammatory studies. [101, 102] In pediatric CPRS patient, fMRI was used to identify transient and persistent pain-induced cerebral connectivity patterns. [103] PET has also been utilized to investigate central aspects of CRPS, but much additional research is needed to establish the optimal application of this imaging modality in CRPS management and research. [37, 104]

Functional MRI has also been utilized to identify central mechanisms of catastrophizing and distraction analgesia in chronic pain. [105] Similarly, this modality has been used to elucidate the neurophysiological underpinnings interconnecting emotions of lust and love with chronic pain. [106] Future research can build on these studies, compare efficacy of this imaging technology with other modalities, further elucidate pathophysiological mechanisms involved in CRPS, and apply this technology for objective prognostication of patient responsiveness to various therapies.

Diagnostics

The current CRPS diagnostic criteria are based on the definitions outlined by the International Association for the Study of Pain, but have been criticized as suboptimal in regards to validation and have been underutilized in research. [107-113] These criteria do not currently incorporate data from functional neuroimaging, but as evidence of distinctive CPRS-specific patterns emerges through functional investigations of pain imaging, such modalities may yield findings to be incorporated into CRPS diagnostic criteria. [99, 101, 103, 114] A major challenge will be the differentiation and isolation of CRPS-specific imaging patters when compared to other pain states. [115, 116]

Assessing Efficacy of Therapy

With the introduction of some of the newer imaging technologies, real-time assessments can be made prior, during, and after therapy. These types of assessments are not only useful as mechanistic studies, identifying neuroanatomical structures within which functional changes occur, but they are also useful for assessing comparative or synergistic efficacy of various therapies. In this manner, functional imaging may become increasingly ubiquitously applied for objective and reproducible assessment or prognostication of almost all other therapeutic modalities pertaining to CRPS management. Of course, different imaging modalities have the potential to yield variable results, thereby also establishing a need for validation studies.

To date, there have been few studies of functional imaging applied to assess the efficacy of therapy of CRPS. Functional MRI has been used to show cortical normalization in human case series of CRPS patients receiving peripheral sympathetic blocks. [117] Similarly, pediatric CRPS patients have shown normalization of intrinsic brain networks following an intensive 3-week physical and psychological treatment program. [118] Static central nervous system imaging has identified several loci in which neuroanatomical changes were present when comparing MRI brain images pre- and post-ketamine therapy. [119] Such findings may be useful in designs of future prospective real-time assessments of therapy.

Imaging as a Therapy

Positron emission tomography has been used for guidance of other therapies, like MCS and DBS. [37] Real-time fMRI has been used as an adjunct to biofeedback therapy and may take on a pivotal role in empowering patients to manage their own pain, self-perception, and psychiatric symptoms. [120-122] Bone scintigraphy has also been use to describe various scintigraphic patterns in CRPS patients and may prove useful for research related to bone changes in this syndrome [123] Transcranial magnetic stimulation has been similarly used for elicitations of motor evoked potentials and assessment of patient responsiveness prior to surgical implantation of MCSs. [124] Transcranial magnetic stimulation, in-and-of itself, has been used for treatment of CRPS (see the above section in this chapter titled, *Transcranial*

Magnetic Stimulation). Real-time fMRI, in particular, appears to be a very actively investigated area or functional imaging research at this time, with implications in the fields of pain, psychiatry, neuroscience, and rehabilitative medicine. Functional imaging has also been proposed as a requisite tool for development of central nervous system medications, and may play a role in the development of new therapies or validation of current therapies for CRPS. [125]

Prognostication Value

With the elucidation of CRPS-specific central neuropathophysiological mechanisms, along with potential new diagnostic criteria and treatment-specific functional imaging data, functional pain imaging tools may become increasingly useful for prognostication of syndrome or treatment progression. While current functional imaging data regarding therapy has largely been limited to investigations of mechanisms of action, other research has focused on empirically identifying effective and ineffective therapy. One case series of CRPS I and II patients, for example, identifies ketamine responders and non-responders. In this report, ketamine ointment was found to be effective in treating CRPS signs and symptoms in some patients, including improvements in dystrophic signs, but only in those patients without atrophy of the affected limb. [126] Although functional imaging may have provided clues to identify the mechanisms discerning ketamine-responders from non-responders, this study did not use any such modality, leaving room for future researchers to perform such investigations. Supporting the notion that neuroimaging may assist in differentiating medication-responsive and non-responsive patients, another study has shown that neuroanatomical changes were identifiable in static MRI imaging at various loci pre- and post-ketamine therapy. [119] This is but one example in which the incorporation of functional neuroimaging into study designs may not only elucidate the mechanisms by which non-responders fail therapy, but provide a new modality for prognostication of treatment. A similar design could be applied to most CRPS therapies and subsets of CRPS patients, thereby providing a plethora of potential future investigational opportunities.

Summary

- Functional pain imaging has started being investigated in CRPS patients.
- Functional pain imaging has potential for future application in identifying central neurological mechanisms underlying CRPS pathophysiology
- These modalities may find purpose in CRPS diagnostics and may have implications as both adjuvants to therapy and tools for assessing efficacy of other therapeutic modalities
- Functional pain imaging may provide prognostication value, but has only begun to be investigated in this regard.

PHARMACEUTICAL OPTIMIZATION: REFINING AND EXPANDING CURRENT EVIDENCE

Pharmaceutical or medical management remains at the forefront of therapy as a pillar for the treatment of CRPS. The pharmaceutical optimization segment has been split into two sections: (a) refining and expanding current evidence, and (b) potential therapeutic agents.

Bisphosphonates

Although bisphosphonates are classically used to treat diseases with pathologic bone metabolism, like osteoporosis or Paget's disease, they have gained popularity and shown efficacy for the treatment of neuropathic bone pain associated with CRPS. [127-136] Despite consistent reports of successful treatment, questions regarding bisphosphonates persist.

Although some would argue that the small number of patients presented in each study limits the generalizability of results, the results are overwhelmingly positive across studies, regardless of study design or choice of bisphosphonate. The small numbers do limit the reliability and generalizability of safety data, however, and safety should remain a concern until it is effectively and prospectively assessed in a larger sample. There is also a paucity of data to provide evidence-based recommendations regarding optimal dose and duration of treatment for each bisphosphonate. There have been no head-to-head studies comparing efficacy of one bisphosphonate to another for treatment of CPRS patients. Lastly, variability in bisphosphonate medications utilized and lack of concordance in data analyzed between studies limits meta-analytical conclusions. [129] Each of these gaps in evidence provides many opportunities for potential investigators to explore future avenues of research.

NMDA Antagonists: Ketamine, Memantine, and New Phencyclidine Derivatives

Although emerging evidence regarding N-methyl-D-aspartic acid (NMDA) receptor subunit variability, activity, neuroanatomical and temporal distributions, and expression suggests a plethora of significant implications for future research in modulating CRPS signs and symptoms, NMDA receptors are primarily discussed herein as they pertain to ketamine therapy. Ketamine has been trialed in many forms for the treatment of CRPS, including isoenantiomeric infusions, subanesthetic infusions (both inpatient and outpatient), and coma-inducing higher doses requiring intensive care admission. [137-148] Results have varied greatly, however, from no effect to complete and lasting remission of not only pain symptoms, but of sympathetic signs as well. This variability in response presents investigators with an expansive field of potential research from basic science studies to large-scale clinical trials.

Potential Mechanisms for Variability in Efficacy of Ketamine Therapy

As NMDA receptor activation is implicated in spinal cord plasticity in the dorsal horn and long-term potentiation of allodynia and hyperalgesia, the variable efficacy of ketamine may be a function of receptor-neuron-cortical pain axis maturation, whereby ketamine therapy may have variable efficacy at different neuroanatomical structures or, noting the plasticity of these structures, at different stages of CRPS. [149, 150] This is further supported by evidence of local anesthetic resistance to the CRPS-affected area in a case of a child with CRPS who received anesthetic doses of local anesthetics through an epidural catheter that resulted in absolution of sympathetic signs, but had no effects on pain. [151] It may be that in such cases, plastic neuronal changes and centralization of pain have already occurred, limiting ketamine efficacy in the dorsal horns of the spinal cord. Supporting this notion, ketamine ointment was found to be effective in treating acute CRPS, but was ineffective when atrophic changes had already taken place. [126] Future research may combine ketamine therapy with imaging techniques to assess centralization of pain and evaluate treatment efficacy with various dose-duration ketamine protocols. It may prove true that treatment of centralized pain may require higher doses or longer duration of therapy for patients who fail low dose infusion trials or topical ointment therapy. An induction period exceeding 1-month was required in a randomized controlled trial of DBS for chronic cluster headaches, suggesting that similarly prolonged induction periods may be required with other therapies when targeting central components of various pain syndromes, including CRPS. [30]

NMDA is also implicated in memory formation, both short and long-term, through variable actions on several subtypes of NMDA receptors in the hippocampus, which may play a role in the supraspinal component of pain centralization and pain-memory formation. [162] Ketamine's effects on short-term and long-term potentiation of pain memory in CRPS require further research, both in the acute setting and in chronic treatment-resistant cases of CRPS, but investigators must consider that empirical evidence exists showing that unlearning of centralized pain is possible. [140, 142, 143, 153, 154]

Wide dynamic range neurons in the dorsal horn are thought to be responsive to a variety of stimuli, from light mechanical stimulation to nociceptive input and involve various fiber types. They have been proposed to play a crucial role in sympathetically maintained pain, with various etiologies that may contribute to allodynia and hyperalgesia. [155] Some of these physiological processes may be ketamine-responsive, while others may not be, but further research is needed to elucidate interactions between ketamine and wide dynamic neurons in CRPS patients.

Pharmacogentics may play a role and further research could help clinicians identify candidates for ketamine trials. [156] For example, a recent meta-analysis found genetic variability to significantly impact human responsiveness to opiates. [157] Along with genetic variability, one must consider NMDA receptor subunit distribution and how that may differ between patients in reference to their symptomatology. In the mid-1990s a differential effect of NMDA activity was identified in various neuronal structures, which led to the discovery of several subtypes NMDA receptors. NMDA receptor morphology was found to possess a heterotetramer structure differentially composed of subunits GluN1, GluN2, and GluN3. [158-161] Each subunit has been shown to have subtypes of its own. These have been described to be differentially expressed across various neuroanatomical structures, both centrally and peripherally, but this is a relatively youthful field of research and a paucity of definitive data exist regarding NMDA receptor subtype distribution, activity, modulation, or pathology specific to CRPS patients. [162-164] For example, the GluN2B subtype has been shown to play an integral role in spinal dorsal horn neurons in the pathophysiological process of pain central sensitization, but this was studied in neuropathic rats, not CRPS patients. [165] GluN3B receptors have been thought to be dominant-negative modulators of NMDA receptor activity, but a variant has recently been found to have NDMA stimulatory properties. [166] Similarly, although some evidence regarding ketamine's effect on select subtypes exists, clinical relevance and a plethora of research to identify and modulate the multitude of NMDA receptor subtype-ketamine tissue-specific interactions in CRPS patients is needed. [167]

It is also possible that dose or duration of infusion hold part of the answer and, while there have been many variations of dose and duration reported, there have been no randomized trials comparing one protocol to another. Infusions of up to 20 days duration have been reported. [142] Several studies describe an individualized patient-centered approach for their protocol, starting an infusion at one dose, and then escalating the dose to positive or adverse effects. [137-139, 142] There also appears to be a second-treatment or second-infusion effect for some patients, with which a partial response to initial infusion is subsequently improved to a substantial or complete response following a second treatment. [142] It has been surmised that this phenomenon may be due to the fact that the initial infusion improved symptoms, allowing the patient to start the second infusion with less pain and, thus, allowing that second infusion to produce the desired effect. This phenomenon may also be a function of neuro-plastic changes reflective of partial decentralization of pain or alteration in gene expression in involved neuroanatomical structures following the first round of therapy, which may be mediated by NMDA receptors, but may be a function of other processes as well. These theories have not been proven, however, and mechanistic pathophysiological investigations along with emerging imaging techniques could benefit clinicians to better select patients for repeat ketamine infusions if initial infusions showed modest effectiveness.

One must also consider what effects opiates have in regard to priming the nervous system prior to ketamine administration. Opiate use can in itself induce hyperalgesia, acute tolerance, and sharp withdrawal symptoms. Furthermore, opiates have a direct effect on NMDA receptors and their pathways, both pre- and post-synaptic. Similarly, NMDA activation also induces activity of opiate receptors. [168, 169] Morphine-3-glucuronide, an active morphine metabolite, has been shown in animal models to induce allodynia by NMDA activation and reduce the sensitivity of NMDA receptors to ketamine. [170, 171] Hydromorphone-3-glucuronide has been shown to have the same effect, but with greater potency than morphine-3-glucuronide. [172] These opiate metabolites have also been shown to suppress supraspinal inhibitory synaptic transmission and activate NMDA currents in the hippocampus, suggesting multiple mechanisms for opiate-induced centralization of pain. [173, 174] Protein kinase C-mediated increases in NMDA receptor activity at the primary afferent neuron terminals in the dorsal horn of the spinal cord have been shown to contribute to the development of opioid-induced hyperalgesia and opiate tolerance. [175] Similarly, NMDA antagonism has been shown to have the capacity to attenuate these phenomena. [175, 176] As CRPS is a variably phenotypic syndrome and many CRPS patients take opiates, there is much potential to study opiate-ketamine interaction in a variety of phenotypically different CRPS patient populations. Furthermore, opiate-induced hyperalgesia, allodynia, and central sensitization of pain may be found to be causal or predictive of treatment failure for non-responders to ketamine therapy.

Similarly, such patients may be found to benefit from ketamine therapy after weaning off opiates, even if prior ketamine therapy failed.

Ketamine and the Sympathetic Nervous System

A recent report assessing sympathoexcitation in rats by means of amygdala stimulation holds some hints to elucidate the answer. This study's authors used ethanol to stimulate the central sulcus of the amygdala, inducing a sympathoexcitatory response in lumbar and splanchnic sympathetics with an increase in mean arterial pressure, which was attenuated with the application of an NMDA antagonist. This study implicated GluN1 NMDA subunit activity in the central sulcus of the amygdala. [177] Although this study elucidated an NMDA-dependent pathway from amygdala to lumbar and splanchnic sympathetics, other pathways may exist. A human case series of CRPS patients receiving peripheral sympathetic blocks showed cortical fMRI changes not confined to the amygdala. [117] Another study identified the ventral hippocampus as a site for NMDA-mediated sympathetic activity. [178] Changes in the prefrontal and motor cortex have also been implicated in CRPS as assessed by fMRI and may play a role in sympathetic processing. [99] More likely than not, each of these structures has some contributions for the supraspinal regulation of the sympathetic nervous system in CRPS. In fact, the contribution of these neuroanatomical structures to CRPS pathophysiology has been corroborated by the findings a study of central opioid processing in patients with unilateral CRPS matched to healthy controls, which showed reduced opioid receptor binding potential in contralateral amygdala and parahippocampal gyri and increased opioid receptor binding potential in contralateral prefrontal cortical areas. Opioid receptor binding potential was used as a surrogate for regional cerebral opioid receptor availability, but this study did not investigate the sympathetic nervous system, specifically. [179]

Although promising, these findings leave multiple questions. For one, some of these studies were done in rats, not humans, necessitating further study to substantiate application of these data to human pathophysiology. Second, CRPS is in many ways a neurological disease state and central processing circuits for sympathetic nervous system pathways may differ considerably from healthy patients. Such differences may involve gross anatomical changes or histological ones (i.e., variability in gene expression products), but these data are yet to be sought. Thirdly, NMDA antagonists used in animal studies often differ from ketamine, limiting the generalizability of findings. Variability in the affinity and clinical effect between NMDA antagonists is evident when comparing ketamine and memantine activity at NMDA receptors, for example, and one must consider that results from application of ketamine to humans may differ to those of application of other NMDA antagonists studied in animal models. [180]

Another theory has been proposed in which ventral root fibers contain sympathetic outflow and may, in part, contribute to the sympathetic signs of CRPS. [36] Differences in responsiveness to ketamine therapy may lie in neuroanatomical differences of sympathetic tract distribution and location of relevant lesions. This too has not been extensively investigated and may involve both central and peripheral mechanisms.

Prognostication of Ketamine Therapy

Pain imaging may become an increasingly useful tool for objective assessment and prognostication of ketamine therapy. Investigations are needed to determine protocols and substantiate current evidence regarding both the central mechanisms of pain and the utility of using these modalities for assessing efficacy of treatment on pain processing prior to, during, and following therapy. Functional MRI has been used to show cortical normalization in human case series of CRPS patients receiving peripheral sympathetic blocks. [117] Central nervous system changes were evident in a number of neuroanatomical loci when comparing patient images pre- and post-ketamine therapy. [119] Future research can build on these studies, compare efficacy of this imaging technology with other modalities, further elucidate pathophysiological mechanisms involved in CRPS, and apply this technology for objective prognostication of patient responsiveness to various therapies. Early application may prove more effective at guiding ketamine (and other) therapy and may even prove useful in avoiding opiate abuse or tolerance if appropriate alternative therapy can be administered in a timely fashion. PET has also been utilized to investigate central aspects of CRPS, but the utility of this technology has not been extensively investigated in regard to ketamine prognostication. [37, 104]

Ketamine-Associated Hepatotoxicity

Ketamine therapy, although often effective for treatment of CRPS, carries the risk of developing associated hepatotoxicity. [142, 181, 182] The mechanisms of ketamine-associated hepatotoxicity are unclear, however, and several factors may contribute to the pathophysiology, which in itself may differ between patients.

Unfortunately, ketamine-inclusive CRPS studies were generally not designed to detect biomarkers of pathophyioslogical mechanisms involved in ketamine-associated hepatotoxicity. Elevated liver enzymes appear to the hallmark of this adverse event, but no fatal reactions or cases of severe hepatic disease were reported. In fact, resolution appears to be generally expected. Antinuclear antibodies were found in one patient and eosinophilia in another, suggesting a potential autoimmune mechanism. [181] When present, transaminase elevation is often not seen during the first infusion of ketamine, but with subsequent infusions. [141, 181] This supports the notion of immune system involvement with a hypersensitivity-type reaction and suggestions have been made to limit repeated ketamine exposure to clinical investigations and to avoid it in clinical practice. [183]

Potential drug interactions and lists of patients' concurrent medications have not generally been reported in CRPS studies, however, and these may play a most critical role in the pathophysiology of ketamine-associated hepatotoxicity. As ketamine is metabolized by hepatic cytochrome P450 enzymes and has been found to have many metabolites, prolonged infusions may affect concurrent drug metabolism and predispose patients to metabolic or drug-drug interactions, which may result in elevation in serum levels of hepatic transaminases. [138, 142, 184, 185]

Future investigations into the causality of ketamine-induced hepatotoxicity may benefit from seeking to identify autoantibodies in patients' sera and use metabolite arrays (i.e., liquid chromatography, high-resolution mass spectrometry) to identify metabolites involved in specific drug-drug interactions, or other causative agents altogether.

Differential Efficacy of Ketamine between CRPS I and CRPS II Patients

This question is rooted in pathophysiology, namely the neuroanatomical structures related to each patient's disease state. It is possible that ketamine has differential efficacy for central as compared to peripheral causalities, especially when one considers evidence for heterogeneity of NMDA receptors. [158-162] Although there does not appear to be strong empirical evidence for this assumption, as both CRPS I and CRPS II patients have had had documented positive effects and failures of therapy, a comparison of ketamine efficacy between the two types of CRPS has never been studied.

Anti-depressive Roles of Ketamine in Resolution of Signs and Symptoms of CRPS

Ketamine has been described as the prototypical glutamatergic antidepressant, with mixed results similar to that described in chronic pain literature: short-term efficacy in many patients with sustained long-term efficacy in only a few individuals. [186] The concurrency of chronic pain with depression or anxiety is frequent and well documented, with interrelated pathophysiology. [187] Hence, there is reason to postulate that the antidepressive effects of ketamine may precede or facilitate its analgesic activity. Ketamine's action is not confined to NMDA receptor inhibition and includes inhibition of the reuptake of serotonin, dopamine, and norepinephrine, weak agonism of the mu-opioid and kappa-opioid receptors, inhibitor of nitric oxide synthase, along with upregulation of gene expression related to mammalian target of rapamycin and brain-derived neurotrophic factor, which are proteins implicated in the antidepressive effects of multiple medications and collectively associated with neuronal growth, differentiation, synaptogenesis, and general maintenance of healthy neuronal functioning. [188-191] Ketamine has also been reported to induce peripheral anti-nociception by stimulating the L-arginine/nitric oxide/cyclic GMP pathway via neuronal nitric oxide synthase. [192] Hence, there are many potential pathways for ketamine to exert its effects and a plethora of future research will be needed to identify the differential contribution of each to the treatment and pathophysiologic understanding of CRPS.

Not all NMDA antagonists share these properties. Memantine, for example, is not an effective antidepressant. [193] Cultured mouse hippocampal neurons were used to show that ketamine was superior in blocking NMDA receptor function because memantine does not inhibit the phosphorylation of eukaryotic elongation factor 2 or augment subsequent expression of brain-derived neurotrophic factor. [180]

It is also worth noting that ketamine is a phencyclidine derivative, but new phencyclidine derivatives have been discovered. They are not available for clinical use, but do present potential avenues for future research. [194, 195] It is also worth noting that ketamine itself may be applied topically, rather than intravenously, and this has been demonstrated to be effective in improving allodynia for some cases, but future research regarding alternate forms of ketamine administration (i.e., oral, nasal) may yield interesting results and may facilitate less invasive therapy as administration would not require placement of an intravenous line. [126, 196]

Magnesium

Magnesium infusions have been widely used in a variety of settings for both acute and chronic pain management, including preemptive analgesia. [197-200] The utility, efficacy, tolerability, and adverse effect profiles in different subsets of CRPS patients have not been exclusively investigated. Glutamate does not induce NMDA currents in the presence of magnesium, despite concurrent activation of acute pain receptors and pathways, thereby presenting an interesting potential therapy for inhibition of central sensitization by magnesium supplementation in CRPS. There is evidence that magnesium supplementation may improve memory and neuropathic pain symptoms by inhibiting tumor necrosis factor (TNF)-alpha expression and reducing NMDA receptor currents in the rat hippocampus. [201] This supports the hypothesis that magnesium supplementation may be beneficial by means of NMDA receptor modulation. Unfortunately there has been significant variability in magnesium treatment protocols and results across trials, but cumulative evidence suggests that success may be related to duration of magnesium therapy.

A pilot study of magnesium therapy for CRPS patients showed that intravenous magnesium significantly improved pain, functional impairment and quality of life and was well tolerated at 1, 3, 6, and 12 weeks follow-up. [202] Subsequently, a randomized placebo-controlled trial of magnesium for CRPS patients employed the same protocol as their pilot study, exposing patients to infusions for 4 hours daily over 5 days, and failed to show analgesic benefit over placebo. [203] Nonetheless, it is noteworthy that trials in other neurpathic pain populations have been successful. Intravenous magnesium was administered for a 2-week period, followed by 4 weeks of oral magnesium supplementation, in a randomized placebo-controlled trial for neuropathic back pain and showed significant benefit at six months post-treatment. [200] There are many possibilities for the variability in results seen herein, not limited to the pathophysiological differences of CRPS and chronic back pain or the dose and duration of magnesium therapy. It is possible that CRPS patients may not be responsive to magnesium therapy in all stages of the syndrome as is suggested by evidence variable efficacy when applying ketamine ointment in early versus late-stage CRPS. [126] This stage-specific responsiveness should be further explored. Animal evidence of rat hippocampal plasticity with magnesium therapy for neuropathic pain suggests that it is still possible to obtain analgesic benefit during chronic pain states, and this may be a function of dose and duration of treatment to attain adequate neuronal extracellular concentrations of magnesium. [201] It is worth noting that the rats in this study received 2 weeks of magnesium therapy, which is significantly longer than that used in the negative randomized control trial of CRPS patients mentioned above.

Summary

- Bisphosphonates they shown efficacy for the treatment of neuropathic bone pain associated with CRPS, but questions regarding safety and optimization remain.

- Ketamine has shown great promise, but its efficacy is profoundly variable between patient and much research is needed to identify the mechanisms responsible for success and failure.
- Ketamine-associated hepatotoxicity remains a concern and its pathophysiological determinants must be identified.
- Magnesium supplementation shows promise as an NMDA inhibitor to glutamate activation. It may have activity at many neuroanatomical structures and may involve immunomodulatory function with TNF-alpha as well.

PHARMACEUTICAL OPTIMIZATION: REFINING AND EXPANDING CURRENT EVIDENCE

Immunoresolvents

Also known as Specialized Pro-resolving Mediators (SRM)

Immunoresolvents are a truly fascinating and increasingly tangible, new and expanding pharmacogenus of lipid metabolites involved in a number of immune-modulating, tissue-regenerative, and analgesic processes. [204-208] They are manifest from the discovery that resolution of inflammation is an active process, not a passive one, and have been identified as the mediators that accelerate resolution of inflammation.

These lipid metabolites are derivatives of omega-3 fatty acids, specifically eicosapentanoic acid (EPA) and docosahexanoic acid (DHA), and display an astounding amount of phylogenetic conservation. These previously undiscovered primordial molecules, now deemed immunoresolvents, are physiologically conserved in a slew of phylogenetically distant organisms, including humans, marine animals like salmon, rainbow trout, and the Peruvian anchovy, along with brown planaria (*D. tigrina*), a simple non-parasitic flatworm that is increasingly used for study of tissue regeneration. [209-214]

Although the first description of omega-3 fatty acids as potentially medically beneficial was published in 1929, this pharmacogenus is in its infancy. [215] From the first reports in the 1990s, new compounds continue to be discovered regularly, including a newly discovered precursor: n-3 docosapentanoic acid (DPA). [204, 205, 216-219] Although the compound n-3 DPA is an intermediate in the conversion of EPA to DHA, it is now considered to be a separate precursor to its own set of immunoresolvents. [204, 205] This is in part because structural differences between EPA, DHA, and n-3 DPA metabolites and stereospecificity of receptor sites for these molecules have been shown to have unique physiologic properties. [205, 209] Moreover, n-3 DPA has been shown to be present at concentrations comparable to DHA and EPA in a variety of mammalian tissues, including heart, plasma, brain, and retina, suggesting that it maintains a considerable physiological purpose beyond that of an intermediate metabolite. [205, 220]

The implications of potential applications of immunoresolvents in CRPS are numerous, but should be considered with caution as investigation of this pharmacogenus is in its infancy and have been sparsely applied to CRPS patients in the published literature. [221] First of all, these molecules possess anti-inflammatory and pro-resolving properties that differ from glucocorticoids in that they do not suppress an inflammatory reaction, but actively promote its resolution. This has obvious therapeutic implications with a wide breadth of investigatory possibilities. Second, past investigators have utilized a number of enzymatic and effect-site inhibitors to corroborate the downstream effects of these lipid metabolites, thereby establishing physiological mechanisms as a basis for investigation of inflammatory processes in CRPS pathophysiology, including peripheral and central mechanisms, and tissue-specific components. [222-224] Third, as CRPS may be characterized in part as a multi-faceted neuroimmunololological disorder, and DHA is stored in the membranes of neurons, where it is released by phospholipases for conversion to immunoresolvents, supply and demand of EPA and DHA may become an interesting field of research for CRPS. [225, 226] Given that low DHA states have been associated with a higher incidence of cardiovascular disease, it is plausible that a similar discordance in the balance of pro-inflammatory arachidonic acid compounds and their respective immunoresolvents counterparts may play a role in not only the onset of CRPS, but its pathophysiology, including centralization. In fact, a pilot study of this nature was published in 2010, leaving a breadth of potential research areas in regard to this specific area. [221] Additionally, single nucleotide polymorphisms have been described as associated with enzymatic mutations that have an effect on lipid metabolomics. One example is the gene encoding for the enzyme fatty acid elongase 2 (ELOVL2), which induces an elevation in n-3 DPA and a reduction in concentration of DHA. [227] The implications of genetic variations of enzymes involved in lipid metabolomics, whether from large-scale mutations or single nucleotide polymorphisms, have not yet been investigated in reference to CRPS pathophysiology and any potential therapeutic target sites.

Currently, four types of immunoresolvents have been defined: resolvins, protectins, neuroprotectins, and maresins. Current evidence for each of these types is discussed below, but CRPS implications are not discussed specific to each type of immunoresolvent as these implications are numerous, the body of knowledge is very rapidly expanding, and there appears to be synergism between of each type of immunoresolvent. It is important to note that when synthesized, exogenous immunoresolvents appear to have equivalent bioactivity as their endogenous native counterparts, which is important as it establishes them as potential clinically applicable therapeutic agents.

Resolvins

Like the other classes, resolvins are lipid metabolites, and are named as such to reflect their role as *resolution phase interaction products*. [207] They are named after their precursor compounds. Derivatives of EPA are denoted as E-series Resolvins (i.e., Resolvin E1 or RvE1) and derivatives of DHA are D-series Resolvins (i.e., Resolvin D1 or RvD1). They have been shown to reduce dermal inflammation and polymorphonuclear leukocyte infiltration in mice in one study and promoted resolution of peritonitis and colitis in two other reports. [218, 219, 228] They were also shown to reduce inflammation-induced bone loss associated with periodontitis after topical application of RvE1 in rabbits, mitigate renal ischemic injury in mouse models, and reduced cytokine expression in inflammatory cells. [229-231] Resolvin E1 was also found to reduce inflammatory pain by inhibiting transient receptor potential vanilloid subtype-1 (TRPV1) and TNF-alpha-evoked NMDA receptor hyperactivity in spinal dorsal horn neurons. [232] This has direct implications for management of CRPS.

Protectins

Similar to resolvins, protectins play an integral role in inflammatory resolution, and are named after their EPA or DHA precursors in the same manner as resolvins (i.e., Protectin E1 or PE1, or Protectin D1 or PD1, respectively). They are synthesized by polymorphonuclear leukocytes. [222] Protectin D1 is a potent regulator of polymorphonuclear leukocyte infiltration during peritonitis, and was found to be effective even when administration was exogenously applied several hours after peritonitis was induced, indicating that it may have clinically relevant utility. Furthermore, when quantifying resolution of inflammation in peritonitis, protectins were shown to induce in an additive effect to that of resolvins. [219, 231] Protectin D1 was also shown to block T-cell migration in vivo and inhibited secretion of TNF-alpha and interferon-gamma. [233]

Neuroprotectins

Neuroprotectins are essentially protectins, but rather than being synthesized by polymorphonuclear leukocytes, they are synthesized in neural tissue, where they take on numerous roles, including protection against oxidative stress, acceleration of tissue healing, and inflammatory modulation. [222, 234] Neuroprotectin D1 was shown to attenuate ischemic cerebral injury in induced stroke in rats, play an anti-apoptotic and anti-inflammatory role in Alzheimers disease, and protect against age-related retinal epithelial cell damage. [235-238]

Maresins

Maresins are a more-recently discovered macrophage-biosynthesized group of lipid mediators. [224] In addition to playing an active role in inflammatory homeostasis, platelet-neutrophil interactions, and macrophage phagocytosis of apoptotic neutrophils, they hace roles in tissue regeneration and analgesia. [223, 239, 240] In a brown planaria (*D. tigrina*) model for tissue regeneration, maresin 1 enhanced the rate of tissue regeneration in a concentration dependent fashion. [223] Maresin 1 was shown to have a potent inhibitory effect on TRPV1 in mouse dorsal root ganglia, significantly reducing capsaicin-induced inflammatory pain. Maresin 1 was also shown to have a significant impact on chemotherapy-induced neuropathic pain, reducing mechanical allodynia in mice following intraperitoneal injection of vincristine. [223] Inflammatory pain mediated by activation of transient receptor potential ankyrin type 1 (TRPA1) was not inhibited by maresin 1, however, with no change in TRPA1 currents even at high concentrations of maresin 1. [237] Findings from a rat model of hyperalgesia showed that local peripheral mechanical hyperalgesia is mediated via activation of peripheral TRPA1 and NMDA receptors, with peripheral production of nitric oxide. [241] As maresins induce inflammatory analgesia by inhibition of TRPV1, with no effect on TRPA1-mediated pain, concurrent therapy with maresins and other medications may prove beneficial in the management of CRPS.

As a final note, metabolites of n-3 DPA are given subscript suffix nomenclature, "n-3 DPA," following the name of the immunoresolvents that was derived from n-3 DPA (i.e.,

$RvD1_{n-3DPA}$). Aspirin treated immunoresolvents have also been described and are denoted with a prefix "AT-" prior to the name of each immunoresolvents (i.e., AT-RvE1). These aspirin treated immunoresolvents appear to undergo an interesting enantiomeric transformation with aspirin treatment, but their potency remains similar to their non-treated counterparts. [207]

Anabolic Steroids

Oxandrolone, a synthetic testosterone analog, has been used to combat the severely catabolic inflammatory state of burn patients with ample evidence that it improves function, lean muscle mass, protein synthesis, induces upregulation in gene expression for products of anabolism, and decreases both ospital length of stay and net nitrogen loss in the acute stage of burns. [242-246] It is generally safe to administer to both males and females as it has no or minimal effects on the endocrine axis. It has safely been administered to adults, children, and the elderly, including prolonged administration following hospital discharge. [247-250] Benefits of a 12-month period of therapy with oxandrolone were found to persist up to 5-years post-burn in children. [248]

It is interesting to consider that oxandrolone, through its pharmaceutical actions, induces a systemic inflammatory state transition from catabolism to anabolism similar to the anabolic physiological changes induced by physical therapy and functionally rehabilitative exercise performed for treatment of CRPS patients or others. [251-254] This convergence in catabolism-anabolism axis physiology between therapeutic modalities introduces oxandrolone as a potential agent for a multitude of new research opportunities in CRPS management, whether it is coupled to other therapy or studied alone. Its anabolic effects may prove particularly useful when atrophic changes have already set in and other therapies fail to be effective. [126]

Carbon-Monoxide

Several studies have investigated the potential beneficial role of low-concentration carbon monoxide in acute inflammatory disease processes. [255-258] Carbon monoxide has also been utilized as an investigational intervention for these syndromes. [256, 259] Several potentially contributory pathophysiological mechanisms are emerging. [255, 256, 259] In a model of acute lung injury, carbon monoxide was shown to mediate signaling in multiple pathways, including mitogen activated protein kinases, hypoxia-inducible factor-1-alpha, caspases, heat shock proteins, and fibrinolytic factors. [255] Others have shown that administered carbon monoxide can protect against the polymorphonuclear leukocyte-mediated acute lung injury from ischemia-reperfusion. [260] In a sepsis model, anti-inflammatory and anti-apoptotic cellular effects were seen with both endogenous and exogenous carbon monoxide, and when it applied at low concentrations to rodents, carbon monoxide was associated with a reduction in morbidity and mortality in vivo. [256, 261] Exogenous carbon monoxide was also shown to effectively accelerate resolution of acute inflammation, enhance macrophage phagocytosis, and temporally regulate local levels of immunoresolvents. [259] With significant evidence of immunomodulatory characteristics, low-concentration carbon monoxide may have a role in modulating the inflammatory aspects of CRPS, but has never been investigated in this regard, in neither humans nor animals.

Novel Local Anesthetic Agents

Local anesthetics inhibit NMDA signaling in the dorsal horn. [252, 253] Local anesthetics have also been shown to have an inhibitory effect on central NMDA receptors in the hippocampal pyramidal neurons, thereby providing possible explanation as to why lidocaine infusions may induce desirable analgesic effects for chronic pain patients. [254] Local anesthetics may become a useful tool for prevention of the centralizing effects of CRPS, but future research will be needed as there is great variability between local anesthetics abilities to block NMDA currents, along with a paucity of data examining local anesthetic effects on various heterotetrameric subunit groupings of different NMDA receptors, and the neuroanatomical differential distribution of these receptors is actively being researched.

Magnetized local anesthetics have recently been presented in a proof of concept study, showing feasibility of producing an ankle nerve block in a rat by application of a magnet to the ankle and concurrent intravenous injection of magnetic nanoparticles associated with ropivacaine. [255] Such nanoanesthesia may allow for better targeting to specific nerve lesions (CRPS II) or painful CRPS-affected areas.

Liposomal bupivacaine has recently been introduced to the market as a long-acting local anesthetic and has gained considerable popularity. [266-269] It has generally been assessed to be well tolerated with a wide margin of safety. [270] Although there is little data for its use in chronic pain management, it may prove to be a useful adjunct in CRPS diagnosis and management since it has been applied as an epidural injection and for peripheral nerve blocks with success, along with one report of its successful use to treat digital ischemia, where it acted in similar fashion to sympathetic blockade used to treat the vasoconstrictive components of CRPS. [271-274]

Summary

- Immunoresolvents are a new pharmacologic genus of lipid metabolites that actively mediate resolution of inflammation in a variety of processes and cell-cell interactions, exert anti-apoptotic functions in neuronal structures, and appear to be effective analgesics for inflammatory and chemotherapy-induced neuropathic pain in animal models.
- Anabolic steroids like oxandrolone may have a role in mediating the inflammatory state transition from catabolism to anabolism, and may find greatest utility in the atrophic stages of CRPS.
- Low-concentration carbon monoxide administration has immunomodulatory effects, but research is its infancy.
- Novel local anesthetics and techniques may be effective adjuncts on a case-by-case basis.

GENETICS, GENOMICS, AND EPIGENETICS

Overview

Long before the Human Genome Project, Mendel's work established the basic evidence for passing of heritable traits to offspring. [275] Over the past two decades, there has been an explosion of research into not only genes and gene sequencing, but genomics (the study of whole genomes) and epigenetics (the study of modification of an organism or its function by changes in gene expression, rather than changes in DNA sequencing). [276, 277] More recently, these fields have started establishing a foothold in pain research with hopes for a plethora of new applications and safer practices. [278-280]

Although identification of gene variants can have direct implications for pain physicians, and others, the field of epigenetics may hold greater applicability for near-future research as it does not require genetic engineering and limits ethical risks involved with DNA sequence manipulations. [281] Reassuringly, epigenetics is a natural process and, by crude example, it describes the mechanisms by which a cell, tissue, or organ (i.e., the human eye) expresses genes pertinent to its function and does not express other genes, while other tissues (i.e., the human quadriceps muscles) express genes pertinent to their own function, despite all tissues in that particular organism containing the same set of genes. Three main processes are involved in governing epigenetic changes: DNA methylation, histone acetylation, or chromatin remodeling, but the enzymes involved in these processes are also differentially expressed between cell types and tissues. [282]

Manipulation of these processes can be physiologic (as mentioned above), pathologic, endogenous, or exogenous. Pathologic mechanisms can begin in utero, or prior to conception, with environmentally induced stressors that can lead to gene expression changes, and the transference thereof, to offspring. [283, 284] Like other organ systems, epigenetic changes impact neurodevelopment, playing a role in pain, memory, stress-response, anxiety, depression, and neurodengenerative processes. It is interesting to note, however, that such changes are not limited to those in-utero or early development and epigenetic modifications happening in adult life may be passed on to gametes to persist in subsequent generations. [285] Similarly, there is evidence that such pathologic changes may be reversible, irrespective of their temporal onset.

The following pages describe some preliminary epigenetic findings specific to various aspects of pain processing and pathogenesis, psychological disease, and CRPS, specifically. This is a rapidly expanding field, however, with approximately 3000 manuscripts published in 2014 alone, and new knowledge may drastically change the findings described herein.

Maternal-Fetal Transference: Environmentally-Induced Epigenetic Modifications

There are now many examples of environmentally mediated heritable processes. Various aspects of the maternal and paternal diet, including both macronutrients and micronutrients, have been shown or associated with changes in gene expression, and some such changes may be genome-wide. Although some such changes are positive (i.e., maternal folic acid intake reducing the risk of fetal neural tube defects), the timing and quantity of nutrient intake has been implicated in the development of pathological processes as well. [284] Human maternal smoking during pregnancy, for example, has been shown to result in infants with persistently attenuated basal and reactive cortisol levels over the first postnatal month when compared to unexposed infants. Maternal smoking during pregnancy was also found to be associated with altered methylation of a placental gene promoter, NR3C1, and the degree of methylation correlated with infant cortisol levels. [286] Maternal behavior in rodents has also been shown to have the capacity to induce epigenetic glucocorticoid changes in offspring. Increased glucocorticoid receptor expression was found to be mediated by increased hippocampal serotonergic tone. Specific epigenetic modifications were found to be mediated by transcription factor NGFI-A, which induced an increase in histone acetylase transferase activity, histone acetylation and DNA demethylation. Moreover, as histone acetylation and DNA methylation are dynamic processes, the authors of this study concluded that, although the epigenetic changes observed were established in early life, they are potentially reversible in adulthood. [283] Although there is no indication at this time to believe that CRPS pathogenesis is rooted in maternal-fetal epigenetic transference, nobody has examined this possibility. The understanding that epigenetic changes can happen at any point in life, however, provides potential for future testing of numerous hypotheses regarding CRPS pathogenesis and therapy.

Anxiety, Depression, and Other Psychiatric Pathology

Epigenetic programming within the amygdala was found to play an important role in the maintenance of chronic anxiety and pain. The process appears to be mediated by histone deacetylation, which was found to contribute to cortisol regulation of glucocorticoid receptors, both of which play a role in amygdala-mediated anxiety. Moreover, infusions of a histone deacetylase inhibitor into the amygdala attenuated signs of anxiety, even with concurrent cortisol exposure. Interestingly, this study found that the same infusion of the histone deacetylase inhibitor also resulted in improvements in somatic and visceral hypersensitivity, establishing implications for potential concurrent treatment of both pain and psychiatric disease. [287] BDNF expression and DNA methylation have been found to be altered in multiple psychiatric disorders associated with early-life adversity. Interestingly, serum BDNF gene methylation has been found to be a useful predictor of brain BDNF DNA methylation and points to another example of genome wide epigenetic modifications predisposing an individual to a variety of pathologies. [288] In another study, mouse hippocampal DNA methylation patterns of prenatally stressed mice were also found to induce a genome-wide promoter methylation-dependent process that led to behavioral changes compared to controls. [289] These propensities for psychiatric pathology may be the result of epigenetic modifications in utero, post-utero, or from past generations who passed such modifications on to their offspring through affected gametes. [290]

The role of epigenetic modification of psychiatric states has many implications for CPRS and other chronic pain conditions. Firstly, most chronic pain conditions have a high incidence of concurrent depression or anxiety, potentially connected by epigenetic mechanisms. Second, as therapies directed at modification of gene expression take on a role in pain, there will be great potential for pharmaceutically targeted modification of gene expression contributing to CRPS signs and symptoms. Of course, there is much potential for conducting safety studies, identification of disease-specific processes, introduction of potential therapies, and building upon the current knowledge base.

Pain Vulnerability

Several studies have shown the contribution of epigenetics to both acute and chronic pain, identifying predisposing factors and pharmacogenetic implications. [280] Multiple potential mechanisms and processes have been proposed to play a role in an individual's vulnerability or resilience for developing chronic pain, including priming effects on a cellular level, alterations in central reward networks, and descending cortico-spinal control, but much additional study is needed before these data can be applied to CRPS care. [291] Perhaps most significantly, data regarding pain vulnerability may be utilized to develop prevention protocols and screening tools prior to any kind of surgery or known dangerous activity.

Pain Perception

Using a mouse model, it was found that through epigenetically regulated spinal pathways, histone modification plays an important role in regulating incision-induced nociceptive sensitization, both in the acute setting and in latent sensitization. [292] Another study found that pain perception in later life may be impacted by perinatal methyl donor dietary content in rodents, an example of epigenetic modification of gene expression. [293] Others found that differential DNA methylation of the promoter of the TRPA1 gene significantly correlates with pain perception. [294] TRPA1 has been implicated to have a role in neuropathic pain. [295] DNA methyltransferase, a key enzyme for epigenetic manipulations of gene expression, has been proposed to play a role in acute inflammatory pain and epigenetic modification of spinal micro-RNA expression has been proposed to regulate chronic inflammatory pain. [296, 297]

Pain perception is a hallmark entity of CRPS, with hyperalgesia and allodynia representing two major components of patient morbidity directly resultant from derangements in pain perception. Thus, future investigations of the epigenetic mechanisms involved in pain perception, the translational research from such data, and the clinical outcomes research to follow will be of great interest to pain physicians and CRPS patients.

Epigenetics Involving Opiates

With many interactions having implications in pain processing, including those specific to CPRS pathology and treatment, opiate-centered epigenetic studies will continue to be of great importance. Epigenetic mechanisms involved in opiate interactions represent a rapidly growing knowledge base, however, and any review on this topic will likely be almost instantly dated at the time of publication. Thus, this segment introduces some of the evidence regarding epigenetics involving mu-receptors and opiate-induced hyperalgesia with hopes of providing some knowledge and ample inspiration to future investigators who may wish to explore opiate-epigenetic interactions in CRPS.

Mu opiate receptors have been found to be differentially expressed in different regions of the brain. In a mouse model, this heterogeneity of receptor expression coincided with DNA methylation and histone modifications within those cells, providing some evidence to for epigenetic mechanisms of receptor transcription, targeting, and delivery. [298] Others have found that this receptor's gene expression is mediated through chromatin remodeling, DNA methylation, and transcriptional factors affecting the gene's promoter region in fully differentiated neuronal cells. [299-301]

Opiate-induced hyperalgesia can cause devastating morbidity for chronic pain patients, especially those dependent on opiates for some modicum of analgesia. Epigenetic mechanisms have also been implicated in the pathophysiology of opiate-induced hyperalgesia. In a mouse model of chronic opiate use, concurrent administration of a histone deacetylase inhibitor increased the incidence of opiate-induced hyperalgesia and two genes were identified to play prominent roles from spinal cord tissue (BDNF and prodynorphin), suggesting possible targets for future therapy. [302] Others have found that a disruption of the CXCL1/CXCR2 signaling pathway by epigenetic mechanisms plays a role in sensitization to incisional pain, suggesting that this pathway might be targeted for treatment of chronic opiate users presenting to surgery. [303]

Neuropathic Pain

Epigenetic modulation has been implicated in several mechanisms involved in neuropathic pain pathophysiology. [304] Inflammatory mediators have been implicated as facilitators of epigenetic mechanisms involved in neuropathic pain pathogenesis. [305, 306] In one study, partial sciatic nerve ligation was found to significantly increase the expression of monocyte chemotactic protein 3 (also known as CCL-7) in the spinal cord neurons (mostly astrocytes) after decreased trimethylation of histone H3 at the promoter region of the monocyte chemotactic protein 3 gene. This effect lasted for a 4-week period in control mice, but no such epigenetic modifications of monocyte chemotactic protein 3 gene expression were observed in interleukin 6 knockout mice. Supporting the integral role of interleukin 6, intrathecal injection of into the knockout mice significantly increased monocyte chemotactic protein 3 mRNA and exhibited a similar decrease in the level of promoter histone trimethylation to that seen in the control mice. [306] Prostaglandin E2 was also found to play a role in the genesis of neuropathic pain through its contribution to upregulation of BDNF expression in dorsal root ganglia neurons following nerve injury. [305]

BDNF is upregulated in the dorsal root ganglion after peripheral nerve injury and contributes to the pathogenesis of neuropathic pain. Despite elevated levels of BDNF mRNA being elevated for 14 days post injury, this BDNF-mediated pathway appears to be time-dependent in that intrathecally administered anti-BDNF antibodies were only found to be effective at attenuating hyperalgesic and allodynic responses to stimuli if given by day 2 following nerve injury. [307] Supporting these temporal findings, another study found BDNF to play an integral role in the initiation of neuropathic pain within the first two days following nerve injury, but noted that activation of NMDA GluN2B receptor subunit played a greater role in maintenance of persistent pain states from 2 to 14 days. Furthermore, with the additional finding that a subtype-specific NMDA receptor antagonist was able to block BDNF-mediated allodynia in all test animals, it suggests that this signaling pathway involves BDNF-facilitated activation of dorsal horn NMDA GluN2B receptors in the pathogenesis of neuropathic pain induced by nerve injury. [308]

Histone deacetylase inhibitors have also shown promise in attenuating neuropathic pain, but data may be conflicting. For example, in one study histone deacetylase inhibitors were able to attenuate mechanical and thermal hyperalgesia, but only if applied prior to the insult and their effects were not seen in dorsal root ganglia, despite being present in other spinal cord structures. [309] These findings are contrasted by another study, which found that epigenetic repression of a specific sodium channel in the dorsal root ganglia was both facilitated by a histone deacetylase inhibitor and that such inhibitors may be able to restore C-fiber sensitivity in a hypoesthesia model. [310]

The cyclin-dependent kinase 5 (Cdk5) gene is another target that has been explored for epigenetic manipulation. Upregulation of Cdk5 in dorsal horn neurons was shown to contribute to the pathogenesis of neuropathic pain in rats. [311] Moreover, the Cdk5 inhibitor roscovitine was shown to downregulate NMDA GluN2A receptor subunit (without action on GluN2B or GluN1 expression) in dorsal root ganglia, thereby attenuating neuropathic pain symptomatology. [312] In another study in which roscovitine was injected intrathecally, significant attenuation of NMDA GluN2B mRNA expression was noted, which correlated with an improvement in cancer-pain symptomatology, but this study used a milieu of spinal cord tissue for RT-PCR identification of genetic material and did not specifically assess expression in dorsal root ganglia. [313] Interestingly, a BDNF-mediated signaling pathway has been implicated in Cdk5-mediated neuropathic pain pathogenesis, suggesting that therapies may be developed to target multiple sites in this pathological epigenetically modulated cascade. [314]

Thus, future research of epigenetic mechanisms and potential interventions for neuropathic pain components of CRPS are numerous. BDNF, NMDA, TRPA1, Cdk5, and inflammatory mediators (interleukin 6, prostaglandin E2) have been identified as modulators of the epigenetics of neuropathic pain. Future investigations may target receptors (i.e., NMDA), subunits, gene promoter regions, signaling pathways, gene transcription and product modifications, the role of inflammatory mediators and various proteins in epigenetic modulation, and the safety of all potential interventions, as there are certainly many hypotheses that have not yet been tested.

Central Sensitization of Pain

Central sensitization of pain can be a highly morbid and difficult-to-treat aspect of CRPS. As one might suspect, the plastic changes necessary for pain processing to shift from acute and peripheral to centralized and pathological likely involve epigenetic mechanisms for reprogramming of gene expression to induce altered neuronal function. Evidence is mounting in this field, which is both young and growing rapidly, with potential for a plethora of future investigations with many implications for CRPS management.

In mice, chronic genome-wide changes were identified in cells of the prefrontal cortex following peripheral nerve injury. [315] BDNF upregulation, which was induced by persistent inflammation, resulted in promoter-enhanced delivery of α-amino-3-hydroxy-5-methyl-4-

isoxazolepropionic acid (AMPA) receptor GluA1 subunits through descending pathways. At their target sites, AMPA receptor phosphorylation of GluA1 subunits plays a pivotal role in descending pain facilitation and provides epigenetic evidence of pain centralization. [316] Central sensitization mechanisms have also been shown to be conserved across species and phyla. [317]

Current Evidence from CRPS-Specific Epigenetic Data

Epigenetics in CRPS is a new field. To date, there has only been one set of manuscripts describing epigenetics in CRPS, specifically, and these were not original studies. [318, 319] Thus, there is a plethora of potential investigatory avenues to explore when considering future studies in epigenetics for CRPS patients or in animal models of CRPS.

Summary

- Epigenetics is the study of modulation of an organism or part of its function by changes in gene expression, rather than changes in the DNA sequence, itself.
- Epigenetic mechanisms may modulate single genes or entire genomes, and such changes may be heritable, environmentally induced, or pharmaceutically altered.
- Epigenetic mechanisms have been implicated in patient vulnerability to developing chronic pain, anxiety, depression, and other psychiatric conditions, along with neurodegenerative diseases.
- Epigenetics play a role in pain perception, development of neuropathic pain, and central sensitization of pain.
- Epigenetic mechanisms have been stipulated to act on a number of processes involved in CRPS, but studies specific to this syndrome will be needed to substantiate theories and conclusions extrapolated from findings among other patient populations or animal models.

SCREENING STRATEGIES

Overview

While many studies have focused on pathophysiology or treatment of CRPS, few studies have been conducted to develop predictive models or screening strategies. Attempts have been made to identify at-risk populations, namely limb-fracture patients, but there is a lack of congruence between studies in identifying significant patient and surgical factors predisposing to development of CRPS. To date, there is no ubiquitously applied screening algorithm or tool for CRPS, and the future development of such a tool may be of great utility.

Recognizing that CRPS pathogenesis and pathophysiology are multifactorial, one study attempted to identify patient and surgical factors predisposing to the development of CRPS by focusing on an apparent at-risk population: limb fracture patients presenting for surgery. [320] In a retrospective review of 185,378 inpatients treated in Japan with an open reduction and internal fixation of a fractured limb between 2007 and 2010, this study identified utilized a multivariate logistic regressions analysis to identify several significant variables. Patients with fractures of the forearm, wrist, or hand were at 2.81 times greater risk of developing CRPS than their reference population of patients with upper arm or shoulder fractures (odds ratio 2.81, 95% confidence interval 1.25 – 6.30, P = 0.012). Femur fractures were negatively associated with CRPS, with an odds ratio of 0.05 (95% confidence interval 0.01 – 0.28, P<0.001). Multiple fractures and other specific limb fracture sites were not found to be significantly associated with development of CRPS. Age and sex were not significantly associated with development of CRPS, nor was the type of anesthesia used (regional versus general anesthesia). Duration of anesthesia was, however, significantly associated with development of CRPS. CRPS developed 3.15 times more frequently in patients for whom anesthesia exceeding 2 hours (odds ratio 3.15, 95% confidence interval 1.24 – 7.97, P=0.016) and 5.73 times more frequently for anesthesia exceeding 3 hours (odds ratio 5.73, 95% confidence interval 2.31 – 14.24, P < 0.001). This duration of anesthesia may reflect greater complexity of surgery and involve longer tourniquet times with greater predisposition to limb ischemia, but these data were not reported. It is also worth noting, however, that the prevalence of CRPS in this population was fairly low (39 cases), which is considerably lower than found in several prospective wrist fracture studies. Nonetheless, these data suggest several avenues for future research regarding perioperative preventative strategies, especially for high-risk cases (wrist or hand surgery, expectantly prolonged operative time)

In a prospective study of 596 single-fracture patients of whom 7.0% developed CRPS I, no psychological factors were found to be significantly associated with the development of CRPS. In fact, this study's authors found that their patients scored similarly to the general population, with less psychiatric morbidity than that found in other pain or psychiatric disease populations. [321] While no psychiatric factors were associated with development of CRPS, this study found that ankle fractures, fracture-dislocations, and intra-articular fractures were predictive of CRPS development.

In another, albeit small (n=27), prospective study of patients with radial fractures, comparisons of sympathetic tone and responsiveness to heat and cold were assessed while monitoring for the development of CRPS. Four of this study's 27 patients showed signs of CPRS, with 2 receiving the official diagnosis. Despite having few CRPS patients, this study's authors were able to find a significant correlation between sympathetic derangements, as measured using laser Doppler flowmetry, and the development of CRPS. [322336] While such positive findings hold promise for screening, early diagnosis and treatment, or prevention of CRPS, larger and more robust studies will be needed both to refine the screening techniques and to validate current findings.

Table 10.1. Summary of Variables Predictive for the Development of CRPS

Study	Sumitani 2014 [320]	Beerthuizen 2011[321]	Zollinger 2007 [323]	Schurmann 2000 [324]
Population	• Limb fracture patients undergoing open reduction internal fixation, Japan	• Single-limb fracture patients presenting to the emergency department, The Netherlands	• Wrist fracture patients, The Netherlands	• Distal radius fracture patients, Germany
Positive Predictive Variables	• Limb fracture location (forearm, wrist, or hand) • Duration of anesthesia	• Ankle fractures • Fracture-dislocations • Intra-articular fractures	• Early postoperative cast-related irritability • Female sex	• Sympathetic nervous system derangements (measured by laser Doppler flowmetry)
Negative Predictive Variables	• Limb fracture location (femur)	• None reported	• None reported	• None reported
Variables with no Predictive Value	• Other limb fracture location • Multiple limb fractures • Age • Sex • Regional versus general anesthesia	• All psychiatric variables analyzed (Symptom Checklist-90) • Age • Sex • Education • Type of fracture treatment • Hand dominance	• Side of the fracture • Hand dominance • Type of fracture • Dislocation • Type of fracture treatment	• None reported

Summary

- Few studies have provided data to identify variables predictive for the development of CRPS.
- There is significant variability in findings between studies.
- To date, there is no ubiquitously applied screening tool for the development of CRPS.
- The development of reliable CRPS screening tools would hold great promise for prevention, early diagnosis, and expedient treatment.

FREE RADICAL SCAVENGERS

Overview

In select situations, the incidence of CRPS may be markedly higher than in the general population. For patients undergoing hand surgery or wrist fracture surgery, the incidence of CRPS has been reported to range from 4.2% - 38.3%. [323-339] For foot and ankle surgery patients, the incidence has been reported to range from 1.7% to 9.6%. [330]

In the 1980s, it was reported that reactive oxygen species likely play a significant role in the pathophysiology of CRPS. [331, 332] Since then, numerous studies have substantiated these results and expanded the body of knowledge pertaining to the roles of inflammation and reactive oxygen radicals in CRPS pathophysiology. [333-335] More recently, free radical scavengers have been proposed as a potential therapy and they may play a dual role in prevention of CRPS and in management during this syndrome's early stages. Ascorbic acid (vitamin C), mannitol, dimethyl-sulfoxide (DMSO) and N-acetyl cysteine (NAC) have been evaluated in this regard.

Vitamin C (Ascorbic Acid)

Vitamin C has been assessed in 2 randomized double-blind placebo-controlled trials and one observational trial. [313, 326, 329] In the first placebo-controlled trial, done in 1999, 500mg oral vitamin C taken orally for 50 days starting on the day of surgery was shown to be significantly associated with a reduction in the incidence of CPRS development (7%, compared to 22% in the placebo group) following wrist fracture surgery. This study's authors also discovered that cast discomfort was significantly associated with development of CRPS and may be of prognostic value for wrist fracture patients. [329] The second study was an observational one in which patients with distal radial fractures were not given vitamin C before 1999 (control group), and then all distal radial fracture patients were given 1 gram of vitamin C daily for 45 days starting on the day of surgery from 1999 to 2002 (intervention group). The incidence was significantly lower in the vitamin C group (2.1%) compared to the control group (10%). [326] The third trial was a multicenter, randomized, double-blinded, placebo-controlled, dose-response study with a significantly larger sample and 3 dosing regimens for the active arms of the study (200mg, 500mg, and 1500mg of daily vitamin C).

All groups (active and placebo) started their dosing regimens on the day of surgery and continued for 50 days. While the 200mg dosing group did not show any significant improvement compared to placebo, both the 500mg and 1500mg dosing regimens had significantly fewer CRPS patients in follow-up, but there was no significant difference between these two dose regimens (relative risk 0.17 for both regimens, each compared to placebo). Thus, this study's authors concluded that 500mg appeared to be an adequate dose to achieve desired effects. This study's authors also found early cast discomfort to be a significant predictor of CRPS development (odds ratio 5.35, 95% confidence interval 2.13 to 13.42), corroborating earlier findings from their 1999 trial. [323, 329]

In 2009, a sizable observational unblended study was undertaken to assess the impact of vitamin C in foot and ankle surgery. Patients from 2002-2003 were not given vitamin C, while patients from 2003 to 2004 received 1 gram of oral vitamin C daily starting on the day of surgery and continuing for 45 days. This study's results correlate with the data from wrist fracture studies noted above, with significantly fewer patients in the vitamin C group developing CRPS as compared to those in the non-treatment group. [330] In 2010, a prospective open label observational study of preoperative oral vitamin C at 500mg daily for patients undergoing basal thumb prostheses surgery also corroborated earlier findings from wrist fracture surgeries. None of this study's 40 patients developed signs or symptoms of CRPS. This was compared to historical reports, citing 5 of 38 patients developing CRPS after undergoing the same procedure. [336]

Taken together, these data support the use of vitamin C, but many questions about the specific mechanisms of action, the timing and duration of therapy, and the determinants of failure of therapy are yet to be adequately investigated. Furthermore, new studies investigating specific subsets of CRPS patients (i.e., acute/chronic, warm/cold) are likely to help optimize efficacy of this preventative therapy.

Mannitol

Like vitamin C, mannitol is a free radical scavenger that has been studied in CRPS patients. It is important to make the distinction, however, that while mannitol has been used in the treatment of CRPS, vitamin C is the only free radical scavenger that has been used as a preventative therapy for CRPS. What follows is a discussion of other free radical scavenging therapies, including mannitol, which have been used for treatment of acute and chronic CPRS, but are yet to have their preventative roles explored with future research.

In 1994, a prospective study of 30 CRPS patients treated for 1 month with daily infusions of mannitol found improvement in hand grip strength and bone density per scintigraphic imaging. [337] In 2008, a prospective open label observational study was conducted in CRPS I patients within 4 months of developing symptoms. All patients were given intravenous mannitol and dexamethasone daily for a 1-week period, with assessments at baseline, at completion of the 1-week course of therapy, and at a mean of 9 months post-treatment. This study's authors found significant and sustained improvement in signs and symptoms, including pain, range-of-motion, and grip strength. [338] The apparent success of this study supports the results from the wrist, hand, foot, and ankle surgery studies noted above, but success of therapy may be a function of timing. All of these studies enrolled patients either prior to development of CRPS or in its early stages ("warm" CRPS).

In 2010, the role of mannitol as salvage therapy in conjunction with an already applied treatment protocol for CRPS was assessed, involving a population of both acute and chronic CRPS I patients. At 1-month follow-up, 79.3% of patients experienced improvement in pain, 85.5% experienced improvements in skin temperature in the affected region, and 61.0% experienced improvements in range of motion. Mannitol treatment appeared to be more effective in "warm" type CRPS (odds ratio = 6.30, 95% confidence interval 2.37-16.75) and acute CRPS (odds ratio = 6.15, 95% confidence interval 1.54–24.50) compared to "cold" type and chronic CPRS, respectively. [339]

In a 2008 randomized, double-blind, placebo-controlled study, a similar infusion of 10% mannitol was not found to be more effective than placebo at alleviating CRPS symptomatology. This trial differed in methodology and had a propensity for inclusion of a greater number of chronic CRPS patients with less intense symptomatology than some other studies. [340] Thus, further research will be needed to substantiate either positive or negative results, and studies designed to elucidate mannitol's potential mechanisms of action in specific subsets of CRPS patient (i.e., warm/cold, acute/chronic) would be helpful in guiding the design of larger clinical trials.

Dimethylsulfoxide (DMSO) and N-Acetyl Cysteine (NAC)

DMSO is a free radical scavenger and has been applied to CRPS patients in the form of a cream at 50% concentration. A prospective, randomized, double-blind, placebo-controlled trial was published in 1996, with report of improvement in pain scores and patient symptomatology in the active group being statistically greater than the placebo group. [341] These findings were substantiated in a 2003 report of another placebo-controlled prospective randomized trial that also included an additional active arm with NAC, which found marginal differences between active groups. Post-hoc patient subgroup analysis identified DMSO as being more effective therapy for "warm" type CRPS patients and NAC for being more effective for "cold" type CPRS patients. [340] In a separate analysis of this study population, DMSO was found to be more cost-effective. [342]

Taken together, these data support the use of either DMSO or NAC, leaving room for a plethora of future research. First, as DMSO and NAC have been reported to have properties in addition to being free radical scavengers, investigations focused on their individual actions may yield greater insight for optimizing CRPS management. While there is significant potential for future investigations targeting specific CPRS subgroups, dose-response studies, and dose-duration optimization, DMSO and NAC efficacy is yet to be compared to that of vitamin C, mannitol, or other free radical scavengers.

Summary

- Free oxygen radicals appear to play a significant role in the pathophysiology of CRPS.
- Vitamin C has been shown to effectively decrease the incidence of CRPS in patients with wrist fractures when administered on the day of surgery and continued for 45-50 days at an oral dose of at least 500mg daily.

- To date, vitamin C is the only investigated preventative therapy used to prevent CRPS.
- Intravenous mannitol has also been administered as a free radical scavenger for the treatment of CRPS. While early evidence showed efficacy, the only blinded, placebo-controlled trial did not show improvement over placebo.
- DMSO and NAC have also been shown to be efficacious at attenuating CPRS symptomatology, and DMSO was found to be more cost-effective.
- Some evidence suggests that mannitol and DMSO may be more effective in treating acute or "warm" type CRPS, while NAC may be more effective in treating "cold" type CRPS.

ANESTHETIC STRATEGIES

Overview

Little has been studied with respect to anesthetic agents, techniques, causal relationships, or protocols in relation to the development of CRPS. This remains a very open field for future investigators to explore various facets of CRPS pathogenesis and pathophysiology. As surgical patients presenting with specific limb fractures have a greater propensity for development of CRPS than the general population, exploring anesthetic implications as they pertain to CRPS development is likely to be a worthwhile endeavor. To date, however, only the type (regional versus general anesthesia) and duration of anesthesia have been assessed.

Type and Duration of Anesthesia

The use of regional anesthesia has been theorized to have a preventative function in CRPS development. [343, 344] Brachial plexus injury from regional anesthesia has also been implicated in a case report as causative in the development of CRPS. [345] In a study of 301 Brazilian carpal tunnel release patients, prospectively randomized to either regional or general anesthesia, the authors found no association between anesthetic technique and CRPS development. The study did not appear to be limited by sample size, as there were 25 total CRPS patients following this procedure, representing an incidence of 8.3%. [327] Similarly, in a Japanese retrospective national database review of limb fracture patients, no association between type of anesthesia and CRPS was revealed, but this study showed a positive correlation between duration of anesthesia and likelihood of CRPS development. Patients with durations of anesthesia exceeding 2 hours and 3 hours were associated with a 3.15 and 5.73 times greater likelihood for development of CRPS, respectively, when compared to anesthetic durations less than 2 hours. This association may be a function of complexity of injury or surgery, duration of tourniquet use, or other factors prolonging anesthetic course, rather than a direct cause-and-effect relationship between anesthesia and CRPS pathogenesis. [320]

Summary

- Anesthetic agents, techniques, causal relationships, and strategies in relation to the pathogenesis of CRPS have not been adequately studied.
- With current available data, there appears to be no difference between general and regional anesthesia in the pathogenesis of CRPS.
- Duration of anesthesia for open reduction and internal fixation surgeries appears to be positively correlated with likelihood of CRPS development, but this association may be a function of complexity of injury or surgery, duration of tourniquet use, or other factors prolonging anesthetic course, rather than a direct cause-and-effect relationship between anesthesia and CRPS pathogenesis. Additional prospective study will be needed to assess the causative factors contributing to these findings.

REFERENCES

[1]   Melzack, R; Wall, PD. Pain mechanisms: a new theory. *Science.* 1965, 150(3699), 971-979. PubMed PMID, 5320816.

[2]   Sarramon, JP; Lazorthes, Y; Buffet, J; Sedan, R; Bourhis, A; Sarrazin, L. [Spinal cord neurostimulation in neurogenic bladder]. *J Urol Nephrol (Paris).* 1974, 80(12 pt 2), 287-289. PubMed PMID, 4469297.

[3]   Smirnov, VM; Iovlev, BV. [Mathematical-statistical analysis of changes in Parkinsonian tremor during diagnostic electric stimulation of deep brain structures]. *Vopr Neirokhir.* 1974(5), 40-46. PubMed PMID, 4420771.

[4]   Dubois, MY; Gallagher, RM; Lippe, PM. Pain medicine position paper. *Pain Med.* 2009, 10(6), 972-1000. doi: 10.1111/j.1526-4637.2009.00696.x. PubMed PMID, 19772540.

[5]   Levy, R; Deer, TR; Henderson, J. Intracranial neurostimulation for pain control: a review. *Pain Physician.* 2010, 13(2), 157-165. PubMed PMID, 20309382.

[6]   Parmar, VK; Gee, L; Smith, H; Pilitsis, JG. Supraspinal stimulation for treatment of refractory pain. *Clin Neurol Neurosurg.* 2014, 123, 155-163. doi: 10.1016/j.clineuro.2014.05.026. PubMed PMID, 24956545.

[7]   Hosobuchi, Y; Adams, JE; Linchitz, R. Pain relief by electrical stimulation of the central gray matter in humans and its reversal by naloxone. *Science.* 1977, 197(4299), 183-186. PubMed PMID, 301658.

[8]   Mazars, GJ. Intermittent stimulation of nucleus ventralis posterolateralis for intractable pain. *Surg Neurol.* 1975, 4(1), 93-95. PubMed PMID, 1080908.

[9]   Richardson, DE; Akil, H. Pain reduction by electrical brain stimulation in man. Part 1: Acute administration in periaqueductal and periventricular sites. *J Neurosurg.* 1977, 47(2), 178-183. doi: 10.3171/jns.1977.47.2.0178. PubMed PMID, 327030.

[10] Richardson, DE; Akil, H. Pain reduction by electrical brain stimulation in man. Part 2: Chronic self-administration in the periventricular gray matter. *J Neurosurg.* 1977, 47(2), 184-194. doi: 10.3171/jns.1977.47.2.0184. PubMed PMID, 301558.

[11] Schvarcz, JR. Chronic self-stimulation of the medial posterior inferior thalamus for the alleviation of deafferentation pain. *Acta Neurochir Suppl (Wien)*. 1980, 30, 295-301. PubMed PMID, 6937110.

[12] Tsubokawa, T; Yamamoto, T; Katayama, Y; Moriyasu, N. Clinical results and physiological basis of thalamic relay nucleus stimulation for relief of intractable pain with morphine tolerance. *Appl Neurophysiol*. 1982, 45(1-2), 143-155. PubMed PMID, 6977315.

[13] Turnbull, IM; Shulman, R; Woodhurst, WB. Thalamic stimulation for neuropathic pain. *J Neurosurg*. 1980, 52(4), 486-493. doi: 10.3171/jns.1980.52.4.0486. PubMed PMID, 6966326.

[14] Young, RF; Kroening, R; Fulton, W; Feldman, RA; Chambi, I. Electrical stimulation of the brain in treatment of chronic pain. Experience over 5 years. *J Neurosurg*. 1985, 62(3), 389-396. doi: 10.3171/jns.1985.62.3.0389. PubMed PMID, 3871844.

[15] Levy, RM; Lamb, S; Adams, JE. Treatment of chronic pain by deep brain stimulation: long term follow-up and review of the literature. *Neurosurgery*. 1987, 21(6), 885-893. PubMed PMID, 3325851.

[16] Boivie, J; Meyerson, BA. A correlative anatomical and clinical study of pain suppression by deep brain stimulation. *Pain*. 1982, 13(2), 113-126. PubMed PMID, 6750509.

[17] Sillery, E; Bittar, RG; Robson, MD; Behrens, TE; Stein, J; Aziz, TZ; Johansen-Berg, H. Connectivity of the human periventricular-periaqueductal gray region. *J Neurosurg*. 2005, 103(6), 1030-1034. doi: 10.3171/jns.2005.103.6.1030. PubMed PMID, 16381189.

[18] Dionne, RA; Mueller, GP; Young, RF; Greenberg, RP; Hargreaves, KM; Gracely, R; Dubner, R. Contrast medium causes the apparent increase in beta-endorphin levels in human cerebrospinal fluid following brain stimulation. *Pain*. 1984, 20(4), 313-321. PubMed PMID, 6097857.

[19] Adams, JE. Naloxone reversal of analgesia produced by brain stimulation in the human. Pain. 1976, 2(2), 161-166. PubMed PMID, 800249.

[20] Hosobuchi, Y; Rossier, J; Bloom, FE; Guillemin, R. Stimulation of human periaqueductal gray for pain relief increases immunoreactive beta-endorphin in ventricular fluid. *Science*. 1979, 203(4377), 279-281. PubMed PMID, 83674.

[21] Hamani, C; Schwalb, JM; Rezai, AR; Dostrovsky, JO; Davis, KD; Lozano, AM. Deep brain stimulation for chronic neuropathic pain, long-term outcome and the incidence of insertional effect. *Pain*. 2006, 125(1-2), 188-196. doi: 10.1016/j.pain.2006.05.019. PubMed PMID, 16797842.

[22] Kumar, K; Toth, C; Nath, RK. Deep brain stimulation for intractable pain: a 15-year experience. *Neurosurgery*. 1997, 40(4), 736-746, discussion 746-737. PubMed PMID, 9092847.

[23] Bittar, RG; Kar-Purkayastha, I; Owen, SL; Bear, RE; Green, A; Wang, S; Aziz, TZ. Deep brain stimulation for pain relief: a meta-analysis. J Clin Neurosci. 2005, 12(5), 515-519. doi: 10.1016/j.jocn.2004.10.005. PubMed PMID, 15993077.

[24] Boccard, SG; Pereira, EA; Moir, L; Aziz, TZ; Green, AL. Long-term outcomes of deep brain stimulation for neuropathic pain. *Neurosurgery*. 2013, 72(2), 221-230, discussion 231. doi: 10.1227/NEU.0b013e31827b97d6. PubMed PMID, 23149975.

[25] Katayama, Y; Yamamoto, T; Kobayashi, K; Kasai, M; Oshima, H; Fukaya, C. Motor cortex stimulation for phantom limb pain: comprehensive therapy with spinal cord and thalamic stimulation. *Stereotact Funct Neurosurg.* 2001, 77(1-4), 159-162. doi: 64593. PubMed PMID, 12378068.

[26] Owen, SL; Green, AL; Nandi, DD; Bittar, RG; Wang, S; Aziz, TZ. Deep brain stimulation for neuropathic pain. *Acta Neurochir Suppl.* 2007, 97(Pt 2), 111-116. PubMed PMID, 17691296.

[27] Hosobuchi, Y. Subcortical electrical stimulation for control of intractable pain in humans. Report of 122 cases (1970-1984). *J Neurosurg.* 1986, 64(4), 543-553. doi: 10.3171/jns.1986.64.4.0543. PubMed PMID, 3485191.

[28] Previnaire, JG; Nguyen, JP; Perrouin-Verbe, B; Fattal, C. Chronic neuropathic pain in spinal cord injury: efficiency of deep brain and motor cortex stimulation therapies for neuropathic pain in spinal cord injury patients. *Ann Phys Rehabil Med.* 2009, 52(2), 188-193. doi: 10.1016/j.rehab.2008.12.002. PubMed PMID, 19909709.

[29] Broggi, G; Franzini, A; Leone, M; Bussone, G. Update on neurosurgical treatment of chronic trigeminal autonomic cephalalgias and atypical facial pain with deep brain stimulation of posterior hypothalamus: results and comments. *Neurol Sci.* 2007, 28 Suppl 2, S138-145. doi: 10.1007/s10072-007-0767-3. PubMed PMID, 17508161.

[30] Fontaine, D; Lazorthes, Y; Mertens, P; Blond, S; Geraud, G; Fabre, N; Navez, M; Lucas, C; Dubois, F; Gonfrier, S; Paquis, P; Lanteri-Minet, M. Safety and efficacy of deep brain stimulation in refractory cluster headache: a randomized placebo-controlled double-blind trial followed by a 1-year open extension. *J Headache Pain.* 2010, 11(1), 23-31. doi: 10.1007/s10194-009-0169-4. PubMed PMID, 19936616.

[31] Leone, M; Franzini, A; Broggi, G; Bussone, G. Hypothalamic stimulation for intractable cluster headache: long-term experience. *Neurology.* 2006, 67(1), 150-152. doi: 10.1212/01.wnl.0000223319. 56699.8a. PubMed PMID, 16832097.

[32] Videnovic, A; Metman, LV. Deep brain stimulation for Parkinson's disease: prevalence of adverse events and need for standardized reporting. *Mov Disord.* 2008, 23(3), 343-349. doi: 10.1002/mds.21753. PubMed PMID, 17987644.

[33] Garcia-Larrea, L; Peyron, R. Motor cortex stimulation for neuropathic pain: From phenomenology to mechanisms. *Neuroimage.* 2007, 37 Suppl 1, S71-79. doi: 10.1016/j.neuroimage.2007.05.062. PubMed PMID, 17644413.

[34] Peyron, R; Faillenot, I; Mertens, P; Laurent, B; Garcia-Larrea, L. Motor cortex stimulation in neuropathic pain. Correlations between analgesic effect and hemodynamic changes in the brain. A PET study. *Neuroimage.* 2007, 34(1), 310-321. doi: 10.1016/j.neuroimage.2006. 08.037. PubMed PMID, 17055297.

[35] Meyerson, B. Motor cortex stimulation--effective for neuropathic pain but the mode of action remains illusive. *Pain.* 2005, 118(1-2), 6-7. doi: 10.1016/j.pain.2005.07.019. PubMed PMID, 16202535.

[36] Velasco, F; Carrillo-Ruiz, JD; Castro, G; Arguelles, C; Velasco, AL; Kassian, A; Guevara, U. Motor cortex electrical stimulation applied to patients with complex regional pain syndrome. *Pain.* 2009, 147(1-3), 91-98. doi: 10.1016/j.pain.2009.08.024. PubMed PMID, 19793621.

[37] Fonoff, ET; Hamani, C; Ciampi, de, Andrade, D; Yeng, LT; Marcolin, MA; Jacobsen, Teixeira, M. Pain relief and functional recovery in patients with complex regional pain

syndrome after motor cortex stimulation. Stereotact *Funct Neurosurg*. 2011, 89(3), 167-172. doi: 10.1159/000324895. PubMed PMID, 21494069.

[38] Garcia-Larrea, L; Peyron, R; Mertens, P; Gregoire, MC; Lavenne, F; Bonnefoi, F; Mauguiere, F; Laurent, B; Sindou, M. Positron emission tomography during motor cortex stimulation for pain control. *Stereotact Funct Neurosurg*. 1997, 68(1-4 Pt 1), 141-148. PubMed PMID, 9711707.

[39] Garcia-Larrea, L; Peyron, R; Mertens, P; Gregoire, MC; Lavenne, F; Le Bars, D; Convers, P; Mauguiere, F; Sindou, M; Laurent, B. Electrical stimulation of motor cortex for pain control: a combined PET-scan and electrophysiological study. *Pain*. 1999, 83(2), 259-273. PubMed PMID, 10534598.

[40] Peyron, R; Garcia-Larrea, L; Deiber, MP; Cinotti, L; Convers, P; Sindou, M; Mauguiere, F; Laurent, B. Electrical stimulation of precentral cortical area in the treatment of central pain: electrophysiological and PET study. *Pain*. 1995, 62(3), 275-286. PubMed PMID, 8657427.

[41] Brown, JA; Barbaro, NM. Motor cortex stimulation for central and neuropathic pain: current status. *Pain*. 2003, 104(3), 431-435. PubMed PMID, 12927615.

[42] Nguyen, JP; Keravel, Y; Feve, A; Uchiyama, T; Cesaro, P; Le Guerinel, C; Pollin, B. Treatment of deafferentation pain by chronic stimulation of the motor cortex: report of a series of 20 cases. *Acta Neurochir Suppl*. 1997, 68, 54-60. PubMed PMID, 9233414.

[43] Nguyen, JP; Lefaucheur, JP; Decq, P; Uchiyama, T; Carpentier, A; Fontaine, D; Brugieres, P; Pollin, B; Feve, A; Rostaing, S; Cesaro, P; Keravel, Y. Chronic motor cortex stimulation in the treatment of central and neuropathic pain. Correlations between clinical, electrophysiological and anatomical data. *Pain*. 1999, 82(3), 245-251. PubMed PMID, 10488675.

[44] Ebel, H; Rust, D; Tronnier, V; Boker, D; Kunze, S. Chronic precentral stimulation in trigeminal neuropathic pain. *Acta Neurochir (Wien)*. 1996, 138(11), 1300-1306. PubMed PMID, 8980733.

[45] Meyerson, BA; Lindblom, U; Linderoth, B; Lind, G; Herregodts, P. Motor cortex stimulation as treatment of trigeminal neuropathic pain. *Acta Neurochir Suppl (Wien)*. 1993, 58, 150-153. PubMed PMID, 8109279.

[46] Rainov, NG; Fels, C; Heidecke, V; Burkert, W. Epidural electrical stimulation of the motor cortex in patients with facial neuralgia. *Clin Neurol Neurosurg*. 1997, 99(3), 205-209. PubMed PMID, 9350402.

[47] Saitoh, Y; Hirano, S; Kato, A; Kishima, H; Hirata, M; Yamamoto, K; Yoshimine, T. Motor cortex stimulation for deafferentation pain. *Neurosurg Focus*. 2001, 11(3), E1. doi: 10.3171/foc.2001.11.3.2. PubMed PMID, 16519421.

[48] Tsubokawa, T; Katayama, Y; Yamamoto, T; Hirayama, T; Koyama, S. Chronic motor cortex stimulation for the treatment of central pain. *Acta Neurochir Suppl (Wien)*. 1991, 52, 137-139. PubMed PMID, 1792954.

[49] Tsubokawa, T; Katayama, Y; Yamamoto, T; Hirayama, T; Koyama, S. Treatment of thalamic pain by chronic motor cortex stimulation. *Pacing Clin Electrophysiol*. 1991, 14(1), 131-134. PubMed PMID, 1705329.

[50] Lefaucheur, JP; Keravel, Y; Nguyen, JP. Treatment of poststroke pain by epidural motor cortex stimulation with a new octopolar lead. *Neurosurgery*. 2011, 68(1 Suppl Operative), 180-187, discussion 187. doi: 10.1227/NEU.0b013e318207f896. PubMed PMID, 21206307.

[51]   Pascual-Leone, A; Tormos, JM; Keenan, J; Tarazona, F; Canete, C; Catala, MD. Study and modulation of human cortical excitability with transcranial magnetic stimulation. *J Clin Neurophysiol.* 1998, 15(4), 333-343. PubMed PMID, 9736467.

[52]   Plow, EB; Pascual-Leone, A; Machado, A. Brain stimulation in the treatment of chronic neuropathic and non-cancerous pain. *J Pain.* 2012, 13(5), 411-424. doi: 10.1016/j.jpain.2012.02.001. PubMed PMID, 22484179.

[53]   Barker, AT; Jalinous, R; Freeston, IL. Non-invasive magnetic stimulation of human motor cortex. *Lancet.* 1985, 1(8437), 1106-1107. PubMed PMID, 2860322.

[54]   de Andrade, DC; Mhalla, A; Adam, F; Texeira, MJ; Bouhassira, D. Neuropharmacological basis of rTMS-induced analgesia: the role of endogenous opioids. *Pain.* 2011, 152(2), 320-326. doi: 10.1016/j.pain. 2010.10.032. PubMed PMID, 21146300.

[55]   Maarrawi, J; Peyron, R; Mertens, P; Costes, N; Magnin, M; Sindou, M; Laurent, B; Garcia-Larrea, L. Motor cortex stimulation for pain control induces changes in the endogenous opioid system. *Neurology.* 2007, 69(9), 827-834. doi: 10.1212/01.wnl. 0000269783.86997.37. PubMed PMID, 17724284.

[56]   Nahmias, F; Debes, C; de Andrade, DC; Mhalla, A; Bouhassira, D. Diffuse analgesic effects of unilateral repetitive transcranial magnetic stimulation (rTMS) in healthy volunteers. *Pain.* 2009, 147(1-3), 224-232. doi: 10.1016/j.pain.2009.09.016. PubMed PMID, 19822394.

[57]   Lorenz, J; Minoshima, S; Casey, KL. Keeping pain out of mind: the role of the dorsolateral prefrontal cortex in pain modulation. *Brain.* 2003, 126(Pt 5), 1079-1091. PubMed PMID, 12690048.

[58]   Mylius, V; Knaack, A; Haag, A; Teepker, M; Oertel, WH; Thut, G; Hamer, HM; Rosenow, F. Effects of paired-pulse transcranial magnetic stimulation of the motor cortex on perception of experimentally induced pain. *Clin J Pain.* 2010, 26(7), 617-623. doi: 10.1097/AJP. 0b013e3181dedf8a. PubMed PMID, 20639733.

[59]   Lefaucheur, JP; Holsheimer, J; Goujon, C; Keravel, Y; Nguyen, JP. Descending volleys generated by efficacious epidural motor cortex stimulation in patients with chronic neuropathic pain. *Exp Neurol.* 2010, 223(2), 609-614. doi: 10.1016/j.expneurol. 2010.02.008. PubMed PMID, 20188091.

[60]   Pagano, RL; Assis, DV; Clara, JA; Alves, AS; Dale, CS; Teixeira, MJ; Fonoff, ET; Britto, LR. Transdural motor cortex stimulation reverses neuropathic pain in rats: a profile of neuronal activation. *Eur J Pain.* 2011, 15(3), 268 e261-214. doi: 10.1016/j.ejpain.2010.08.003. PubMed PMID, 20817578.

[61]   Kishima, H; Saitoh, Y; Osaki, Y; Nishimura, H; Kato, A; Hatazawa, J; Yoshimine, T. Motor cortex stimulation in patients with deafferentation pain: activation of the posterior insula and thalamus. *J Neurosurg.* 2007, 107(1), 43-48. doi: 10.3171/JNS-07/07/0043. PubMed PMID, 17639872.

[62]   Ciampi de Andrade, D; Mhalla, A; Adam, F; Texeira, MJ; Bouhassira, D. Repetitive transcranial magnetic stimulation induced analgesia depends on N-methyl-D-aspartate glutamate receptors. *Pain.* 2014, 155(3), 598-605. doi: 10.1016/j.pain.2013.12.022. PubMed PMID, 24342462.

[63]   George, MS; Wassermann, EM; Williams, WA; Callahan, A; Ketter, TA; Basser, P; Hallett, M; Post, RM. Daily repetitive transcranial magnetic stimulation (rTMS)

improves mood in depression. *Neuroreport.* 1995, 6(14), 1853-1856. PubMed PMID, 8547583.

[64] Pascual-Leone, A; Rubio, B; Pallardo, F; Catala, MD. Rapid-rate transcranial magnetic stimulation of left dorsolateral prefrontal cortex in drug-resistant depression. *Lancet.* 1996, 348(9022), 233-237. PubMed PMID, 8684201.

[65] Pascual-Leone, A; Valls-Sole, J; Wassermann, EM; Hallett, M. Responses to rapid-rate transcranial magnetic stimulation of the human motor cortex. *Brain.* 1994, 117 (Pt 4), 847-858. PubMed PMID, 7922470.

[66] Lefaucheur, JP; Drouot, X; Keravel, Y; Nguyen, JP. Pain relief induced by repetitive transcranial magnetic stimulation of precentral cortex. *Neuroreport.* 2001, 12(13), 2963-2965. PubMed PMID, 11588611.

[67] Lefaucheur, JP; Drouot, X; Nguyen, JP. Interventional neurophysiology for pain control: duration of pain relief following repetitive transcranial magnetic stimulation of the motor cortex. *Neurophysiol Clin.* 2001, 31(4), 247-252. PubMed PMID, 11601430.

[68] Brigo, F; Storti, M; Nardone, R; Fiaschi, A; Bongiovanni, LG; Tezzon, F; Manganotti, P. Transcranial magnetic stimulation of visual cortex in migraine patients: a systematic review with meta-analysis. *J Headache Pain.* 2012, 13(5), 339-349. doi: 10.1007/s10194-012-0445-6. PubMed PMID, 22535147.

[69] Tzabazis, A; Aparici, CM; Rowbotham, MC; Schneider, MB; Etkin, A; Yeomans, DC. Shaped magnetic field pulses by multi-coil repetitive transcranial magnetic stimulation (rTMS) differentially modulate anterior cingulate cortex responses and pain in volunteers and fibromyalgia patients. *Mol Pain.* 2013, 9, 33. doi: 10.1186/1744-8069-9-33. PubMed PMID, 23819466.

[70] Onesti, E; Gabriele, M; Cambieri, C; Ceccanti, M; Raccah, R; Di, Stefano, G; Biasiotta, A; Truini, A; Zangen, A; Inghilleri, M. H-coil repetitive transcranial magnetic stimulation for pain relief in patients with diabetic neuropathy. *Eur J Pain.* 2013, 17(9), 1347-1356. doi: 10.1002/j.1532-2149.2013.00320.x. PubMed PMID, 23629867.

[71] Berlim, MT; van den Eynde, F; Tovar-Perdomo, S; Daskalakis, ZJ. Response, remission and drop-out rates following high-frequency repetitive transcranial magnetic stimulation (rTMS) for treating major depression: a systematic review and meta-analysis of randomized, double-blind and sham-controlled trials. *Psychol Med.* 2014, 44(2), 225-239. doi: 10.1017/S0033291713000512. PubMed PMID, 23507264.

[72] Xie, J; Chen, J; Wei, Q. Repetitive transcranial magnetic stimulation versus electroconvulsive therapy for major depression: a meta-analysis of stimulus parameter effects. *Neurol Res.* 2013, 35(10), 1084-1091. doi: 10.1179/1743132813Y.0000000245. PubMed PMID, 23889926.

[73] De Raedt, R; Vanderhasselt, MA; Baeken, C. Neurostimulation as an intervention for treatment resistant depression: From research on mechanisms towards targeted neurocognitive strategies. *Clin Psychol Rev.* 2014. doi: 10.1016/j.cpr.2014.10.006. PubMed PMID, 25468571.

[74] Liu, B; Zhang, Y; Zhang, L; Li, L. Repetitive transcranial magnetic stimulation as an augmentative strategy for treatment-resistant depression, a meta-analysis of randomized, double-blind and sham-controlled study. *BMC Psychiatry.* 2014, 14(1), 342. doi: 10.1186/s12888-014-0342-4. PubMed PMID, 25433539.

[75] Gaynes, BN; Lloyd, SW; Lux, L; Gartlehner, G; Hansen, RA; Brode, S; Jonas, DE; Swinson, Evans, T; Viswanathan, M; Lohr, KN. Repetitive transcranial magnetic

stimulation for treatment-resistant depression: a systematic review and meta-analysis. *J Clin Psychiatry.* 2014, 75(5), 477-489, quiz 489. doi: 10.4088/JCP.13r08815. PubMed PMID, 24922485.

[76] Kang, BS; Shin, HI; Bang, MS. Effect of repetitive transcranial magnetic stimulation over the hand motor cortical area on central pain after spinal cord injury. *Arch Phys Med Rehabil.* 2009, 90(10), 1766-1771. doi: 10.1016/j.apmr.2009.04.008. PubMed PMID, 19801069.

[77] Passard, A; Attal, N; Benadhira, R; Brasseur, L; Saba, G; Sichere, P; Perrot, S; Januel, D; Bouhassira, D. Effects of unilateral repetitive transcranial magnetic stimulation of the motor cortex on chronic widespread pain in fibromyalgia. *Brain.* 2007, 130(Pt 10), 2661-2670. doi: 10.1093/brain/awm189. PubMed PMID, 17872930.

[78] Galhardoni, R; Correia, GS; Araujo, H; Fernandes, DT; Kaziyama, HH; Marcolin, MA; Bouhassira, D; Teixeira, MJ; de Andrade, DC. Repetitive Transcranial Magnetic Stimulation (rTMS) in Chronic Pain: a review of the literature. *Arch Phys Med Rehabil.* 2014. doi: 10.1016/j.apmr.2014.11.010. PubMed PMID, 25437106.

[79] de Oliveira, RA; de, Andrade, DC; Mendonca, M; Barros, R; Luvisoto, T; Myczkowski, ML; Marcolin, MA; Teixeira, MJ. Repetitive transcranial magnetic stimulation of the left premotor/dorsolateral prefrontal cortex does not have analgesic effect on central poststroke pain. *J Pain.* 2014, 15(12), 1271-1281. doi: 10.1016/j.jpain.2014.09.009. PubMed PMID, 25267523.

[80] Hosomi, K; Shimokawa, T; Ikoma, K; Nakamura, Y; Sugiyama, K; Ugawa, Y; Uozumi, T; Yamamoto, T; Saitoh, Y. Daily repetitive transcranial magnetic stimulation of primary motor cortex for neuropathic pain: a randomized, multicenter, double-blind, crossover, sham-controlled trial. *Pain.* 2013, 154(7), 1065-1072. doi: 10.1016/ j.pain.2013.03.016. PubMed PMID, 23623156.

[81] Eisenberg, E; Chistyakov, AV; Yudashkin, M; Kaplan, B; Hafner, H; Feinsod, M. Evidence for cortical hyperexcitability of the affected limb representation area in CRPS: a psychophysical and transcranial magnetic stimulation study. *Pain.* 2005, 113(1-2), 99-105. doi: 10.1016/j.pain.2004.09.030. PubMed PMID, 15621369.

[82] Picarelli, H; Teixeira, MJ; de Andrade, DC; Myczkowski, ML; Luvisotto, TB; Yeng, LT; Fonoff, ET; Pridmore, S; Marcolin, MA. Repetitive transcranial magnetic stimulation is efficacious as an add-on to pharmacological therapy in complex regional pain syndrome (CRPS) type I. *J Pain.* 2010, 11(11), 1203-1210. doi: 10.1016/j.jpain.2010.02. 006. PubMed PMID, 20430702.

[83] Turton, AJ; McCabe, CS; Harris, N; Filipovic, SR. Sensorimotor integration in Complex Regional Pain Syndrome: a transcranial magnetic stimulation study. *Pain.* 2007, 127(3), 270-275. doi: 10.1016/j.pain.2006.08.021. PubMed PMID, 17011705.

[84] Krause, P; Forderreuther, S; Straube, A. TMS motor cortical brain mapping in patients with complex regional pain syndrome type I. *Clin Neurophysiol.* 2006, 117(1), 169-176. doi: 10.1016/j.clinph.2005. 09.012. PubMed PMID, 16326140.

[85] Krause, P; Forderreuther, S; Straube, A. [Motor cortical representation in patients with complex regional pain syndrome: a TMS study]. *Schmerz.* 2006, 20(3), 181-184, 186-188. doi: 10.1007/s00482-005-0417-8. PubMed PMID, 16047170.

[86] Schwenkreis, P; Janssen, F; Rommel, O; Pleger, B; Volker, B; Hosbach, I; Dertwinkel, R; Maier, C; Tegenthoff, M. Bilateral motor cortex disinhibition in complex regional

pain syndrome (CRPS) type I of the hand. *Neurology.* 2003, 61(4), 515-519. Epub 2003/08/27. PubMed PMID, 12939426.

[87] Pleger, B; Janssen, F; Schwenkreis, P; Volker, B; Maier, C; Tegenthoff, M. Repetitive transcranial magnetic stimulation of the motor cortex attenuates pain perception in complex regional pain syndrome type I. *Neurosci Lett.* 2004, 356(2), 87-90. PubMed PMID, 14746870.

[88] Berlim, MT; Broadbent, HJ; Van den Eynde, F. Blinding integrity in randomized sham-controlled trials of repetitive transcranial magnetic stimulation for major depression: a systematic review and meta-analysis. *Int J Neuropsychopharmacol.* 2013, 16(5), 1173-1181. doi: 10.1017/S1461145712001691. PubMed PMID, 23399312.

[89] Mhalla, A; Baudic, S; Ciampi de Andrade, D; Gautron, M; Perrot, S; Teixeira, MJ; Attal, N; Bouhassira, D. Long-term maintenance of the analgesic effects of transcranial magnetic stimulation in fibromyalgia. *Pain.* 2011, 152(7), 1478-1485. doi: 10.1016/j.pain.2011.01.034. PubMed PMID, 21397400.

[90] Boyer, L; Dousset, A; Roussel, P; Dossetto, N; Cammilleri, S; Piano, V; Khalfa, S; Mundler, O; Donnet, A; Guedj, E. rTMS in fibromyalgia: a randomized trial evaluating QoL and its brain metabolic substrate. *Neurology.* 2014, 82(14), 1231-1238. doi: 10.1212/WNL. 0000000000000280. PubMed PMID, 24670891.

[91] Ware, JE; Jr. Sherbourne, CD. The MOS 36-item short-form health survey (SF-36). I. Conceptual framework and item selection. *Med Care.* 1992, 30(6), 473-483. PubMed PMID, 1593914.

[92] Dubois, PE; Ossemann, M; de, Fays, K; De Bue, P; Gourdin, M; Jamart, J; Vandermeeren, Y. Postoperative analgesic effect of transcranial direct current stimulation in lumbar spine surgery: a randomized control trial. *Clin J Pain.* 2013, 29(8), 696-701. doi: 10.1097/ AJP.0b013e31826fb302. PubMed PMID, 23719070.

[93] Chung, SW; Hoy, KE; Fitzgerald, PB. Theta-Burst Stimulation: A New Form of Tms Treatment for Depression? *Depress Anxiety.* 2014. doi: 10.1002/da.22335. PubMed PMID, 25450537.

[94] Jelic, MB; Milanovic, SD; Filipovic, SR. Differential effects of facilitatory and inhibitory theta burst stimulation of the primary motor cortex on motor learning. *Clin Neurophysiol.* 2014. doi: 10.1016/j.clinph.2014.09.003. PubMed PMID, 25281475.

[95] Moisset, X; Goudeau, S; Poindessous-Jazat, F; Baudic, S; Clavelou, P; Bouhassira, D. Prolonged Continuous Theta-burst Stimulation is More Analgesic Than 'Classical' High Frequency Repetitive Transcranial Magnetic *Stimulation. Brain Stimul.* 2014. doi: 10.1016/j.brs.2014. 10.006. PubMed PMID, 25456979.

[96] Baudic, S; Attal, N; Mhalla, A; Ciampi, de, Andrade, D; Perrot, S; Bouhassira, D. Unilateral repetitive transcranial magnetic stimulation of the motor cortex does not affect cognition in patients with fibromyalgia. *J Psychiatr Res.* 2013, 47(1), 72-77. doi: 10.1016/j.jpsychires. 2012.09.003. PubMed PMID, 23079535.

[97] Lefaucheur, JP; Drouot, X; Menard-Lefaucheur, I; Zerah, F; Bendib, B; Cesaro, P; Keravel, Y; Nguyen, JP. Neurogenic pain relief by repetitive transcranial magnetic cortical stimulation depends on the origin and the site of pain. *J Neurol Neurosurg Psychiatry.* 2004, 75(4), 612-616. PubMed PMID, 15026508.

[98] Lefaucheur, JP; Hatem, S; Nineb, A; Menard-Lefaucheur, I; Wendling, S; Keravel, Y; Nguyen, JP. Somatotopic organization of the analgesic effects of motor cortex rTMS in

neuropathic pain. *Neurology*. 2006, 67(11), 1998-2004. doi: 10.1212/01.wnl. 0000247138.85330.88. PubMed PMID, 17159107.

[99] Pleger, B; Draganski, B; Schwenkreis, P; Lenz, M; Nicolas, V; Maier, C; Tegenthoff, M. Complex regional pain syndrome type I affects brain structure in prefrontal and motor cortex. *PLoS One*. 2014, 9(1), e85372. doi: 10.1371/journal.pone.0085372. PubMed PMID, 24416397.

[100] Schwenkreis, P; Maier, C; Tegenthoff, M. Functional imaging of central nervous system involvement in complex regional pain syndrome. *AJNR Am J Neuroradiol*. 2009, 30(7), 1279-1284. doi: 10.3174/ajnr.A1630. PubMed PMID, 19386737.

[101] Baliki, MN; Mansour, AR; Baria, AT; Apkarian, AV. Functional reorganization of the default mode network across chronic pain conditions. *PLoS One*. 2014, 9(9), e106133. doi: 10.1371/journal.pone.0106133. PubMed PMID, 25180885.

[102] Linnman, C; Becerra, L; Borsook, D. Inflaming the brain: CRPS a model disease to understand neuroimmune interactions in chronic pain. *J Neuroimmune Pharmacol*. 2013, 8(3), 547-563. doi: 10.1007/s11481-012-9422-8. PubMed PMID, 23188523.

[103] Linnman, C; Becerra, L; Lebel, A; Berde, C; Grant, PE; Borsook, D. Transient and persistent pain induced connectivity alterations in pediatric complex regional pain syndrome. *PLoS One*. 2013, 8(3), e57205. doi: 10.1371/journal.pone.0057205. PubMed PMID, 23526938.

[104] Shiraishi, S; Kobayashi, H; Nihashi, T; Kato, K; Iwano, S; Nishino, M; Ishigaki, T; Ikeda, M; Kato, T; Ito, K; Kimura, T. Cerebral glucose metabolism change in patients with complex regional pain syndrome: a PET study. *Radiat Med*. 2006, 24(5), 335-344. doi: 10.1007/s11604-006-0035-0. PubMed PMID, 16958411.

[105] Schreiber, KL; Campbell, C; Martel, MO; Greenbaum, S; Wasan, AD; Borsook, D; Jamison, RN; Edwards, RR. Distraction analgesia in chronic pain patients: the impact of catastrophizing. *Anesthesiology*. 2014, 121(6), 1292-1301. doi: 10.1097/ALN.0000000000000465. PubMed PMID, 25264596.

[106] Younger, J; Aron, A; Parke, S; Chatterjee, N; Mackey, S. Viewing pictures of a romantic partner reduces experimental pain: involvement of neural reward systems. *PLoS One*. 2010, 5(10), e13309. doi: 10.1371/journal.pone.0013309. PubMed PMID, 20967200.

[107] Galer, BS; Bruehl, S; Harden, RN. IASP diagnostic criteria for complex regional pain syndrome: a preliminary empirical validation study. International Association for the Study of Pain. *Clin J Pain*. 1998, 14(1), 48-54. Epub 1998/04/16. PubMed PMID, 9535313.

[108] Reinders, MF; Geertzen, JH; Dijkstra, PU. Complex regional pain syndrome type I: use of the International Association for the Study of Pain diagnostic criteria defined in 1994. *Clin J Pain*. 2002, 18(4), 207-215. PubMed PMID, 12131062.

[109] Harden, RN; Bruehl, S; Stanton-Hicks, M; Wilson, PR. Proposed new diagnostic criteria for complex regional pain syndrome. *Pain Med*. 2007, 8(4), 326-331. doi: 10.1111/j.1526-4637.2006.00169.x. PubMed PMID, 17610454.

[110] Harden, RN; Bruehl, S; Galer, BS; Saltz, S; Bertram, M; Backonja, M; Gayles, R; Rudin, N; Bhugra, MK; Stanton-Hicks, M. Complex regional pain syndrome: are the IASP diagnostic criteria valid and sufficiently comprehensive? *Pain*. 1999, 83(2), 211-219. Epub 1999/10/27. PubMed PMID, 10534592.

[111] Harden, RN; Bruehl, S; Perez, RS; Birklein, F; Marinus, J; Maihofner, C; Lubenow, T; Buvanendran, A; Mackey, S; Graciosa, J; Mogilevski, M; Ramsden, C; Chont, M; Vatine, JJ. Validation of proposed diagnostic criteria (the "Budapest Criteria") for Complex Regional Pain Syndrome. *Pain.* 2010, 150(2), 268-274. doi: 10.1016/j.pain.2010. 04.030. PubMed PMID, 20493633.

[112] Harden, RN; Bruehl, SP. Diagnosis of complex regional pain syndrome: signs, symptoms, and new empirically derived diagnostic criteria. *Clin J Pain.* 2006, 22(5), 415-419. doi: 10.1097/01.ajp.0000194279.36261.3e. PubMed PMID, 16772794.

[113] Bruehl, S; Harden, RN; Galer, BS; Saltz, S; Bertram, M; Backonja, M; Gayles, R; Rudin, N; Bhugra, MK; Stanton-Hicks, M. External validation of IASP diagnostic criteria for Complex Regional Pain Syndrome and proposed research diagnostic criteria. International Association for the Study of Pain. *Pain.* 1999, 81(1-2), 147-154. PubMed PMID, 10353502.

[114] Bolwerk, A; Seifert, F; Maihofner, C. Altered resting-state functional connectivity in complex regional pain syndrome. *J Pain.* 2013, 14(10), 1107-1115 e1108. doi: 10.1016/j.jpain.2013.04.007. PubMed PMID, 23791136.

[115] Peyron, R; Schneider, F; Faillenot, I; Convers, P; Barral, FG; Garcia-Larrea, L; Laurent, B. An fMRI study of cortical representation of mechanical allodynia in patients with neuropathic pain. *Neurology.* 2004, 63(10), 1838-1846. PubMed PMID, 15557499.

[116] Tseng, MT; Chiang, MC; Chao, CC; Tseng, WY; Hsieh, ST. fMRI evidence of degeneration-induced neuropathic pain in diabetes: enhanced limbic and striatal activations. *Hum Brain Mapp.* 2013, 34(10), 2733-2746. doi: 10.1002/hbm.22105. PubMed PMID, 22522975.

[117] Stude, P; Enax-Krumova, EK; Lenz, M; Lissek, S; Nicolas, V; Peters, S; Westermann, A; Tegenthoff, M; Maier, C. Local anesthetic sympathectomy restores fMRI cortical maps in CRPS I after upper extremity stellate blockade: a prospective case study. *Pain Physician.* 2014, 17(5), E637-644. PubMed PMID, 25247914.

[118] Becerra, L; Sava, S; Simons, LE; Drosos, AM; Sethna, N; Berde, C; Lebel, AA; Borsook, D. Intrinsic brain networks normalize with treatment in pediatric complex regional pain syndrome. *Neuroimage Clin.* 2014, 6, 347-369. Doi: 10.1016/j.nicl.2014.07.012. PubMed PMID, 25379449.

[119] Becerra, L; Schwartzman, RJ; Kiefer, RT; Rohr, P; Moulton, EA; Wallin, D; Pendse, G; Morris, S; Borsook, D. CNS Measures of Pain Responses Pre- and Post-Anesthetic Ketamine in a Patient with Complex Regional Pain Syndrome. *Pain Med.* 2009. doi: 10.1111/j.1526-4637.2009.00559.x. PubMed PMID, 19254342.

[120] Chapin, H; Bagarinao, E; Mackey, S. Real-time fMRI applied to pain management. *Neurosci Lett.* 2012, 520(2), 174-181. doi: 10.1016/j.neulet.2012.02.076. PubMed PMID, 22414861.

[121] deCharms, RC; Maeda, F; Glover, GH; Ludlow, D; Pauly, JM; Soneji, D; Gabrieli, JD; Mackey, SC. Control over brain activation and pain learned by using real-time functional MRI. *Proc Natl Acad Sci U S A.* 2005, 102(51), 18626-18631. doi: 10.1073/pnas.0505210102. PubMed PMID, 16352728.

[122] Zotev, V; Phillips, R; Young, KD; Drevets, WC; Bodurka, J. Prefrontal control of the amygdala during real-time fMRI neurofeedback training of emotion regulation. *PLoS*

One. 2013, 8(11), e79184. doi: 10.1371/journal.pone.0079184. PubMed PMID, 24223175.

[123] Pachowicz, M; Nocun, A; Postepski, J; Olesinska, E; Emeryk, A; Chrapko, B. Complex Regional Pain Syndrome type I with atypical scintigraphic pattern--diagnosis and evaluation of the entity with three phase bone scintigraphy. A case report. *Nucl Med Rev Cent East Eur.* 2014, 17(2), 115-119. doi: 10.5603/NMR.2014.0029. PubMed PMID, 25088114.

[124] Lefaucheur, JP; Menard-Lefaucheur, I; Goujon, C; Keravel, Y; Nguyen, JP. Predictive value of rTMS in the identification of responders to epidural motor cortex stimulation therapy for pain. *J Pain.* 2011, 12(10), 1102-1111. doi: 10.1016/j.jpain.2011.05.004. PubMed PMID, 21807565.

[125] Borsook, D; Becerra, L; Fava, M. Use of functional imaging across clinical phases in CNS drug development. *Transl Psychiatry.* 2013, 3, e282. doi: 10.1038/tp.2013.43. PubMed PMID, 23860483.

[126] Ushida, T; Tani, T; Kanbara, T; Zinchuk, VS; Kawasaki, M; Yamamoto, H. Analgesic effects of ketamine ointment in patients with complex regional pain syndrome type 1. *Reg Anesth Pain Med.* 2002, 27(5), 524-528. PubMed PMID, 12373705.

[127] Yanow, J; Pappagallo, M; Pillai, L. Complex regional pain syndrome (CRPS/RSD) and neuropathic pain: role of intravenous bisphosphonates as analgesics. *ScientificWorldJournal.* 2008, 8, 229-236. doi: 10.1100/tsw.2008.33. PubMed PMID, 18661047.

[128] Breuer, B; Pappagallo, M; Ongseng, F; Chen, CI; Goldfarb, R. An open-label pilot trial of ibandronate for complex regional pain syndrome. *Clin J Pain.* 2008, 24(8), 685-689. doi: 10.1097/AJP.0b013e318175920f. PubMed PMID, 18806533.

[129] Brunner, F; Schmid, A; Kissling, R; Held, U; Bachmann, LM. Biphosphonates for the therapy of complex regional pain syndrome I--systematic review. *Eur J Pain.* 2009, 13(1), 17-21. doi: 10.1016/j.ejpain.2008.03.005. PubMed PMID, 18440845.

[130] Cortet, B; Flipo, RM; Coquerelle, P; Duquesnoy, B; Delcambre, B. Treatment of severe, recalcitrant reflex sympathetic dystrophy, assessment of efficacy and safety of the second generation bisphosphonate pamidronate. *Clin Rheumatol.* 1997, 16(1), 51-56. PubMed PMID, 9132326.

[131] Kubalek, I; Fain, O; Paries, J; Kettaneh, A; Thomas, M. Treatment of reflex sympathetic dystrophy with pamidronate: 29 cases. *Rheumatology* (Oxford). 2001, 40(12), 1394-1397. PubMed PMID, 11752511.

[132] Maillefert, JF; Chatard, C; Owen, S; Peere, T; Tavernier, C; Tebib, J. Treatment of refractory reflex sympathetic dystrophy with pamidronate. *Ann Rheum Dis.* 1995, 54(8), 687. PubMed PMID, 7677451.

[133] Robinson, JN; Sandom, J; Chapman, PT. Efficacy of pamidronate in complex regional pain syndrome type I. *Pain Med.* 2004, 5(3), 276-280. doi: 10.1111/j.1526-4637.2004.04038.x. PubMed PMID, 15367305.

[134] Varenna, M; Adami, S; Rossini, M; Gatti, D; Idolazzi, L; Zucchi, F; Malavolta, N; Sinigaglia, L. Treatment of complex regional pain syndrome type I with neridronate: a randomized, double-blind, placebo-controlled study. *Rheumatology (Oxford).* 2013, 52(3), 534-542. doi: 10.1093/rheumatology/kes312. PubMed PMID, 23204550.

[135] Varenna, M; Zucchi, F; Ghiringhelli, D; Binelli, L; Bevilacqua, M; Bettica, P; Sinigaglia, L. Intravenous clodronate in the treatment of reflex sympathetic dystrophy

syndrome. A randomized, double blind, placebo controlled study. *J Rheumatol.* 2000, 27(6), 1477-1483. PubMed PMID, 10852274.

[136] Kosharskyy, B; Almonte, W; Shaparin, N; Pappagallo, M; Smith, H. Intravenous infusions in chronic pain management. *Pain Physician.* 2013, 16(3), 231-249. PubMed PMID, 23703410.

[137] Patil, S; Anitescu, M. Efficacy of outpatient ketamine infusions in refractory chronic pain syndromes: a 5-year retrospective analysis. *Pain Med.* 2012, 13(2), 263-269. doi: 10.1111/j.1526-4637.2011.01241.x. PubMed PMID, 21939497.

[138] Goldberg, ME; Torjman, MC; Schwartzman, RJ; Mager, DE; Wainer, IW. Pharmacodynamic profiles of ketamine (R)- and (S)- with 5-day inpatient infusion for the treatment of complex regional pain syndrome. *Pain Physician.* 2010, 13(4), 379-387. PubMed PMID, 20648207.

[139] Kapural, L; Kapural, M; Bensitel, T; Sessler, DI. Opioid-sparing effect of intravenous outpatient ketamine infusions appears short-lived in chronic-pain patients with high opioid requirements. *Pain Physician.* 2010, 13(4), 389-394. PubMed PMID, 20648208.

[140] Koffler, SP; Hampstead, BM; Irani, F; Tinker, J; Kiefer, RT; Rohr, P; Schwartzman, RJ. The neurocognitive effects of 5 day anesthetic ketamine for the treatment of refractory complex regional pain syndrome. *Arch Clin Neuropsychol.* 2007, 22(6), 719-729. doi: 10.1016/j.acn.2007.05.005. PubMed PMID, 17611073.

[141] Bell, RF. Ketamine for chronic non-cancer pain. *Pain.* 2009, 141(3), 210-214. doi: 10.1016/j.pain.2008.12.003. PubMed PMID, 19128879.

[142] Correll, GE; Maleki, J; Gracely, EJ; Muir, JJ; Harbut, RE. Subanesthetic ketamine infusion therapy: a retrospective analysis of a novel therapeutic approach to complex regional pain syndrome. *Pain Med.* 2004, 5(3), 263-275. doi: 10.1111/j.1526-4637.2004.04043.x. PubMed PMID, 15367304.

[143] Sigtermans, MJ; van, Hilten, JJ; Bauer, MC; Arbous, MS; Marinus, J; Sarton, EY; Dahan, A. Ketamine produces effective and long-term pain relief in patients with Complex Regional Pain Syndrome Type 1. *Pain.* 2009, 145(3), 304-311. doi: 10.1016/j.pain.2009.06.023. PubMed PMID, 19604642.

[144] Kiefer, RT; Rohr, P; Ploppa, A; Dieterich, HJ; Grothusen, J; Koffler, S; Altemeyer, KH; Unertl, K; Schwartzman, RJ. Efficacy of ketamine in anesthetic dosage for the treatment of refractory complex regional pain syndrome: an open label phase II study. *Pain Med.* 2008, 9(8), 1173-1201. doi: 10.1111/j.1526-4637.2007.00402.x. PubMed PMID, 18266808.

[145] Schwartzman, RJ; Alexander, GM; Grothusen, JR; Paylor, T; Reichenberger, E; Perreault, M. Outpatient intravenous ketamine for the treatment of complex regional pain syndrome: a double-blind placebo controlled study. *Pain.* 2009, 147(1-3), 107-115. doi: 10.1016/j.pain.2009.08.015. PubMed PMID, 19783371.

[146] Dahan, A; Olofsen, E; Sigtermans, M; Noppers, I; Niesters, M; Aarts, L; Bauer, M; Sarton, E. Population pharmacokinetic-pharmacodynamic modeling of ketamine-induced pain relief of chronic pain. *Eur J Pain.* 2011, 15(3), 258-267. doi: 10.1016/j.ejpain.2010.06.016. PubMed PMID, 20638877.

[147] Sigtermans, M; Noppers, I; Sarton, E; Bauer, M; Mooren, R; Olofsen, E; Dahan, A. An observational study on the effect of S+-ketamine on chronic pain versus experimental acute pain in Complex Regional Pain Syndrome type 1 patients. *Eur J Pain.* 2010, 14(3), 302-307. doi: 10.1016/j.ejpain.2009.05.012. PubMed PMID, 19540140.

[148] Kiefer, RT; Rohr, P; Ploppa, A; Nohe, B; Dieterich, HJ; Grothusen, J; Altemeyer, KH; Unertl, K; Schwartzman, RJ. A pilot open-label study of the efficacy of subanesthetic isomeric S(+)-ketamine in refractory CRPS patients. *Pain Med.* 2008, 9(1), 44-54. doi: 10.1111/j.1526-4637.2006.00223.x. PubMed PMID, 18254766.

[149] Youn, DH; Gerber, G; Sather, WA. Ionotropic glutamate receptors and voltage-gated Ca(2)(+) channels in long-term potentiation of spinal dorsal horn synapses and pain hypersensitivity. *Neural Plast.* 2013, 2013, 654257. doi: 10.1155/2013/654257. PubMed PMID, 24224102.

[150] Liu, XG; Zhou, LJ. Long-Term Potentiation at Spinal C-Fiber Synapses: a Target for Pathological Pain. *Curr Pharm Des.* 2014. PubMed PMID, 25345608.

[151] Maneksha, FR; Mirza, H; Poppers, PJ. Complex regional pain syndrome (CRPS) with resistance to local anesthetic block: a case report. *J Clin Anesth.* 2000, 12(1), 67-71. PubMed PMID, 10773513.

[152] Volianskis, A; Bannister, N; Collett, VJ; Irvine, MW; Monaghan, DT; Fitzjohn, SM; Jensen, MS; Jane, DE; Collingridge, GL. Different NMDA receptor subtypes mediate induction of long-term potentiation and two forms of short-term potentiation at CA1 synapses in rat hippocampus in vitro. *J Physiol.* 2013, 591(Pt 4), 955-972. doi: 10.1113/jphysiol.2012.247296. PubMed PMID, 23230236.

[153] Shirani, P; Salamone, AR; Schulz, PE; Edmondson, EA. Ketamine treatment for intractable pain in a patient with severe refractory complex regional pain syndrome: a case report. *Pain Physician.* 2008, 11(3), 339-342. PubMed PMID, 18523505.

[154] Kiefer, RT; Rohr, P; Ploppa, A; Altemeyer, KH; Schwartzman, RJ. Complete recovery from intractable complex regional pain syndrome, CRPS-type I, following anesthetic ketamine and midazolam. *Pain Pract.* 2007, 7(2), 147-150. doi: 10.1111/j.1533-2500.2007.00123.x. PubMed PMID, 17559485.

[155] Roberts, WJ. A hypothesis on the physiological basis for causalgia and related pains. *Pain.* 1986, 24(3), 297-311. PubMed PMID, 3515292.

[156] Sabia, M; Hirsh, RA; Torjman, MC; Wainer, IW; Cooper, N; Domsky, R; Goldberg, ME. Advances in translational neuropathic research: example of enantioselective pharmacokinetic-pharmacodynamic modeling of ketamine-induced pain relief in complex regional pain syndrome. *Curr Pain Headache Rep.* 2011, 15(3), 207-214. doi: 10.1007/s11916-011-0185-3. PubMed PMID, 21360034.

[157] Ren, ZY; Xu, XQ; Bao, YP; He, J; Shi, L; Deng, JH; Gao, XJ; Tang, HL; Wang, YM; Lu, L. The impact of genetic variation on sensitivity to opioid analgesics in patients with postoperative pain: a systematic review and meta-analysis. *Pain Physician.* 2015, 18(2), 131-152. PubMed PMID, 25794200.

[158] Yao, Y; Belcher, J; Berger, AJ; Mayer, ML; Lau, AY. Conformational analysis of NMDA receptor GluN1, GluN2, and GluN3 ligand-binding domains reveals subtype-specific characteristics. *Structure.* 2013, 21(10), 1788-1799. doi: 10.1016/j.str.2013.07.011. PubMed PMID, 23972471.

[159] Bresink, I; Danysz, W; Parsons, CG; Mutschler, E. Different binding affinities of NMDA receptor channel blockers in various brain regions--indication of NMDA receptor heterogeneity. *Neuropharmacology.* 1995, 34(5), 533-540. PubMed PMID, 7566488.

[160] Wenzel, A; Fritschy, JM; Mohler, H; Benke, D. NMDA receptor heterogeneity during postnatal development of the rat brain: differential expression of the NR2A, NR2B, and NR2C subunit proteins. *J Neurochem.* 1997, 68(2), 469-478. PubMed PMID, 9003031.

[161] Glasgow, NG; Siegler, Retchless, B; Johnson, JW. Molecular bases of NMDA receptor subtype-dependent properties. *J Physiol.* 2014. doi: 10.1113/jphysiol.2014.273763. PubMed PMID, 25107930.

[162] Kehoe, LA; Bernardinelli, Y; Muller, D. GluN3A: an NMDA receptor subunit with exquisite properties and functions. *Neural Plast.* 2013, 2013: 145387. doi: 10.1155/2013/145387. PubMed PMID, 24386575.

[163] Sanz-Clemente, A; Nicoll, RA; Roche, KW. Diversity in NMDA receptor composition: many regulators, many consequences. *Neuroscientist.* 2013, 19(1), 62-75. doi: 10.1177/1073858411435129. PubMed PMID, 22343826.

[164] Paoletti, P; Bellone, C; Zhou, Q. NMDA receptor subunit diversity: impact on receptor properties, synaptic plasticity and disease. *Nat Rev Neurosci.* 2013, 14(6), 383-400. doi: 10.1038/nrn3504. PubMed PMID, 23686171.

[165] Qu, XX; Cai, J; Li, MJ; Chi, YN; Liao, FF; Liu, FY; Wan, Y; Han, JS; Xing, GG. Role of the spinal cord NR2B-containing NMDA receptors in the development of neuropathic pain. *Exp Neurol.* 2009, 215(2), 298-307. doi: 10.1016/j.expneurol.2008.10.018. PubMed PMID, 19046970.

[166] Pachernegg, S; Strutz-Seebohm, N; Hollmann, M. GluN3 subunit-containing NMDA receptors: not just one-trick ponies. *Trends Neurosci.* 2012, 35(4), 240-249. doi: 10.1016/j.tins.2011.11.010. PubMed PMID, 22240240.

[167] Miller, OH; Yang, L; Wang, CC; Hargroder, EA; Zhang, Y; Delpire, E; Hall, BJ. GluN2B-containing NMDA receptors regulate depression-like behavior and are critical for the rapid antidepressant actions of ketamine. *Elife.* 2014, 3. doi: 10.7554/eLife.03581. PubMed PMID, 25340958.

[168] Finck, AD; Samaniego, E; Ngai, SH. Morphine tolerance decreases the analgesic effects of ketamine in mice. *Anesthesiology.* 1988, 68(3), 397-400. PubMed PMID, 3344994.

[169] Cai, YC; Ma, L; Fan, GH; Zhao, J; Jiang, LZ; Pei, G. Activation of N-methyl-D-aspartate receptor attenuates acute responsiveness of delta-opioid receptors. *Mol Pharmacol.* 1997, 51(4), 583-587. PubMed PMID, 9106622.

[170] Smith, MT. Neuroexcitatory effects of morphine and hydromorphone: evidence implicating the 3-glucuronide metabolites. *Clin Exp Pharmacol Physiol.* 2000, 27(7), 524-528. PubMed PMID, 10874511.

[171] Bartlett, SE; Cramond, T; Smith, MT. The excitatory effects of morphine-3-glucuronide are attenuated by LY274614, a competitive NMDA receptor antagonist, and by midazolam, an agonist at the benzodiazepine site on the GABAA receptor complex. *Life Sci.* 1994, 54(10), 687-694. PubMed PMID, 8107513.

[172] Wright, AW; Mather, LE; Smith, MT. Hydromorphone-3-glucuronide: a more potent neuro-excitant than its structural analogue, morphine-3-glucuronide. *Life Sci.* 2001, 69(4), 409-420. PubMed PMID, 11459432.

[173] Hemstapat, K; Monteith, GR; Smith, D; Smith, MT. Morphine-3-glucuronide's neuro-excitatory effects are mediated via indirect activation of N-methyl-D-aspartic acid receptors: mechanistic studies in embryonic cultured hippocampal neurones. *Anesth Analg.* 2003, 97(2), 494-505, table of contents. PubMed PMID, 12873944.

[174] Moran, TD; Smith, PA. Morphine-3beta-D-glucuronide suppresses inhibitory synaptic transmission in rat substantia gelatinosa. *J Pharmacol Exp Ther.* 2002, 302(2), 568-576. doi: 10.1124/jpet.102.035626. PubMed PMID, 12130717.

[175] Zhao, YL; Chen, SR; Chen, H; Pan, HL. Chronic opioid potentiates presynaptic but impairs postsynaptic N-methyl-D-aspartic acid receptor activity in spinal cords: implications for opioid hyperalgesia and tolerance. *J Biol Chem.* 2012, 287(30), 25073-25085. doi: 10.1074/jbc.M112.378737. PubMed PMID, 22679016.

[176] Ahmadi, S; Golbaghi, H; Azizbeigi, R; Esmailzadeh, N. N-methyl-D-aspartate receptors involved in morphine-induced hyperalgesia in sensitized mice. *Eur J Pharmacol.* 2014, 737, 85-90. doi: 10.1016/j.ejphar.2014.04.048. PubMed PMID, 24842190.

[177] Chapp, AD; Gui, L; Huber, MJ; Liu, J; Larson, RA; Zhu, J; Carter, JR; Chen, QH. Sympathoexcitation and pressor responses induced by ethanol in the central nucleus of amygdala involves activation of NMDA receptors in rats. *Am J Physiol Heart Circ Physiol.* 2014, 307(5), H701-709. doi: 10.1152/ajpheart.00005.2014. PubMed PMID, 24993048.

[178] Santini, CO; Fassini, A; Scopinho, AA; Busnardo, C; Correa, FM; Resstel, LB. The ventral hippocampus NMDA receptor/nitric oxide/guanylate cyclase pathway modulates cardiovascular responses in rats. *Auton Neurosci.* 2013, 177(2), 244-252. doi: 10.1016/j.autneu.2013.05.008. PubMed PMID, 23735844.

[179] Klega, A; Eberle, T; Buchholz, HG; Maus, S; Maihofner, C; Schreckenberger, M; Birklein, F. Central opioidergic neurotransmission in complex regional pain syndrome. *Neurology.* 2010, 75(2), 129-136. doi: 10.1212/WNL.0b013e3181e7ca2e. PubMed PMID, 20625165.

[180] Gideons, ES; Kavalali, ET; Monteggia, LM. Mechanisms underlying differential effectiveness of memantine and ketamine in rapid antidepressant responses. *Proc Natl Acad Sci U S A.* 2014, 111(23), 8649-8654. doi: 10.1073/pnas.1323920111. PubMed PMID, 24912158.

[181] Noppers, IM; Niesters, M; Aarts, LP; Bauer, MC; Drewes, AM; Dahan, A; Sarton, EY. Drug-induced liver injury following a repeated course of ketamine treatment for chronic pain in CRPS type 1 patients: a report of 3 cases. *Pain.* 2011, 152(9), 2173-2178. doi: 10.1016/j.pain.2011. 03.026. PubMed PMID, 21546160.

[182] Niesters, M; Martini, C; Dahan, A. Ketamine for chronic pain: risks and benefits. *Br J Clin Pharmacol.* 2014, 77(2), 357-367. doi: 10.1111/bcp.12094. PubMed PMID, 23432384.

[183] Bell, RF. Ketamine for chronic noncancer pain: concerns regarding toxicity. *Curr Opin Support Palliat Care.* 2012, 6(2), 183-187. doi: 10.1097/SPC.0b013e328352812c. PubMed PMID, 22436323.

[184] Moaddel, R; Venkata, SL; Tanga, MJ; Bupp, JE; Green, CE; Iyer, L; Furimsky, A; Goldberg, ME; Torjman, MC; Wainer, IW. A parallel chiral-achiral liquid chromatographic method for the determination of the stereoisomers of ketamine and ketamine metabolites in the plasma and urine of patients with complex regional pain syndrome. *Talanta.* 2010, 82(5), 1892-1904. doi: 10.1016/j.talanta.2010.08.005. PubMed PMID, 20875593.

[185] Kharasch, ED; Labroo, R. Metabolism of ketamine stereoisomers by human liver microsomes. *Anesthesiology.* 1992, 77(6), 1201-1207. PubMed PMID, 1466470.

[186] Caddy, C; Giaroli, G; White, TP; Shergill, SS; Tracy, DK. Ketamine as the prototype glutamatergic antidepressant: pharmacodynamic actions, and a systematic review and meta-analysis of efficacy. *Ther Adv Psychopharmacol.* 2014, 4(2), 75-99. doi: 10.1177/2045125313507739. PubMed PMID, 24688759.

[187] Yalcin, I; Barthas, F; Barrot, M. Emotional consequences of neuropathic pain: Insight from preclinical studies. *Neurosci Biobehav Rev.* 2014, 47C, 154-164. doi: 10.1016/j.neubiorev.2014.08.002. PubMed PMID, 25148733.

[188] Belujon, P; Grace, AA. Restoring Mood Balance in Depression: Ketamine Reverses Deficit in Dopamine-Dependent Synaptic Plasticity. Biol *Psychiatry.* 2014, 76(12), 927-936. doi: 10.1016/j.biopsych. 2014.04.014. PubMed PMID, 24931705.

[189] Jernigan, CS; Goswami, DB; Austin, MC; Iyo, AH; Chandran, A; Stockmeier, CA; Karolewicz, B. The mTOR signaling pathway in the prefrontal cortex is compromised in major depressive disorder. *Prog Neuropsychopharmacol Biol Psychiatry.* 2011, 35(7), 1774-1779. doi: 10.1016/j.pnpbp.2011.05.010. PubMed PMID, 21635931.

[190] Yang, C; Hu, YM; Zhou, ZQ; Zhang, GF; Yang, JJ. Acute administration of ketamine in rats increases hippocampal BDNF and mTOR levels during forced swimming test. *Ups J Med Sci.* 2013, 118(1), 3-8. doi: 10.3109/03009734.2012.724118. PubMed PMID, 22970723.

[191] Kohrs, R; Durieux, ME. Ketamine: teaching an old drug new tricks. *Anesth Analg.* 1998, 87(5), 1186-1193. PubMed PMID, 9806706.

[192] Romero, TR; Galdino, GS; Silva, GC; Resende, LC; Perez, AC; Cortes, SF; Duarte, ID. Ketamine activates the L-arginine/Nitric oxide/cyclic guanosine monophosphate pathway to induce peripheral antinociception in rats. *Anesth Analg.* 2011, 113(5), 1254-1259. doi: 10.1213/ANE.0b013e3182285dda. PubMed PMID, 21788321.

[193] Lee, SY; Chen, SL; Chang, YH; Chen, PS; Huang, SY; Tzeng, NS; Wang, YS; Wang, LJ; Lee, IH; Wang, TY; Yeh, TL; Yang, YK; Hong, JS; Lu, RB. The effects of add-on low-dose memantine on cytokine levels in bipolar II depression: a 12-week double-blind, randomized controlled trial. *J Clin Psychopharmacol.* 2014, 34(3), 337-343. doi: 10.1097/JCP.0000000000000109. PubMed PMID, 24717258.

[194] Ahmadi, A; Khalili, M; Marami, S; Ghadiri, A; Nahri-Niknafs, B. Synthesis and pain perception of new analogues of phencyclidine in NMRI male mice. *Mini Rev Med Chem.* 2014, 14(1), 64-71. PubMed PMID, 24251803.

[195] Roth, BL; Gibbons, S; Arunotayanun, W; Huang, XP; Setola, V; Treble, R; Iversen, L. The ketamine analogue methoxetamine and 3- and 4-methoxy analogues of phencyclidine are high affinity and selective ligands for the glutamate NMDA receptor. *PLoS One.* 2013, 8(3), e59334. doi: 10.1371/journal.pone.0059334. PubMed PMID, 23527166.

[196] Finch, PM; Knudsen, L; Drummond, PD. Reduction of allodynia in patients with complex regional pain syndrome: A double-blind placebo-controlled trial of topical ketamine. *Pain.* 2009, 146(1-2), 18-25. doi: 10.1016/j.pain.2009.05.017. PubMed PMID, 19703730.

[197] De Oliveira, GS; Jr. Castro-Alves, LJ; Khan, JH; McCarthy, RJ. Perioperative systemic magnesium to minimize postoperative pain: a meta-analysis of randomized controlled trials. *Anesthesiology.* 2013, 119(1), 178-190. doi: 10.1097/ALN.0b013e318297630d. PubMed PMID, 23669270.

[198] Kathuria, B; Luthra, N; Gupta, A; Grewal, A; Sood, D. Comparative efficacy of two different dosages of intrathecal magnesium sulphate supplementation in subarachnoid block. *J Clin Diagn Res.* 2014, 8(6), GC01-05. doi: 10.7860/JCDR/2014/8295.4510. PubMed PMID, 25120997.

[199] Kumar, M; Dayal, N; Rautela, RS; Sethi, AK. Effect of intravenous magnesium sulphate on postoperative pain following spinal anesthesia. A randomized double blind controlled study. *Middle East J Anaesthesiol.* 2013, 22(3), 251-256. PubMed PMID, 24649780.

[200] Yousef, AA; Al-deeb, AE. A double-blinded randomised controlled study of the value of sequential intravenous and oral magnesium therapy in patients with chronic low back pain with a neuropathic component. *Anaesthesia.* 2013, 68(3), 260-266. doi: 10.1111/anae.12107. PubMed PMID, 23384256.

[201] Wang, J; Liu, Y; Zhou, LJ; Wu, Y; Li, F; Shen, KF; Pang, RP; Wei, XH; Li, YY; Liu, XG. Magnesium L-threonate prevents and restores memory deficits associated with neuropathic pain by inhibition of TNF-alpha. *Pain Physician.* 2013, 16(5), E563-575. PubMed PMID, 24077207.

[202] Collins, S; Zuurmond, WW; de, Lange, JJ; van Hilten, BJ; Perez, RS. Intravenous magnesium for complex regional pain syndrome type 1 (CRPS 1) patients: a pilot study. *Pain Med.* 2009, 10(5), 930-940. doi: 10.1111/j.1526-4637.2009.00639.x. PubMed PMID, 19496957.

[203] Fischer, SG; Collins, S; Boogaard, S; Loer, SA; Zuurmond, WW; Perez, RS. Intravenous magnesium for chronic complex regional pain syndrome type 1 (CRPS-1). *Pain Med.* 2013, 14(9), 1388-1399. doi: 10.1111/pme.12211. PubMed PMID, 23889940.

[204] Dalli, J; Colas, RA; Serhan, CN. CORRIGENDUM: Novel n-3 Immunoresolvents, Structures and Actions. *Sci Rep.* 2014, 4, 6726. doi: 10.1038/srep06726. PubMed PMID, 25342442.

[205] Dalli, J; Colas, RA; Serhan, CN. Novel n-3 immunoresolvents: structures and actions. *Sci Rep.* 2013, 3, 1940. doi: 10.1038/srep01940. PubMed PMID, 23736886.

[206] Levy, BD; Serhan, CN. Resolution of acute inflammation in the lung. *Annu Rev Physiol.* 2014, 76, 467-492. doi: 10.1146/annurev-physiol-021113-170408. PubMed PMID, 24313723.

[207] Serhan, CN; Arita, M; Hong, S; Gotlinger, K. Resolvins, docosatrienes, and neuroprotectins, novel omega-3-derived mediators, and their endogenous aspirin-triggered epimers. *Lipids.* 2004, 39(11), 1125-1132. PubMed PMID, 15726828.

[208] Serhan, CN; Chiang, N. Endogenous pro-resolving and anti-inflammatory lipid mediators: a new pharmacologic genus. *Br J Pharmacol.* 2008, 153 Suppl 1, S200-215. doi: 10.1038/sj.bjp.0707489. PubMed PMID, 17965751.

[209] Crawford, MA; Broadhurst, CL; Guest, M; Nagar, A; Wang, Y; Ghebremeskel, K; Schmidt, WF. A quantum theory for the irreplaceable role of docosahexaenoic acid in neural cell signalling throughout evolution. *Prostaglandins Leukot Essent Fatty Acids.* 2013, 88(1), 5-13. doi: 10.1016/j.plefa.2012.08.005. PubMed PMID, 23206328.

[210] Hong, S; Tjonahen, E; Morgan, EL; Lu, Y; Serhan, CN; Rowley, AF. Rainbow trout (Oncorhynchus mykiss) brain cells biosynthesize novel docosahexaenoic acid-derived resolvins and protectins-Mediator lipidomic analysis. *Prostaglandins Other Lipid*

Mediat. 2005, 78(1-4), 107-116. doi: 10.1016/j.prostaglandins.2005.04.004. PubMed PMID, 16303609.

[211] Oh, SF; Vickery, TW; Serhan, CN. Chiral lipidomics of E-series resolvins, aspirin and the biosynthesis of novel mediators. *Biochim Biophys Acta.* 2011, 1811(11), 737-747. doi: 10.1016/j.bbalip. 2011.06.007. PubMed PMID, 21712098.

[212] Pellettieri, J; Fitzgerald, P; Watanabe, S; Mancuso, J; Green, DR; Sanchez, Alvarado, A. Cell death and tissue remodeling in planarian regeneration. *Dev Biol.* 2010, 338(1), 76-85. doi: 10.1016/j.ydbio. 2009.09.015. PubMed PMID, 19766622.

[213] Psychogios, N; Hau, DD; Peng, J; Guo, AC; Mandal, R; Bouatra, S; Sinelnikov, I; Krishnamurthy, R; Eisner, R; Gautam, B; Young, N; Xia, J; Knox, C; Dong, E; Huang, P; Hollander, Z; Pedersen, TL; Smith, SR; Bamforth, F; Greiner, R; McManus, B; Newman, JW; Goodfriend, T; Wishart, DS. The human serum metabolome. *PLoS One.* 2011, 6(2), e16957. doi: 10.1371/journal.pone.0016957. PubMed PMID, 21359215.

[214] Raatz, SK; Golovko, MY; Brose, SA; Rosenberger, TA; Burr, GS; Wolters, WR; Picklo, MJ; Sr. Baking reduces prostaglandin, resolvin, and hydroxy-fatty acid content of farm-raised Atlantic salmon (Salmo salar). *J Agric Food Chem.* 2011, 59(20), 11278-11286. doi: 10.1021/jf202576k. PubMed PMID, 21919483.

[215] Burr, GO; Burr, MM. Nutrition classics from The Journal of Biological Chemistry 82, 345-67, 1929. A new deficiency disease produced by the rigid exclusion of fat from the diet. *Nutr Rev.* 1973, 31(8), 248-249. PubMed PMID, 4586201.

[216] Claria, J; Serhan, CN. Aspirin triggers previously undescribed bioactive eicosanoids by human endothelial cell-leukocyte interactions. *Proc Natl Acad Sci U S A.* 1995, 92(21), 9475-9479. PubMed PMID, 7568157.

[217] Clish, CB; O'Brien, JA; Gronert, K; Stahl, GL; Petasis, NA; Serhan, CN. Local and systemic delivery of a stable aspirin-triggered lipoxin prevents neutrophil recruitment in vivo. *Proc Natl Acad Sci U S A.* 1999, 96(14), 8247-8252. PubMed PMID, 10393980.

[218] Serhan, CN; Clish, CB; Brannon, J; Colgan, SP; Chiang, N; Gronert, K. Novel functional sets of lipid-derived mediators with antiinflammatory actions generated from omega-3 fatty acids via cyclooxygenase 2-nonsteroidal antiinflammatory drugs and transcellular processing. *J Exp Med.* 2000, 192(8), 1197-1204. PubMed PMID, 11034610.

[219] Serhan, CN; Hong, S; Gronert, K; Colgan, SP, Devchand, PR; Mirick, G; Moussignac, RL. Resolvins: a family of bioactive products of omega-3 fatty acid transformation circuits initiated by aspirin treatment that counter proinflammation signals. *J Exp Med.* 2002, 196(8), 1025-1037. PubMed PMID, 12391014.

[220] Hussein, N; Fedorova, I; Moriguchi, T; Hamazaki, K; Kim, HY; Hoshiba, J; Salem, N; Jr. Artificial rearing of infant mice leads to n-3 fatty acid deficiency in cardiac, neural and peripheral tissues. *Lipids.* 2009, 44(8), 685-702. doi: 10.1007/s11745-009-3318-2. PubMed PMID, 19588181.

[221] Ramsden, C; Gagnon, C; Graciosa, J; Faurot, K; David, R; Bralley, JA; Harden, RN. Do omega-6 and trans fatty acids play a role in complex regional pain syndrome? A pilot study. *Pain Med.* 2010, 11(7), 1115-1125. doi: 10.1111/j.1526-4637.2010. 00882.x. PubMed PMID, 20545870.

[222] Serhan, CN. Novel chemical mediators in the resolution of inflammation, resolvins and protectins. *Anesthesiol Clin.* 2006, 24(2), 341-364. PubMed PMID, 16927933.

[223] Serhan, CN; Dalli, J; Karamnov, S; Choi, A; Park, CK; Xu, ZZ; Ji, RR; Zhu, M; Petasis, NA. Macrophage proresolving mediator maresin 1 stimulates tissue regeneration and controls pain. *FASEB J.* 2012, 26(4), 1755-1765. doi: 10.1096/fj.11-201442. PubMed PMID, 22253477.

[224] Serhan, CN; Yang, R; Martinod, K; Kasuga, K; Pillai, PS; Porter, TF; Oh, SF; Spite, M. Maresins: novel macrophage mediators with potent antiinflammatory and proresolving actions. *J Exp Med.* 2009, 206(1), 15-23. doi: 10.1084/jem.20081880. PubMed PMID, 19103881.

[225] Bazan, NG. Cell survival matters: docosahexaenoic acid signaling, neuroprotection and photoreceptors. *Trends Neurosci.* 2006, 29(5), 263-271. doi: 10.1016/ j.tins.2006.03.005. PubMed PMID, 16580739.

[226] Salem, N; Jr. Litman, B; Kim, HY; Gawrisch, K. Mechanisms of action of docosahexaenoic acid in the nervous system. *Lipids.* 2001, 36(9), 945-959. PubMed PMID, 11724467.

[227] Lemaitre, RN; Tanaka, T; Tang, W; Manichaikul, A; Foy, M; Kabagambe, EK; Nettleton, JA; King, IB; Weng, LC; Bhattacharya, S; Bandinelli, S; Bis, JC; Rich, SS; Jacobs, DR; Jr.; Cherubini, A; McKnight, B; Liang, S; Gu, X; Rice, K; Laurie, CC; Lumley, T; Browning, BL; Psaty, BM; Chen, YD; Friedlander, Y; Djousse, L; Wu, JH; Siscovick, DS; Uitterlinden, AG; Arnett, DK; Ferrucci, L; Fornage, M; Tsai, MY; Mozaffarian, D; Steffen, LM. Genetic loci associated with plasma phospholipid n-3 fatty acids: a meta-analysis of genome-wide association studies from the CHARGE Consortium. *PLoS Genet.* 2011, 7(7), e1002193. doi: 10.1371/journal.pgen.1002193. PubMed PMID, 21829377.

[228] Arita, M; Yoshida, M; Hong, S; Tjonahen, E; Glickman, JN; Petasis, NA; Blumberg, RS; Serhan, CN. Resolvin E1, an endogenous lipid mediator derived from omega-3 eicosapentaenoic acid, protects against 2,4,6-trinitrobenzene sulfonic acid-induced colitis. *Proc Natl Acad Sci USA.* 2005, 102(21), 7671-7676. doi: 10.1073/ pnas.0409271102. PubMed PMID, 15890784.

[229] Hasturk, H; Kantarci, A; Ohira, T; Arita, M; Ebrahimi, N; Chiang, N; Petasis, NA; Levy, BD; Serhan, CN; Van, Dyke, TE. RvE1 protects from local inflammation and osteoclast- mediated bone destruction in periodontitis. *FASEB J.* 2006, 20(2), 401-403. doi: 10.1096/fj.05-4724fje. PubMed PMID, 16373400.

[230] Duffield, JS; Hong, S; Vaidya, VS; Lu, Y; Fredman, G; Serhan, CN; Bonventre, JV. Resolvin D series and protectin D1 mitigate acute kidney injury. *J Immunol.* 2006, 177(9), 5902-5911. PubMed PMID, 17056514.

[231] Hong, S; Gronert, K; Devchand, PR; Moussignac, RL; Serhan, CN. Novel docosatrienes and 17S-resolvins generated from docosahexaenoic acid in murine brain, human blood, and glial cells. Autacoids in anti-inflammation. *J Biol Chem.* 2003, 278(17), 14677-14687. doi: 10.1074/jbc.M300218200. PubMed PMID, 12590139.

[232] Xu, ZZ; Zhang, L; Liu, T; Park, JY; Berta, T; Yang, R; Serhan, CN; Ji, RR. Resolvins RvE1 and RvD1 attenuate inflammatory pain via central and peripheral actions. *Nat Med.* 2010, 16(5), 592-597, 591p following 597. doi: 10.1038/nm.2123. PubMed PMID, 20383154.

[233] Ariel, A; Li, PL; Wang, W; Tang, WX; Fredman, G; Hong, S; Gotlinger, KH; Serhan, CN. The docosatriene protectin D1 is produced by TH2 skewing and promotes human

T cell apoptosis via lipid raft clustering. *J Biol Chem.* 2005, 280(52), 43079-43086. doi: 10.1074/jbc.M509796200. PubMed PMID, 16216871.

[234] Mukherjee, PK; Marcheselli, VL; Serhan, CN; Bazan, NG. Neuroprotectin D1: a docosahexaenoic acid-derived docosatriene protects human retinal pigment epithelial cells from oxidative stress. *Proc Natl Acad Sci U S A.* 2004, 101(22), 8491-8496. doi: 10.1073/pnas.0402531101. PubMed PMID, 15152078.

[235] Bazan, NG. Neurotrophins induce neuroprotective signaling in the retinal pigment epithelial cell by activating the synthesis of the anti-inflammatory and anti-apoptotic neuroprotectin D1. *Adv Exp Med Biol.* 2008, 613, 39-44. PubMed PMID, 18188926.

[236] Bazan, NG; Eady, TN; Khoutorova, L; Atkins, KD; Hong, S; Lu, Y; Zhang, C; Jun, B; Obenaus, A; Fredman, G; Zhu, M; Winkler, JW; Petasis, NA; Serhan, CN; Belayev, L. Novel aspirin-triggered neuroprotectin D1 attenuates cerebral ischemic injury after experimental stroke. *Exp Neurol.* 2012, 236(1), 122-130. doi: 10.1016/j.expneurol. 2012.04.007. PubMed PMID, 22542947.

[237] Lukiw, WJ; Cui, JG; Marcheselli, VL; Bodker, M; Botkjaer, A; Gotlinger, K; Serhan, CN; Bazan, NG. A role for docosahexaenoic acid-derived neuroprotectin D1 in neural cell survival and Alzheimer disease. *J Clin Invest.* 2005, 115(10), 2774-2783. doi: 10.1172/JCI25420. PubMed PMID, 16151530.

[238] Bazan, NG. Neuroprotectin D1 (NPD1), a DHA-derived mediator that protects brain and retina against cell injury-induced oxidative stress. *Brain Pathol.* 2005, 15(2), 159-166. PubMed PMID, 15912889.

[239] Abdulnour, RE; Dalli, J; Colby, JK; Krishnamoorthy, N; Timmons, JY; Tan, SH; Colas, RA; Petasis, NA; Serhan, CN; Levy, BD. Maresin 1 biosynthesis during platelet-neutrophil interactions is organ-protective. *Proc Natl Acad Sci U S A.* 2014, 111(46), 16526-16531. doi: 10.1073/pnas.1407123111. PubMed PMID, 25369934.

[240] Chatterjee, A; Sharma, A; Chen, M; Toy, R; Mottola, G; Conte, MS. The Pro-Resolving Lipid Mediator Maresin 1 (MaR1) Attenuates Inflammatory Signaling Pathways in Vascular Smooth Muscle and Endothelial Cells. *PLoS One.* 2014, 9(11), e113480. doi: 10.1371/journal.pone.0113480. PubMed PMID, 25409514.

[241] Srebro, DP; Vuckovic, SM; Savic, Vujovic, KR; Prostran, MS. TRPA1, NMDA receptors and nitric oxide mediate mechanical hyperalgesia induced by local injection of magnesium sulfate into the rat hind paw. *Physiol Behav.* 2014, 139C, 267-273. doi: 10.1016/j.physbeh. 2014.11.042. PubMed PMID, 25449407.

[242] Real, DS; Reis, RP; Piccolo, MS; Okamoto, RH; Gragnani, A; Ferreira, LM. Oxandrolone use in adult burn patients. Systematic review and meta-analysis. *Acta Cir Bras.* 2014, 29 Suppl 3, 68-76. PubMed PMID, 25351160.

[243] Diaz, EC; Herndon, DN; Porter, C; Sidossis, LS; Suman, OE; Borsheim, E. Effects of pharmacological interventions on muscle protein synthesis and breakdown in recovery from burns. *Burns.* 2014. doi: 10.1016/j.burns.2014.10.010. PubMed PMID, 25468473.

[244] Hart, DW; Wolf, SE; Ramzy, PI; Chinkes, DL; Beauford, RB; Ferrando, AA; Wolfe, RR; Herndon, DN. Anabolic effects of oxandrolone after severe burn. *Ann Surg.* 2001, 233(4), 556-564. PubMed PMID, 11303139.

[245] Cochran, A; Thuet, W; Holt, B; Faraklas, I; Smout, RJ; Horn, SD. The impact of oxandrolone on length of stay following major burn injury: a clinical practice evaluation. *Burns.* 2013, 39(7), 1374-1379. doi: 10.1016/j.burns.2013.04.002. PubMed PMID, 23663900.

[246] Wolf, SE; Thomas, SJ; Dasu, MR; Ferrando, AA; Chinkes, DL; Wolfe, RR; Herndon, DN. Improved net protein balance, lean mass, and gene expression changes with oxandrolone treatment in the severely burned. *Ann Surg.* 2003, 237(6), 801-810, discussion 810-801. doi: 10.1097/01.SLA.0000071562.12637.3E. PubMed PMID, 12796576.

[247] Tuvdendorj, D; Chinkes, DL; Zhang, XJ; Suman, OE; Aarsland, A; Ferrando, A; Kulp, GA; Jeschke, MG; Wolfe, RR; Herndon, DN. Long-term oxandrolone treatment increases muscle protein net deposition via improving amino acid utilization in pediatric patients 6 months after burn injury. *Surgery.* 2011, 149(5), 645-653. doi: 10.1016/j.surg.2010.12.006. PubMed PMID, 21333314.

[248] Porro, LJ; Herndon, DN; Rodriguez, NA; Jennings, K; Klein, GL; Mlcak, RP; Meyer, WJ; Lee, JO; Suman, OE; Finnerty, CC. Five-year outcomes after oxandrolone administration in severely burned children: a randomized clinical trial of safety and efficacy. *J Am Coll Surg.* 2012, 214(4), 489-502, discussion 502-484. doi: 10.1016/j.jamcollsurg.2011.12.038. PubMed PMID, 22463890.

[249] Gherondache, CN; Dowling, WJ; Pincus, G. Metabolic changes induced in elderly patients with an anabolic steroid (oxandrolone). *J Gerontol.* 1967, 22(3), 290-300. PubMed PMID, 6028497.

[250] Schroeder, ET; Vallejo, AF; Zheng, L; Stewart, Y; Flores, C; Nakao, S; Martinez, C; Sattler, FR. Six-week improvements in muscle mass and strength during androgen therapy in older men. *J Gerontol A Biol Sci Med Sci.* 2005, 60(12), 1586-1592. PubMed PMID, 16424293.

[251] Anandkumar, S; Manivasagam, M. Multimodal physical therapy management of a 48-year-old female with post-stroke complex regional pain syndrome. *Physiother Theory Pract.* 2014, 30(1), 38-48. doi: 10.3109/09593985.2013.814186. PubMed PMID, 23879307.

[252] Cucchiaro, G; Craig, K; Marks, K; Middleton, M. Diffuse complex regional pain syndrome in an adolescent: a novel treatment approach. *Clin J Pain.* 2013, 29(12), e42-45. doi: 10.1097/AJP.0b013e31829d676a. PubMed PMID, 23823251.

[253] Austin, T; Franklin, A. Outpatient rehabilitation of pediatric complex regional pain syndrome. *J Clin Anesth.* 2013, 25(6), 514-515. doi: 10.1016/j.jclinane.2013.03.015. PubMed PMID, 24008189.

[254] Schwingshackl, L; Dias, S; Strasser, B; Hoffmann, G. Impact of different training modalities on anthropometric and metabolic characteristics in overweight/obese subjects: a systematic review and network meta-analysis. *PLoS One.* 2013, 8(12), e82853. doi: 10.1371/journal.pone.0082853. PubMed PMID, 24358230.

[255] Faller, S; Hoetzel, A. Carbon monoxide in acute lung injury. *Curr Pharm Biotechnol.* 2012, 13(6), 777-786. PubMed PMID, 22201607.

[256] Hoetzel, A; Dolinay, T; Schmidt, R; Choi, AM; Ryter, SW. Carbon monoxide in sepsis. *Antioxid Redox Signal.* 2007, 9(11), 2013-2026. doi: 10.1089/ars.2007.1762. PubMed PMID, 17822362.

[257] Loop, T; Schlensak, C; Goebel, U. Cytoprotection by inhaled carbon monoxide before cardiopulmonary bypass in preclinical models. *Curr Pharm Biotechnol.* 2012, 13(6), 797-802. PubMed PMID, 22201608.

[258] Ryter, SW; Choi, AM. Therapeutic applications of carbon monoxide in lung disease. *Curr Opin Pharmacol.* 2006, 6(3), 257-262. doi: 10.1016/j.coph.2006.03.002. PubMed PMID, 16580257.

[259] Chiang, N; Shinohara, M; Dalli, J; Mirakaj, V; Kibi, M; Choi, AM; Serhan, CN. Inhaled carbon monoxide accelerates resolution of inflammation via unique proresolving mediator-heme oxygenase-1 circuits. *J Immunol.* 2013, 190(12), 6378-6388. doi: 10.4049/jimmunol.1202969. PubMed PMID, 23650615.

[260] Shinohara, M; Kibi, M; Riley, IR; Chiang, N; Dalli, J; Kraft, BD; Piantadosi, CA; Choi, AM; Serhan, CN. Cell-cell interactions and bronchoconstrictor eicosanoid reduction with inhaled carbon monoxide and resolvin D1. *Am J Physiol Lung Cell Mol Physiol.* 2014, 307(10), L746-757. doi: 10.1152/ajplung.00166.2014. PubMed PMID, 25217660.

[261] Ryter, SW; Choi, AM. Cytoprotective and anti-inflammatory actions of carbon monoxide in organ injury and sepsis models. *Novartis Found Symp.* 2007, 280, 165-175, discussion 175-181. PubMed PMID, 17380794.

[262] Furutani, K; Kohno, T. [Local anesthetics inhibit NMDA-mediated glutamatergic transmission in spinal dorsal horn neurons]. *Masui.* 2011, 60 Suppl, S151-158. PubMed PMID, 22458033.

[263] Furutani, K; Ikoma, M; Ishii, H; Baba, H; Kohno, T. Bupivacaine inhibits glutamatergic transmission in spinal dorsal horn neurons. *Anesthesiology.* 2010, 112(1), 138-143. doi: 10.1097/01.anes.0000365964.97138.9a. PubMed PMID, 20032703.

[264] Nishizawa, N; Shirasaki, T; Nakao, S; Matsuda, H; Shingu, K. The inhibition of the N-methyl-D-aspartate receptor channel by local anesthetics in mouse CA1 pyramidal neurons. *Anesth Analg.* 2002, 94(2), 325-330, table of contents. PubMed PMID, 11812692.

[265] Mantha, VR; Nair, HK; Venkataramanan, R; Gao, YY; Matyjaszewski, K; Dong, H; Li, W; Landsittel, D; Cohen, E; Lariviere, WR. Nanoanesthesia: a novel, intravenous approach to ankle block in the rat by magnet-directed concentration of ropivacaine-associated nanoparticles. *Anesth Analg.* 2014, 118(6), 1355-1362. doi: 10.1213/ANE.0000000000000175. PubMed PMID, 24722259.

[266] Surdam, JW; Licini, DJ; Baynes, NT; Arce, BR. The Use of Exparel (Liposomal Bupivacaine) to Manage Postoperative Pain in Unilateral Total Knee Arthroplasty Patients. *J Arthroplasty.* 2014. doi: 10.1016/j.arth.2014.09.004. PubMed PMID, 25282071.

[267] Herbst, SA. Local infiltration of liposome bupivacaine in foot and ankle surgery: case-based reviews. *Am J Orthop (Belle Mead NJ).* 2014, 43(10 Suppl), S10-12. PubMed PMID, 25303454.

[268] Hutchinson, HL. Local infiltration of liposome bupivacaine in orthopedic trauma patients: case-based reviews. *Am J Orthop (Belle Mead NJ).* 2014, 43(10 Suppl), S13-16. PubMed PMID, 25303455.

[269] Vogel, JD. Liposome bupivacaine (EXPAREL(R)) for extended pain relief in patients undergoing ileostomy reversal at a single institution with a fast-track discharge protocol: an IMPROVE Phase IV health economics trial. *J Pain Res.* 2013, 6, 605-610. doi: 10.2147/JPR.S46950. PubMed PMID, 23935387.

[270] Portillo, J; Kamar, N; Melibary, S; Quevedo, E; Bergese, S. Safety of liposome extended-release bupivacaine for postoperative pain control. *Front Pharmacol.* 2014, 5, 90. doi: 10.3389/fphar.2014.00090. PubMed PMID, 24817851.

[271] McAlvin, JB; Padera, RF; Shankarappa, SA; Reznor, G; Kwon, AH; Chiang, HH; Yang, J; Kohane, DS. Multivesicular liposomal bupivacaine at the sciatic nerve. *Biomaterials.* 2014, 35(15), 4557-4564. doi: 10.1016/j.biomaterials.2014.02.015. PubMed PMID, 24612918.

[272] Raul, Soberon, J; Duncan, SF; Sternbergh, WC. Treatment of digital ischemia with liposomal bupivacaine. *Case Rep Anesthesiol.* 2014, 2014, 853243. doi: 10.1155/2014/853243. PubMed PMID, 24653844.

[273] Yin, C; Matchett, G. Intercostal administration of liposomal bupivacaine as a prognostic nerve block prior to phenol neurolysis for intractable chest wall pain. *J Pain Palliat Care Pharmacother.* 2014, 28(1), 33-36. doi: 10.3109/15360288.2013.876485. PubMed PMID, 24476569.

[274] Viscusi, ER; Candiotti, KA; Onel, E; Morren, M; Ludbrook, GL. The pharmacokinetics and pharmacodynamics of liposome bupivacaine administered via a single epidural injection to healthy volunteers. *Reg Anesth Pain Med.* 2012, 37(6), 616-622. doi: 10.1097/AAP. 0b013e318269d29e. PubMed PMID, 23080351.

[275] Lander, ES. Initial impact of the sequencing of the human genome. *Nature.* 2011, 470(7333), 187-197. doi: 10.1038/nature09792. PubMed PMID, 21307931.

[276] Der Sarkissian, C; Allentoft, ME; Avila-Arcos, MC; Barnett, R; Campos, PF; Cappellini, E; Ermini, L; Fernandez, R; da Fonseca, R; Ginolhac, A; Hansen, AJ; Jonsson, H; Korneliussen, T; Margaryan, A; Martin, MD; Moreno-Mayar, JV; Raghavan, M; Rasmussen, M; Velasco, MS; Schroeder, H; Schubert, M; Seguin-Orlando, A; Wales, N; Gilbert, MT; Willerslev, E; Orlando, L. Ancient genomics. *Philos Trans R Soc Lond B Biol Sci.* 2015, 370(1660). doi: 10.1098/rstb.2013.0387. PubMed PMID, 25487338.

[277] Felsenfeld, G. A brief history of epigenetics. *Cold Spring Harb Perspect Biol.* 2014, 6(1). doi: 10.1101/cshperspect.a018200. PubMed PMID, 24384572.

[278] Svetlik, S; Hronova, K; Bakhouche, H; Matouskova, O; Slanar, O. Pharmacogenetics of chronic pain and its treatment. *Mediators Inflamm.* 2013, 2013, 864319. doi: 10.1155/2013/864319. PubMed PMID, 23766564.

[279] Cohen, M; Sadhasivam, S; Vinks, AA. Pharmacogenetics in perioperative medicine. *Curr Opin Anaesthesiol.* 2012, 25(4), 419-427. doi: 10.1097/ACO.0b013e3283556129. PubMed PMID, 22673786.

[280] Crow, M; Denk, F; McMahon, SB. Genes and epigenetic processes as prospective pain targets. *Genome Med.* 2013, 5(2), 12. doi: 10.1186/gm416. PubMed PMID, 23409739.

[281] Seo, S; Grzenda, A; Lomberk, G; Ou, XM; Cruciani, RA; Urrutia, R. Epigenetics: a promising paradigm for better understanding and managing pain. *J Pain.* 2013, 14(6), 549-557. doi: 10.1016/j.jpain.2013.01.772. PubMed PMID, 23602266.

[282] Pollema-Mays, SL; Centeno, MV; Apkarian, AV; Martina, M. Expression of DNA methyltransferases in adult dorsal root ganglia is cell-type specific and up regulated in a rodent model of neuropathic pain. *Front Cell Neurosci.* 2014, 8, 217. doi: 10.3389/fncel.2014.00217. PubMed PMID, 25152711.

[283] Weaver, IC. Epigenetic programming by maternal behavior and pharmacological intervention. Nature versus nurture: let's call the whole thing off. *Epigenetics.* 2007, 2(1), 22-28. PubMed PMID, 17965624.

[284] Vanhees, K; Vonhogen, IG; van Schooten, FJ; Godschalk, RW. You are what you eat, and so are your children: the impact of micronutrients on the epigenetic programming of offspring. *Cell Mol Life Sci.* 2014, 71(2), 271-285. doi: 10.1007/s00018-013-1427-9. PubMed PMID, 23892892.

[285] Desplats, PA. Perinatal programming of neurodevelopment: epigenetic mechanisms and the prenatal shaping of the brain. *Adv Neurobiol.* 2015, 10, 335-361. doi: 10.1007/978-1-4939-1372-5_16. PubMed PMID, 25287548.

[286] Stroud, LR; Papandonatos, GD; Rodriguez, D; McCallum, M; Salisbury, AL; Phipps, MG; Lester, B; Huestis, MA; Niaura, R; Padbury, JF; Marsit, CJ. Maternal smoking during pregnancy and infant stress response: test of a prenatal programming hypothesis. *Psychoneuroendocrinology.* 2014, 48, 29-40. doi: 10.1016/j.psyneuen.2014.05.017. PubMed PMID, 24999830.

[287] Tran, L; Schulkin, J; Ligon, CO; Greenwood-Van, Meerveld, B. Epigenetic modulation of chronic anxiety and pain by histone deacetylation. *Mol Psychiatry.* 2014, doi: 10.1038/mp.2014.122. PubMed PMID, 25288139.

[288] Kundakovic, M; Gudsnuk, K; Herbstman, JB; Tang, D; Perera, FP; Champagne, FA. DNA methylation of BDNF as a biomarker of early-life adversity. *Proc Natl Acad Sci USA.* 2014. doi: 10.1073/pnas.1408355111. PubMed PMID, 25385582.

[289] Schraut, KG; Jakob, SB; Weidner, MT; Schmitt, AG; Scholz, CJ; Strekalova, T; El Hajj, N; Eijssen, LM; Domschke, K; Reif, A; Haaf, T; Ortega, G; Steinbusch, HW; Lesch, KP; Van den Hove, DL. Prenatal stress-induced programming of genome-wide promoter DNA methylation in 5-HTT-deficient mice. *Transl Psychiatry.* 2014, 4, e473. doi: 10.1038/tp.2014.107. PubMed PMID, 25335169.

[290] Lester, BM; Conradt, E; Marsit, CJ. Epigenetic basis for the development of depression in children. *Clin Obstet Gynecol.* 2013, 56(3), 556-565. doi: 10.1097/GRF.0b013e318299d2a8. PubMed PMID, 23751878.

[291] Denk, F; McMahon, SB; Tracey, I. Pain vulnerability: a neurobiological perspective. *Nat Neurosci.* 2014, 17(2), 192-200. doi: 10.1038/nn.3628. PubMed PMID, 24473267.

[292] Sun, Y; Sahbaie, P; Liang, DY, Li, WW; Li, XQ; Shi, XY; Clark, JD. Epigenetic regulation of spinal CXCR2 signaling in incisional hypersensitivity in mice. *Anesthesiology.* 2013, 119(5), 1198-1208. doi: 10.1097/ALN.0b013e31829ce340. PubMed PMID, 23756451.

[293] Sun, Y; Liang, D; Sahbaie, P; Clark, JD. Effects of methyl donor diets on incisional pain in mice. *PLoS One.* 2013, 8(10), e77881. doi: 10.1371/journal.pone.0077881. PubMed PMID, 24205011.

[294] Bell, JT; Loomis, AK; Butcher, LM; Gao, F; Zhang, B; Hyde, CL; Sun, J; Wu, H; Ward, K; Harris, J; Scollen, S; Davies, MN; Schalkwyk, LC; Mill, J; Mu, TC; Williams, FM; Li, N; Deloukas, P; Beck, S; McMahon, SB; Wang, J; John, SL; Spector, TD. Differential methylation of the TRPA1 promoter in pain sensitivity. *Nat Commun.* 2014, 5, 2978. doi: 10.1038/ncomms3978. PubMed PMID, 24496475.

[295] Pinheiro, FD; Villarinho, JG; da, Silva, CR; de, Oliveira, SM; Pinheiro, KD; Petri, D; Rossato, MF; Guerra, GP; Trevisan, G; Antonello, Rubin, M; Geppetti, P; Ferreira, J; Andre, E. The involvement of the TRPA1 receptor in a mouse model of sympathetically

maintained neuropathic pain. *Eur J Pharmacol*. 2014. doi: 10.1016/j. ejphar. 2014.11.039. PubMed PMID, 25498793.

[296] Abzianidze, E; Kvaratskhelia, E; Tkemaladze, T; Kankava, K; Gurtskaia, G; Tsagareli, M. Epigenetic regulation of acute inflammatory pain. *Georgian Med News*. 2014(235), 78-81. PubMed PMID, 25416223.

[297] Pan, Z; Zhu, LJ; Li, YQ; Hao, LY; Yin, C; Yang, JX; Guo, Y; Zhang, S; Hua, L; Xue, ZY; Zhang, H; Cao, JL. Epigenetic modification of spinal miR-219 expression regulates chronic inflammation pain by targeting CaMKIIgamma. *J Neurosci*. 2014, 34(29), 9476-9483. doi: 10.1523/JNEUROSCI.5346-13.2014. PubMed PMID, 25031391.

[298] Hwang, CK; Song, KY; Kim, CS; Choi, HS; Guo, XH; Law, PY; Wei, LN; Loh, HH. Epigenetic programming of mu-opioid receptor gene in mouse brain is regulated by MeCP2 and Brg1 chromatin remodelling factor. *J Cell Mol Med*. 2009, 13(9B), 3591-3615. doi: 10.1111/j.1582-4934.2008.00535.x. PubMed PMID, 19602036.

[299] Hwang, CK; Kim, CS; Kim do, K; Law, PY; Wei, LN; Loh, HH. Up-regulation of the mu-opioid receptor gene is mediated through chromatin remodeling and transcriptional factors in differentiated neuronal cells. *Mol Pharmacol*. 2010, 78(1), 58-68. doi: 10.1124/mol.110.064311. PubMed PMID, 20385708.

[300] Hwang, CK; Song, KY; Kim, CS; Choi, HS; Guo, XH; Law, PY; Wei, LN; Loh, HH. Evidence of endogenous mu opioid receptor regulation by epigenetic control of the promoters. *Mol Cell Biol*. 2007, 27(13), 4720-4736. doi: 10.1128/MCB.00073-07. PubMed PMID, 17452465.

[301] Hwang, CK; Wagley, Y; Law, PY; Wei, LN; Loh, HH. Analysis of epigenetic mechanisms regulating opioid receptor gene transcription. *Methods Mol Biol*. 2015, 1230, 39-51. doi: 10.1007/978-1-4939-1708-2_3. PubMed PMID, 25293314.

[302] Liang, DY; Sun, Y; Shi, XY; Sahbaie, P; Clark, JD. Epigenetic regulation of spinal cord gene expression controls opioid-induced hyperalgesia. *Mol Pain*. 2014, 10, 59. doi: 10.1186/1744-8069-10-59. PubMed PMID, 25217253.

[303] Sun, Y; Sahbaie, P; Liang, D; Li, W; Clark, JD. opioids enhance CXCL1 expression and function after incision in mice. *J Pain*. 2014, 15(8), 856-866. doi: 10.1016/j.jpain.2014.05.003. PubMed PMID, 24887006.

[304] Ueda, H; Uchida, H. Epigenetic Modification in Neuropathic Pain. *Curr Pharm Des*. 2014. PubMed PMID, 25345610.

[305] Cruz, Duarte, P; St-Jacques, B; Ma, W. Prostaglandin E2 contributes to the synthesis of brain-derived neurotrophic factor in primary sensory neuron in ganglion explant cultures and in a neuropathic pain model. *Exp Neurol*. 2012, 234(2), 466-481. doi: 10.1016/j.expneurol.2012.01.021. PubMed PMID, 22309829.

[306] Imai, S; Ikegami, D; Yamashita, A; Shimizu, T; Narita, M; Niikura, K; Furuya, M; Kobayashi, Y; Miyashita, K; Okutsu, D; Kato, A; Nakamura, A; Araki, A; Omi, K; Nakamura, M; James, Okano, H; Okano, H; Ando, T; Takeshima, H; Ushijima, T; Kuzumaki, N; Suzuki, T; Narita, M. Epigenetic transcriptional activation of monocyte chemotactic protein 3 contributes to long-lasting neuropathic pain. *Brain*. 2013, 136(Pt 3), 828-843. doi: 10.1093/brain/aws330. PubMed PMID, 23364351.

[307] Uchida, H; Matsushita, Y; Ueda, H. Epigenetic regulation of BDNF expression in the primary sensory neurons after peripheral nerve injury: implications in the development

of neuropathic pain. *Neuroscience.* 2013, 240, 147-154. doi: 10.1016/j. neuroscience. 2013.02.053. PubMed PMID, 23466809.

[308] Geng, SJ; Liao, FF; Dang, WH; Ding, X; Liu, XD; Cai, J; Han, JS; Wan, Y; Xing, GG. Contribution of the spinal cord BDNF to the development of neuropathic pain by activation of the NR2B-containing NMDA receptors in rats with spinal nerve ligation. *Exp Neurol.* 2010, 222(2), 256-266. doi: 10.1016/j.expneurol.2010.01.003. PubMed PMID, 20079352.

[309] Denk, F; Huang, W; Sidders, B; Bithell, A; Crow, M; Grist, J; Sharma, S; Ziemek, D; Rice, AS; Buckley, NJ; McMahon, SB. HDAC inhibitors attenuate the development of hypersensitivity in models of neuropathic pain. *Pain.* 2013, 154(9), 1668-1679. doi: 10.1016/j.pain.2013.05.021. PubMed PMID, 23693161.

[310] Matsushita, Y; Araki, K; Omotuyi, O; Mukae, T; Ueda, H. HDAC inhibitors restore C-fibre sensitivity in experimental neuropathic pain model. *Br J Pharmacol.* 2013, 170(5), 991-998. doi: 10.1111/bph.12366. PubMed PMID, 24032674.

[311] Li, K; Zhao, GQ; Li, LY; Wu, GZ; Cui, SS. Epigenetic upregulation of Cdk5 in the dorsal horn contributes to neuropathic pain in rats. *Neuroreport.* 2014, 25(14), 1116-1121. doi: 10.1097/WNR.0000000000000237. PubMed PMID, 25055140.

[312] Yang, L; Gu, X; Zhang, W; Zhang, J; Ma, Z. Cdk5 inhibitor roscovitine alleviates neuropathic pain in the dorsal root ganglia by downregulating N-methyl-D-aspartate receptor subunit 2A. *Neurol Sci.* 2014, 35(9), 1365-1371. doi: 10.1007/s10072-014-1713-9. PubMed PMID, 24659417.

[313] Zhang, R; Liu, Y; Zhang, J; Zheng, Y; Gu, X; Ma, Z. Intrathecal administration of roscovitine attenuates cancer pain and inhibits the expression of NMDA receptor 2B subunit mRNA. *Pharmacol Biochem Behav.* 2012, 102(1), 139-145. doi: 10.1016/j.pbb.2012.03.025. PubMed PMID, 22503970.

[314] Zhang, HH; Zhang, XQ; Xue, QS; Yan, L; Huang, JL; Zhang, S; Shao, HJ; Lu, H; Wang, WY; Yu, BW. The BDNF/TrkB signaling pathway is involved in heat hyperalgesia mediated by Cdk5 in rats. *PLoS One.* 2014, 9(1), e85536. doi: 10.1371/journal.pone.0085536. PubMed PMID, 24465591.

[315] Alvarado, S; Tajerian, M; Millecamps, M; Suderman, M; Stone, LS; Szyf, M. Peripheral nerve injury is accompanied by chronic transcriptome-wide changes in the mouse prefrontal cortex. *Mol Pain.* 2013, 9, 21. doi: 10.1186/1744-8069-9-21. PubMed PMID, 23597049.

[316] Tao, W; Chen, Q; Zhou, W; Wang, Y; Wang, L; Zhang, Z. Persistent inflammation-induced up-regulation of brain-derived neurotrophic factor (BDNF) promotes synaptic delivery of alpha-amino-3-hydroxy-5-methyl-4-isoxazolepropionic acid receptor GluA1 subunits in descending pain modulatory circuits. *J Biol Chem.* 2014, 289(32), 22196-22204. doi: 10.1074/jbc.M114.580381. PubMed PMID, 24966334.

[317] Rahn, EJ; Guzman-Karlsson, MC; David, Sweatt, J. Cellular, molecular, and epigenetic mechanisms in non-associative conditioning: implications for pain and memory. *Neurobiol Learn Mem.* 2013, 105, 133-150. doi: 10.1016/j.nlm.2013.06.008. PubMed PMID, 23796633.

[318] Wang, F; Stefano, GB; Kream, RM. Epigenetic modification of DRG neuronal gene expression subsequent to nerve injury: etiological contribution to complex regional pain syndromes (Part II). *Med Sci Monit.* 2014, 20, 1188-1200. doi: 10.12659/MSM.890707. PubMed PMID, 25027291.

[319] Wang, F; Stefano, GB; Kream, RM. Epigenetic modification of DRG neuronal gene expression subsequent to nerve injury: etiological contribution to complex regional pain syndromes (Part I). *Med Sci Monit*. 2014, 20, 1067-1077. doi: 10.12659/MSM.890702. PubMed PMID, 24961509.

[320] Sumitani, M; Yasunaga, H; Uchida, K; Horiguchi, H; Nakamura, M; Ohe, K; Fushimi, K; Matsuda, S; Yamada, Y. Perioperative factors affecting the occurrence of acute complex regional pain syndrome following limb bone fracture surgery: data from the Japanese Diagnosis Procedure Combination database. *Rheumatology* (Oxford). 2014, 53(7), 1186-1193. doi: 10.1093/rheumatology/ket431. PubMed PMID, 24369418.

[321] Beerthuizen, A; Stronks, DL; Huygen, FJ; Passchier, J; Klein, J; Spijker, AV. The association between psychological factors and the development of complex regional pain syndrome type 1 (CRPS1)--a prospective multicenter study. *Eur J Pain*. 2011, 15(9), 971-975. doi: 10.1016/j.ejpain.2011.02.008. PubMed PMID, 21459637.

[322] Schurmann, M; Gradl, G; Zaspel, J; Kayser, M; Lohr, P; Andress, HJ. Peripheral sympathetic function as a predictor of complex regional pain syndrome type I (CRPS I) in patients with radial fracture. *Auton Neurosci*. 2000, 86(1-2), 127-134. doi: 10.1016/S1566-0702(00)00250-2. PubMed PMID, 11269918.

[323] Zollinger, PE; Tuinebreijer, WE; Breederveld, RS; Kreis, RW. Can vitamin C prevent complex regional pain syndrome in patients with wrist fractures? A randomized, controlled, multicenter dose-response study. *J Bone Joint Surg Am*. 2007, 89(7), 1424-1431. doi: 10.2106/JBJS.F.01147. PubMed PMID, 17606778.

[324] Atkins, RM; Duckworth, T; Kanis, JA. Features of algodystrophy after Colles' fracture. *J Bone Joint Surg Br*. 1990, 72(1), 105-110. PubMed PMID, 2298766.

[325] Camelot, C; Ramare, S; Lemoine, J; Saillant, G. [Orthopedic treatment of fractures of the lower extremity of the radius by the Judet technique. Anatomic results in function of the type of lesion: apropos of 280 cases]. *Rev Chir Orthop Reparatrice Appar Mot*. 1998, 84(2), 124-135. PubMed PMID, 9775056.

[326] Cazeneuve, JF; Leborgne, JM; Kermad, K; Hassan, Y. [Vitamin C and prevention of reflex sympathetic dystrophy following surgical management of distal radius fractures]. *Acta Orthop Belg*. 2002, 68(5), 481-484. PubMed PMID, 12584978.

[327] da, Costa, VV; de, Oliveira, SB; Fernandes, Mdo, C; Saraiva, RA. Incidence of regional pain syndrome after carpal tunnel release. Is there a correlation with the anesthetic technique? *Rev Bras Anestesiol*. 2011, 61(4), 425-433. doi: 10.1016/S0034-7094(11)70050-2. PubMed PMID, 21724005.

[328] Jellad, A; Salah, S; Ben, Salah, Frih, Z. Complex regional pain syndrome type I: incidence and risk factors in patients with fracture of the distal radius. *Arch Phys Med Rehabil*. 2014, 95(3), 487-492. doi: 10.1016/j.apmr.2013.09.012. PubMed PMID, 24080349.

[329] Zollinger, PE; Tuinebreijer, WE; Kreis, RW; Breederveld, RS. Effect of vitamin C on frequency of reflex sympathetic dystrophy in wrist fractures: a randomised trial. *Lancet*. 1999, 354(9195), 2025-2028. doi: 10.1016/S0140-6736(99)03059-7. PubMed PMID, 10636366.

[330] Besse, JL; Gadeyne, S; Galand-Desme, S; Lerat, JL; Moyen, B. Effect of vitamin C on prevention of complex regional pain syndrome type I in foot and ankle surgery. *Foot Ankle Surg*. 2009, 15(4), 179-182. doi: 10.1016/j.fas.2009.02.002. PubMed PMID, 19840748.

[331] Goris, RJ. Treatment of reflex sympathetic dystrophy with hydroxyl radical scavengers. *Unfallchirurg.* 1985, 88(7), 330-332. PubMed PMID, 3931223.

[332] Goris, RJ; Dongen, LM; Winters, HA. Are toxic oxygen radicals involved in the pathogenesis of reflex sympathetic dystrophy? *Free Radic Res Commun.* 1987, 3(1-5), 13-18. PubMed PMID, 3508426.

[333] Fischer, SG; Perez, RS; Nouta, J; Zuurmond, WW; Scheffer, PG. Oxidative Stress in Complex Regional Pain Syndrome (CRPS): No Systemically Elevated Levels of Malondialdehyde, F2-Isoprostanes and 8OHdG in a Selected Sample of Patients. *Int J Mol Sci.* 2013, 14(4), 7784-7794. doi: 10.3390/ijms14047784. PubMed PMID, 23574939.

[334] Parkitny, L; McAuley, JH; Di, Pietro, F. Inflammation in Complex Regional Pain Syndrome: A Systematic Review and Meta-Analysis. *Journal of Vascular Surgery.* 2013, 58(2), 550. doi:http: //dx.doi.org/10.1016/j.jvs.2013.06.010.

[335] Tan, EC; van, Goor, H; Bahrami, S; Kozlov, AV; Leixnering, M; Redl, H; Goris, RJ. Intra-arterial tert-Butyl-hydroperoxide infusion induces an exacerbated sensory response in the rat hind limb and is associated with an impaired tissue oxygen uptake. *Inflammation.* 2011, 34(1), 49-57. doi:10.1007/s10753-010-9207-2. PubMed PMID, 20386971.

[336] Zollinger, PE; Unal, H; Ellis, ML; Tuinebreijer, WE. Clinical Results of 40 Consecutive Basal Thumb Prostheses and No CRPS Type I After Vitamin C Prophylaxis. *Open Orthop J.* 2010, 4, 62-66. Epub 2010/03/13. doi: 10.2174/1874325001004020062. PubMed PMID, 20224742.

[337] Zyluk, A. [Clinical estimation of late treatment results in posttraumatic Sudeck's dystrophy treated with mannitol, calcitonin and exercise therapy]. *Ann Acad Med Stetin.* 1994, 40, 133-144. PubMed PMID, 7503442.

[338] Zyluk, A; Puchalski, P. Treatment of early complex regional pain syndrome type 1 by a combination of mannitol and dexamethasone. *J Hand Surg Eur Vol.* 2008, 33(2), 130-136. doi: 10.1177/1753193408087034. PubMed PMID, 18443050.

[339] Tan, EC; Tacken, MC; Groenewoud, JM; van Goor, H; Frolke, JP. Mannitol as salvage treatment for Complex Regional Pain Syndrome Type I. *Injury.* 2010, 41(9), 955-959. doi: 10.1016/j.injury.2009.11.013. PubMed PMID, 20018281.

[340] Perez, RS; Pragt, E; Geurts, J; Zuurmond, WW; Patijn, J; van Kleef, M. Treatment of patients with complex regional pain syndrome type I with mannitol: a prospective, randomized, placebo-controlled, double-blinded study. *J Pain.* 2008, 9(8), 678-686. doi: 10.1016/j.jpain.2008.02.005. PubMed PMID, 18403271.

[341] Zuurmond, WW; Langendijk, PN; Bezemer, PD; Brink, HE; de Lange, JJ; van loenen, AC. Treatment of acute reflex sympathetic dystrophy with DMSO 50% in a fatty cream. *Acta Anaesthesiol Scand.* 1996, 40(3), 364-367. PubMed PMID, 8721469.

[342] van Dieten, HE; Perez, RS; van Tulder, MW; de Lange, JJ; Zuurmond, WW; Ader, HJ; Vondeling, H; Boers, M. Cost effectiveness and cost utility of acetylcysteine versus dimethyl sulfoxide for reflex sympathetic dystrophy. *Pharmacoeconomics.* 2003, 21(2), 139-148. PubMed PMID, 12515575.

[343] Viel, E; Esteve, M; Draussin, G; Eledjam, JJ. [Reflex sympathetic algodystrophies. Preventive and therapeutic aspects]. *Cah Anesthesiol.* 1995, 43(6), 565-571. PubMed PMID, 8745649.

[344] Viel, E; Pelissier, J; Draussin, G; Bechier, JG; Eledjam, JJ. [Algodystrophies of the limbs: physiopathology, preventive aspects]. *Cah Anesthesiol.* 1993, 41(2), 163-168. PubMed PMID, 8389227.
[345] Gillespie, JH; Menk, EJ; Middaugh, RE. Reflex sympathetic dystrophy, a complication of interscalene block. *Anesth Analg.* 1987, 66(12), 1316-1317. PubMed PMID, 3688504.

In: Complex Regional Pain Syndrome
Editors: Nader D. Nader and Ognjen Visnjevac

ISBN: 978-1-63483-130-7
© 2015 Nova Science Publishers, Inc.

APPENDIX: SPECIAL CONSIDERATIONS CRPS AFTER FOOT AND ANKLE SURGERY

Mark Finkelstein*, DPM

Chief of Podiatric medicine at the Western New York Healthcare System,
Buffalo, NY, US

DIAGNOSTIC CRITERIA

Complex Regional Pain Syndrome (CRPS) is an uncommon complication after foot and ankle surgery. Complex Regional Pain Syndrome currently is known as a neuropathic pain syndrome that can occur postoperatively as a complication of surgery or injury. The diagnosis of CPRS is made clinically with no one diagnostic test being confirmatory.

The incidence of Complex Regional Pain Syndrome after foot and ankle surgery is difficult to measure due to the lack of consensus on the definition of Complex Regional Pain Syndrome. Estimates based on historic literature review had varying results ranging from 1 in 2000 to 1 in 20 after discrete accident, although most current literature suggests less than 5% overall incidence after extremity injury or surgery. [1] A recent study on the incidence of Complex Regional Pain Syndrome after foot and ankle surgery by Rewhorn et al reported that a retrospective cohort study of 390 patients who underwent elective foot and/or ankle surgery had a 4.3% rate of Complex Regional Pain Syndrome as defined by the International Association for the Study of Pain criteria for the diagnosis of CPRS. The mean age was reported as 47.2 ± 9.7 years and 82% were female. 47% had a pre-existing diagnosis of anxiety or depression. [2]

A detailed clinical approach to the diagnosis of Complex Regional Pain Syndrome is important for proper diagnosis and initiation of treatment. An understanding of the subjective signs of patients who presented with atypical pain is critical to the foundation of ruling out or confirming the diagnosis of Complex Regional Pain Syndrome. The ultimate diagnosis of CRPS is a clinical entity and no single test is sufficient to make a diagnosis. There are several recommended diagnostic criteria reported in the medical literature. The most commonly used

---

* Chief of Podiatric medicine at the Western New York Healthcare System, Buffalo, NY 14215..
mark.finkelstein@va.gov.

criteria for diagnosing Complex Regional Pain Syndrome are those recommended by the International Association for the Study of Pain (IASP) 1994 and the 2007 Proposed New Diagnostic Criteria for Complex Regional Pain Syndrome by Harden et al known as the "Budapest criteria." It is important to utilize only 1 set of criteria when diagnosing complex regional pain syndrome. The updated "Budapest criteria" was developed after validation studies suggested that the IASP/CRPS diagnostic criteria were adequately sensitive however utilization of the criteria caused problems of over diagnosis due to poor specificity.

The IASP diagnostic criteria for Complex Regional Pain Syndrome components include:

1. The presence of an initiating noxious event, or a cause of immobilization.
2. Continuing pain, allodynia, or hyperalgesia in which the pain is disproportionate to any known inciting event.
3. Evidence at some time of edema, changes in skin blood flow, or abnormal sudomotor activity in the region of pain (can be sign or symptom).
4. This diagnosis is excluded by the existence of other conditions that would otherwise account for the degree of pain and dysfunction.

The 2007 "Budapest criteria" recommends that the following criteria must be met:

1. Continuing pain, which is disproportionate to the inciting event.
2. Most reported at least 1 symptom in 3 of the 4 following categories
   Sensory: Reports of hyperesthesia and/or allodynia
   Vasomotor: Reports of temperature asymmetry and /or skin color changes and/or skin color asymmetry
   Sudomotor/edema: Reports of edema and/or sweating changes and/ or sweating asymmetry
   Motor/trophic: Reports of decreased range of motion and/or motor dysfunction (weakness, tremor, dystonia) and/or trophic changes (hair, nail, skin)
3. Must display at least 1 sign at time of evaluation in 2 or more of the following categories:
   Sensory: Evidence of hyperalgesia (to pinprick) and/ or allodynia (to light touch and/or temperature sensation and /or deep somatic pressure and/or joint movement)
   Vasomotor: Evidence of temperature asymmetry ($> 1°C$) and/or skin color changes and/or asymmetry
   Sudomotor/edema: Evidence of edema and/ or sweating changes and/or sweating asymmetry
   Motor/Trophic: Evidence of decreased range of motion and/or motor dysfunction (weakness, tremor, dystonia) and/or trophic changes (hair, nail, skin)
4. There is no other diagnosis that better explains the signs and symptoms. [3]

The presentation of the patient who has Chronic Regional Pain Syndrome includes subjective signs given by the patient and objective clinical findings. In addition to the diagnostic criteria identifying the disorder, chronic regional pain syndrome may be staged by the predominant physiologic alterations or characterize its evolution. The early, acute/hyperemic stage of CRPS (stage I) is characterized by hyperalgesia, sudomotor and vasomotor dysfunction and edema. The dystrophic stage (stage II) is characterized more by increasing pain and sensory dysfunction, with the addition of motor and early trophic alterations. Stage III (atrophic stage) is characterized by decreased pain but increased motor and trophic alterations. The most current studies suggested these 3 stages by not necessarily develop in a sequential fashion but may be 3 distinct subtypes.

Both the IASP and "Budapest criteria" include subjective symptoms and physical examination findings. Pain out of proportion to the inciting event is historically the criteria that almost all clinicians agree his prerequisite to the diagnosis. Hyperesthesia /allodynia by history may present with the patient describing light touch or thermal stimulation is being intolerable. The patient often describes vasomotor alteration as involving color change or swelling. Later in the disease course the patient may report reduced muscle bulk. Motor/trophic alterations may present as subjective weakness or tremor and atrophic alterations present within the skin or nails. The second portion of the criteria involves findings on the physical examination of the patient. These physical findings at the time of evaluation include evidence of hyperalgesia and/or allodynia, evidence of temperature asymmetry, color change, edema or sweating changes or asymmetry and motor trophic changes.

In addition to the subjective and physical findings laboratory testing may assist in ruling out coexistent inflammatory or infectious causes of the patient's condition. Radiographic and imaging studies are complementary to the diagnostic criteria. The radiographic and imaging studies include plain radiographs, 3-phase bone scanning, and MRI. The use of photography is also important in documenting the clinical findings. In addition thermal regulatory and nutritional blood flow testing permits assessment of the distal extremity autonomic function. Isolated cold stress testing using both temperature and laser Doppler Fluxmetry has been described to assess dynamic sympathetic response of the extremity to changes and environmental temperature. Isolated cold stress testing is sensitive to vasomotor disturbances that occur in 80-90% of patients with complex regional pain syndrome; however, it is not specific for complex regional pain syndrome. [1]

TREATMENT

The treatment of Complex Regional Pain Syndrome should include a multidisciplinary approach. This may include initiation of physical medicine, pain management consultation, local or sympathetic nerve blocks, oral pharmacologic agents, behavioral medicine and interventional treatments including spinal cord stimulation and transcutaneous electrical nerve stimulation. It is generally agreed that early initiation of treatment is better than later with the avoidance of advanced, trophic limb alterations being a high priority.

After podiatry surgery, the surgeon needs to be aware of signs and symptoms associated with the condition. The trauma of foot surgery is sufficient to result in such a complication. An alert surgeon will recognize a change in expected normal postoperative progress. Once CRPS concerns enter into the postoperative differential diagnosis, the following approach is recommended. Consultation with other medical disciplines is encouraged from a treatment perspective as well as a medical legal standpoint. This can be a life changing condition. Physical Medicine and Therapy consult will assess and recommend modalities for functional rehabilitation including range of motion and desensitization techniques. Pain management specialists will provide the patient with much needed control of pain and may provide local or sympathetic nerve block therapy and possibly spinal cord stimulation. Intervention via Behavioral Medicine consultation is often required due to the high preexistence of anxiety and depression as well as to address the psychological component of chronic pain.

MEDICO-LEGAL CONSIDERATIONS

The patient who has Complex Regional Pain Syndrome requires a detailed approach and chart documentation to avoid medical legal issues. The physician needs to listen to the patient and take a thorough history. The physician needs to allow the patient to describe what they perceived may have been the inciting event or stimulus. The physician should not discount any part of the history or interpret any subjective symptoms as exaggeration or embellishment of the relative discomfort. The physician should document in detail the history and physical findings, diagnostic testing, and treatment modalities and plans for timely follow-up. It is important to not only document the positive findings that suggest Chronic Regional Pain Syndrome but also the negative findings in patients for whom the diagnosis is excluded. The physician should note the patient's affect. Patients who have Chronic Regional Pain Syndrome often exhibit significant emotional distress that is out of proportion compared to the expected emotions associated with the original injury or surgery. Once the diagnosis of Complex Regional Pain Syndrome is suspected or confirmed, the physician should act in a timely, deliberate and aggressive manner to get the patient to appropriate care. It is recommended that along with consultation in the multidisciplinary setting, the original treating physician should continue to see the patient through the remainder of his or her care. Once multidisciplinary care is initiated reassessment should be frequent enough to allow the patient to communicate the relative success or failure of the therapeutic interventions to the surgeon. This continued evaluation by the surgeon can provide the patient with additional reassurance and avoid a sense of being referred out or abandonment.

Frequent reevaluation is suggested, as not all symptoms of CRPS may be present at each evaluation. Many of the symptoms of Complex Regional Pain Syndrome can come and go over time and the patient will be described as having "good" days and "bad" days. Frequent reevaluation will aid in documentation of all associated symptoms and objective findings. Findings may vary from examination to examination. This is how to build the diagnosis.

Consideration must also be taken in the medical legal arena for patients whose Complex Regional Pain Syndrome is permanent. An article in the Journal of Surgical Orthopedic Advances in 2011 by Crick et al noted that the percentage of verdicts or settlements in favor of the plaintiff in physician malpractice/hospital malpractice was 50% regarding Complex Regional Pain Syndrome. The average award or settlement in these cases was over $500,000. These patient's considerations include Life care plans that include electrical implants (spinal cord stimulators, peripheral stimulators, intrathecal pumps), prescription medications and the use of "off label medications." These life care plan therapies may increase the settlement or verdict decisions. [4]

In summary, Complex Regional Pain Syndrome is an uncommon complication after injury or surgery of the foot and ankle. Any patient who presents with subjective complaints of pain out of proportion requires a detailed history and physical examination to be aware of Complex Regional Pain Syndrome. Early consideration of the diagnosis followed by timely intervention by a multidisciplinary team is critical to the proper treatment of the patient and to minimize medical legal questions in the care of the patient.

REFERENCES

[1] Pontell D. A clinical approach to complex regional pain syndrome. *Clinics in podiatric medicine and surgery.* 2008;25(3):361-80; vi.

[2] Rewhorn MJ, Leung AH, Gillespie A, Moir JS, Miller R. Incidence of complex regional pain syndrome after foot and ankle surgery. *The Journal of foot and ankle surgery: official publication of the American College of Foot and Ankle Surgeons.* 2014;53(3):256-8.

[3] Harden RN, Bruehl S, Stanton-Hicks M, Wilson PR. Proposed new diagnostic criteria for complex regional pain syndrome. *Pain medicine.* 2007;8(4):326-31.

[4] Crick BC, Crick JC. Lawsuit verdicts and settlements involving reflex sympathetic dystrophy and complex regional pain syndrome. *Journal of surgical orthopaedic advances.* 2011;20(3):153-7.

INDEX

B

C

G

H

I

internal consistency, 81
internal environment, 3
internal fixation, 238, 239, 244
internal validity, 78
interneurons, 40, 121
intervention, 11, 23, 24, 67, 82, 108, 117, 118, 122, 129, 133, 136, 138, 152, 155, 156, 174, 200, 201, 208, 210, 212, 230, 240, 249, 267, 277
intracellular calcium, 98
ion channels, 32, 33, 72, 96, 97, 98
ipsilateral, 5, 53, 98, 113, 127, 133, 155, 156, 157
irritability, 239
ischemia, 4, 27, 28, 32, 43, 54, 62, 69, 72, 172, 177, 192, 230, 231, 238, 266
ischemia reperfusion injury, 27, 62
isolation, 23, 152, 176, 218

J

joints, 112, 150, 151

K

keratinocytes, 25, 26, 27, 32, 38
kidney, 262
knee arthroplasty, 154, 181

L

labeling, 190
laboratory studies, 171
lactic acid, 97
Langerhans cells, 38
L-arginine, 225, 259
latency, 22
later life, 234
laterality, 163, 187
LC, 171, 172, 259, 262, 267
lead, 23, 31, 33, 36, 37, 42, 54, 58, 60, 64, 78, 97, 119, 123, 128, 129, 133, 141, 155, 158, 169, 175, 207, 210, 211, 215, 232, 247
leakage, 69
learning, 39, 170, 173, 174, 188, 192, 251
legs, 114, 189
lesions, 4, 15, 20, 24, 58, 112, 139, 171, 184, 223, 231
leukocytes, 58, 61, 229
leukotrienes, 44
ligand, 28, 36, 37, 40, 42, 58, 70, 72, 94, 256
light, 11, 21, 29, 31, 32, 40, 44, 84, 146, 154, 167, 221, 274, 275
limbic system, 171, 172, 202

lipid peroxidation, 148
liquid chromatography, 225
lithium, 99
liver, 100, 106, 224, 258
liver enzymes, 100, 224
liver failure, 100
local anesthesia, 119
local anesthetic, 6, 82, 91, 96, 108, 109, 110, 111, 113, 114, 115, 118, 120, 122, 131, 135, 137, 221, 231, 256, 265
localization, 22, 110, 128, 154, 155, 207
loci, 46, 47, 218, 219, 224, 262
locus, 22, 171, 190, 191, 192, 213
love, 217
lumbar spine, 215, 251
lung disease, 265
lymph, 199, 203
lymphocytes, 26

M

M1, 158
macronutrients, 232
macrophage inflammatory protein (MIP), 25, 26, 37
macrophages, 25, 26, 35, 38, 41, 53, 55, 56, 58, 59, 60, 61, 63, 65, 66, 68, 70, 97
magnesium, 98, 100, 226, 259, 260, 263
magnet, 231, 265
magnetic field(s), 154, 157, 201, 212, 249
magnetic resonance imaging (MRI), 84, 85, 100, 128, 141, 143, 149, 156, 157, 159, 179, 187, 201, 207, 217, 218, 219, 224, 275
magnetoencephalography, 156
magnitude, 81, 118, 157, 171
major depression, 99, 191, 249, 251
major depressive disorder, 213, 259
malingering, 168
mammalian tissues, 227
mammals, 171
manipulation, 121, 152, 198, 236
mannitol, 240, 241, 242, 243, 271
mapping, 141, 142, 167, 184, 202, 250
marrow, 2, 84
mass spectrometry, 225
mast cells, 38, 55
maternal smoking, 233
MCP-1, 37
mean arterial pressure, 172, 223
measurement(s), 18, 26, 114, 180
mediation, 26, 37
medical, 1, 3, 10, 12, 52, 99, 120, 130, 149, 151, 157, 161, 173, 196, 197, 206, 210, 212, 220, 273, 275, 276, 277

N

O

P

Q

R

S

T

U

V